150

Anaesthesiologie und Intensivmedizin
Anaesthesiology
and Intensive Care Medicine

vormals „Anaesthesiologie und Wiederbelebung"
begründet von R. Frey, F. Kern und O. Mayrhofer

Herausgeber:
H. Bergmann · Linz (Schriftleiter)
J.B. Brückner · Berlin   M. Gemperle · Genève
W.F. Henschel · Bremen   O. Mayrhofer · Wien
K. Peter · München

150

Anaesthesiologie und Intensivmedizin
Anaesthesiology
and Intensive Care Medicine

vormals Anaesthesiologie und Wiederbelebung
begründet von R. Frey, F. Kern und H. Mayrhofer

Herausgeber:
H. Bergmann · Linz (Schriftleiter)
J.B. Brückner · Berlin · M. Gemperle · Genève
W.F. Henschel · Bremen · O. Mayrhofer · Wien
K. Peter · München

Inhalation Anaesthesia Today and Tomorrow

Edited by
K. Peter and F. Jesch

With 126 Figures and 19 Tables

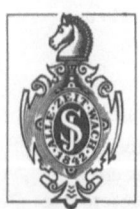

Springer-Verlag Berlin Heidelberg GmbH 1982

Prof. Dr. K. Peter
Ludwig-Maximilians-Universität München
Klinikum Großhadern
Institut für Anaesthesiologie
Marchioninistraße 15
D-8000 München 70
Federal Republic of Germany

PD Dr. F. Jesch
Ludwig-Maximilians-Universität München
Klinikum Großhadern
Institut für Anaesthesiologie
Marchioninistraße 15
D-8000 München 70
Federal Republic of Germany

ISBN 978-3-662-38979-9   ISBN 978-3-662-39944-6 (eBook)
DOI 10.1007/978-3-662-39944-6
Library of Congress Cataloging in Publication Data
Main entry under title: Inhalation Anaesthesia Today and Tomorrow.
(Anaesthesiologie und Intensivmedizin; 150)
Bibliography: p. Includes index.

© Springer-Verlag Berlin Heidelberg 1982
Originally published by Springer-Verlag Berlin Heidelberg New York in 1982

Typesetting: Schreibsatz Service Weihrauch, Würzburg

2119/3321-543210

Preface

In clinical anaesthesiology the inhalation anaesthetics halothane
(fluothane), enflurane and – in recent times – forane got a
renaissance in clinical application. The reasons are not only the advantages of volatile anaesthetics, but also the fact that the investigations of pharmacodynamics and pharmacokinetics of i.v. narcotics showed negative aspects. It was the aim of the organizers of the
symposium to give a survey of the present state of knowledge on
inhalation anaesthetics, which is as up-to-date, critical as well as
detailed as possible. Furthermore it was the intention to evaluate
the recent advances made in the field of basic research. The first
section of the symposium in particular enters into the question
of the toxicity of volatile anaesthetics as well as their mechanisms
of action. In a second main part the influences on cardiovascular
system and on microcirculation are discussed. Apart from the
extensive discussion of the advances in knowledge in the field of
cardiovascular pathophysiology, the focal point of the contribut-
ions is made up of those with anaesthesia in coronary heart disease
and cardiac insufficieny as well as the contribution on interactions
of inhalation anaesthetics with cardiovascular drugs.

In the third and fourth section the influences of volatile
anaesthetics on cerebral, hepatic, renal and pulmonary function are
dealt with as well as questions concerning the clinical application.
Particular attention is given to the important problems of indication in patients belonging to the extreme age groups. The article
"Balanced anaesthesia as an alternative concept" evaluates the role
of volatile anaesthetics retrospectively as well as their future status.

The editors appreciate the work of the chairman and the
speakers of the various sessions.

For their valuable assistance in the completion of this book
the editors are particularly grateful to Dr. C. Brendel, to Dr. C.
Sirtl, and to Mrs. B. Seidel. We are also indebted to Springer-Verlag
for the cooperation in preparing this book and to Deutsche Abbott
GmbH, Wiesbaden, for generously sponsoring the symposium.

K. Peter, F. Jesch

Table of Contents

Contributing Authors

Van Ackern, K., Professor, Institut für Anaesthesiologie, Klinikum Großhadern, D-8000 München 70, Federal Republic of Germany

Bjaertnaes, L., M.D., Institut of Physik, University of Oslo, Karl-Johans-Gate 47, Oslo 1/Norway

Black, G.W., M.D., FRCPI, FFARCS, Consultant Anaesthetist, The Royal Belfast Hospital for Sick Children, Belfast BT 12 6BE Northern Ireland

Brown, B.R., Jr., M.D., Ph.D., Professor and Head, Department of Anaesthesiology, University of Arizona, Health Sciences Center, Tucson, Arizona 85724/USA

Brückner, U., Professor, Abteilung für Experimentelle Chirurgie, Chirurgisches Zentrum, Ruprecht-Karls-Universität Heidelberg, Im Neuenheimer Feld 347, D-6900 Heidelberg 1, Federal Republic of Germany

Campbell, D., Professor, Institut of Anaesthesia, University of Glasgow, Hon. Consultant Anaesthesist, Royal Infirmary, Glasgow, Great Britain

Crul, J.F., M.D., Professor and Head, Dept. of Anaesthesiology, Akademisch Ziekehuis, Radbout, Geert Grooteplein zuid 12 Nijmegen, N-6525 GA-Nijmegen, Netherlands

Cunitz, G., Professor, Knappschaftskrankenhaus, Klinikum der Ruhr-Universität, Bochum-Langendreer, D-4630 Bochum 7, Federal Republic of Germany

Dudziak, R., Professor, Zentrum für Anaesthesiologie der Universitätskliniken Frankfurt, Theodor-Stern-Kai 7, D-6000 Frankfurt 70, Federal Republic of Germany

Dundee, J.W., Professor, Institut of Anaesthetics, Queen's University of Belfast, Northern Ireland

Endrich, B., M.D., Institut für Chirurgische Forschung der Universität München, Klinikum Großhadern, D-8000 München 70, Federal Republic of Germany

Fee, J.P.H., M.D., FFARCS, The Royal Belfast Hospital for Sick Children, Belfast BT12 6BE Northern Ireland

Fitch, W., M.D., FFARCS, Institut of Anaesthesia, University of Glasgow, Royal Infirmary, Glasgow/Great Britain

Foëx, P., M.D., Nuffield Dept. of Anaesthesiology, Radcliffe Infirmary, Oxford/Great Britain

Franke, N., M.D., Institut für Anaesthesiologie der Universität München, Klinikum Großhadern, D-8000 München 70, Federal Republic of Germany

Gemperle, M., Professor, Institut universitaire d'Anesthesiologie, Hôpital Cantonale de Genève, CH-1211 Genève, Switzerland

Göthert, M., Professor, Universitätsklinikum der Gesamthochschule Essen, Pharmakologisches Institut, D-4300 Essen 1, Federal Republic of Germany

Haldemann, G., M.D., Institut für Anaesthesiologie und Intensivmedizin, Kantonspital Aarau, CH-5000 Aarau, Switzerland

Hilfiker, O., M.D., Zentrum für Anaesthesiologie der Universität Göttingen, Robert-Koch-Straße 40, D-3400 Göttingen, Federal Republic of Germany

Irestedt, L., M.D., Department of Anaesthesia, Karolinska Institutet, S-10401 Stockholm, Sweden

Jaernberg, P.O., M.D., Department of Anaesthesia, Karolinska Institutet S-10401 Stockholm, Sweden

Jeretin, St., M.D., Klinik Center Ljubljana, Ferberjeva 37, Ljubljana/Jugoslavia

Kettler, D., Professor, Institut für Anaesthesiologie d. Universität Göttingen, Robert-Koch-Straße 40, D-3400 Göttingen, Federal Republic of Germany

Lappas, D., Professor and Head, Department of Anaesthesiology, Medical School, Aristoteles University, Thessaloniki/Greece

Larsen, R., Professor, Institut für Anaesthesiologie der Universität Göttingen, Robert-Koch-Str. 40, D-3400 Göttingen, Federal Republic of Germany

Lauven, P., M.D., Institut für Anaesthesiologie, Universität Bonn, Rheindorfer Straße 50, D-5300 Bonn, Federal Republic of Germany

Madler, Ch., Dr., Institut für Anaesthesiologie der Universität München, Klinikum Großhadern, D-8000 München 70, Federal Republic of Germany

Martani, C., Dr., Ospedale San Raffaele, Via Olgettina, I-20134 Milano, Italy

Meßmer, K., Professor, Abteilung für Experimentelle Chirurgie, Chirurgisches Zentrum, Ruprecht-Karls-Universität Heidelberg, Im Neuenheimer Feld 347, D-6900 Heidelberg 1, Federal Republic of Germany

Mittmann, U., Professor, Fa. Dr. Karl Thomae GmbH, Biologische Forschung, Birkendorferstr. 65, D-7950 Biberach a.d. Riß, Federal Republic of Germany

Norlander, O., M.D., Professor and Chairman, Department of Anaesthesia, Karolinska Institutet, S-10401 Stockholm, Sweden

Perotti, V., Dr., Ospedale San Raffaele, Via Olgettina, I-20134 Milano, Italy

Rietbrock, I., Professor, Institut für Anaesthesiologie, Universität Würzburg, Josef-Schneider-Straße 2, D-8700 Würzburg, Federal Republic of Germany

Rouge, J.C., M.D., Institut universitaire d'Anesthesiologie, Hôpital Cantonal de Genève, CH-1211 Genève 4, Switzerland

Schmidt, H., Privatdozent, Zentrum für Anaesthesiologie der Universitätskliniken Frankfurt, Theodor-Stern-Kai 7, D-6000 Frankfurt 70, Federal Republic of Germany

Schwilden, H., M.D., Institut für Anaesthesiologie, Universität Bonn, Rheindorfer Straße 50, D-5300 Bonn, Federal Republic of Germany

Smith, G., M.D., Professor of Anaesthesia, Leicester General Hospital, University of Leicester, Leicester/Great Britain

Sonntag, H., Professor, Institut für Anaesthesiologie der Universität Göttingen, Robert-Koch-Str. 40, D-3400 Göttingen, Federal Republic of Germany

Steen, P.A., M.D., Ullevaal Hospital, Bjerkebakken 69 E, Oslo 7/ Norway

Stoeckel, H., Professor, Institut für Anaesthesiologie der Universität Bonn, D-5300 Bonn-Venusberg, Federal Republic of Germany

Strauer, B., Professor, Medizinische Klinik I, Klinikum Großhadern, D-8000 München 70, Federal Republic of Germany

Taeger, K., M.D., Institut für Anaesthesiologie, Klinikum Großhadern, D-8000 München 70, Federal Republic of Germany

Teichmann, J., Professor, Institut für Anaesthesiologie der Universität Göttingen, Robert-Koch-Str. 40, D-3400 Göttingen,
Federal Republic of Germany

Torri, G., Professor, Ospedale San Raffaele, Via Olgettina,
I-20134 Milano, Italy

Trudell, J.R., M.D., Department of Anaesthesiology, Stanford
University, School of Medicine, Stanford, California 94305/USA

Vetter, H.O., Dr., Institut für Anaesthesiologie der Universität München, Klinikum Großhadern, D-8000 München 70, Federal Republic of Germany

Victor, H., Dipl.-Phys., Abteilung für Experimentelle Chirurgie,
Chirurgisches Zentrum, Ruprecht-Karls-Universität Heidelberg, Im
Neuenheimer Feld 347, D-6900 Heidelberg 1, Federal Republic of
Germany

Basics of Biotransformation

I. Rietbrock

Summary

Interindividual differences in response to drug administration can often be related to differences in metabolic rates and/or pharmacological activity and quantitiy of each metabolite produced. Adverse effects observed in the post-operative phase may be due to the extent of accumulation of intravenous anaesthetics, which depends exclusively on their metabolic clearance. On the other hand, toxic reactions after inhalation anaesthetics may be attributed to reactive intermediates of their metabolic degradation. This review of the basic concepts of drug metabolism will present three areas where the mono-oxygenase system is involved:
1. In addition to specific hepatic enzyme activity a number of factors may control the rate of drug oxidation. Depending on the drug's physico-chemical properties, alterations caused by disease may lead to high interindividual differences in metabolic rate. There is however, also a lack of correlation between biotransformation rates of different drugs in healthy individuals. One explanation for this observation focuses on the cytochrome P_{450} heterogeneity, both qualitative and quantitative.
2. A brief outline of anaesthetic chemical modification and of the main features of the mono-oxygenase system is given. This system is involved in the oxidative and reductive pathways, leading to radicals and carbene complexes responsible for lipid peroxidation.
3. The reductive pathway, e.g. of halothane is principally more toxic than the oxidative route. Because the former occurs at a low oxygen concentration, the question arises as to which clinical conditions lead to a higher level of liver toxic reductive intermediates. Normally, regulation mechanisms of liver blood flow provide for a sufficient oxygen supply to hepatic cells even in pathological situations and to a great extent prevent a reductive metabolism.

Introduction

Without a biochemical change to more water-soluble derivatives, lipophilic anaesthetics could not be excreted and would accumulate in body fat or membranes. Here they would persist for long periods of time and possibly disturb normal cell metabolism. Even those anaesthetics which are exhaled to a great extent undergo a certain degree of metabolism depending on their lipid solubilities. Inhalation anaesthetics with high lipid solubility are metabolized to a greater extent than more polar drugs. Metabolism therefore plays a role in both drug distribution in body tissues and excretion.

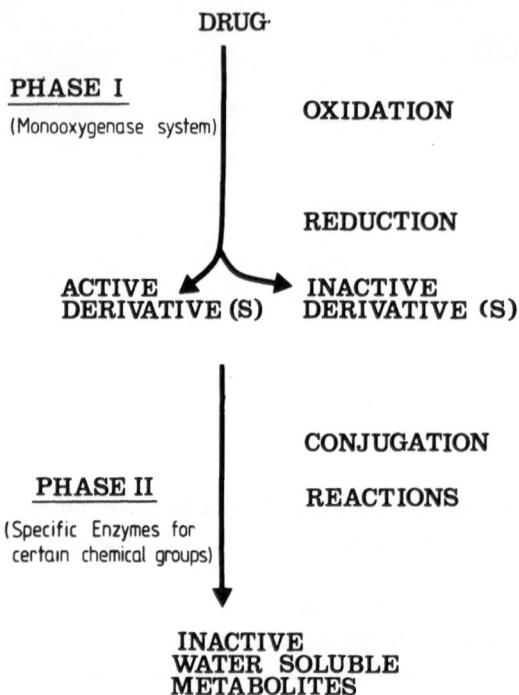

DRUG

PHASE I
(Monooxygenase system)

OXIDATION

REDUCTION

ACTIVE
DERIVATIVE (S)   INACTIVE
DERIVATIVE (S)

CONJUGATION

PHASE II

REACTIONS

(Specific Enzymes for
certain chemical groups)

INACTIVE
WATER SOLUBLE
METABOLITES

Fig. 1. The two phases of drug metabolism

The Two Phases of Drug Metabolism

The degradation of most drugs including anaesthetics follows a two-step process (Fig. 1).
The most common reaction in phase I is oxidation [3]. The molecular structure of the drug
is changed, facilitating the conjugation reactions of phase II. Phase I reactions can lead to
either active or inactive intermediates. The products of phase II reactions are nearly always
inactive. There is now much evidence indicating that the interindividual differences in response to anaesthetic application are often related to differences in the rate of drug metabolism [1, 26]. This means that unusually rapid or slow metabolism can cause adverse reactions, depending on the pharmacological activity of the metabolites. Phase I plays the most
important role in determining the appearance of adverse effects. The microsomal mono-oxygenase system contains the key enzymes for phase I. This system consists of several iron-con-
taining enzymes present mainly in liver, but also in the lungs, intestines and kidneys [36, 37].

Factors Controlling the Drug Oxidation Rate in Man

Let us first consider the factors which can change enzymic drug oxidation in man. In addition to substances which can change the quantity of enzymes in the body (e.g. inducers such
as phenobarbital) there are also those which can alter the specific enzyme activity, that is
the catalytic activity per mg of protein. Results from cytochrome P_{450} studies using broken
cell preparations cannot easily be extrapolated to the intact organism. These studies cannot
possibly indicate the effect of changes in liver blood flow, which control drug metabolism by

determining availability of oxygen and the rate of drug transport to the cell. Drug oxidation in man is therefore dependent on changes in both liver blood flow and intrinsic activity [46].

Different rates of drug oxidation due to variations in the severity, intensity or duration of the disease, can change from day to day, and can be altered by the drug therapy applied. It is a well-known fact that the number of drugs employed increases exponentially with the severity of the disease [26, 32]. To illustrate these phenomena I will use hexobarbitone as an example [2, 14, 27, 48] (Fig. 2). Hexobarbitone clearance, which is related to its metabolism, is reduced 30%−60% in patients with liver disease. This reduction in clearance is greatest in the more severe cases, such as decompensated liver cirrhosis. In contrast to intensive care patients, these patients are clinically stable and the hexobarbitone clearances are relatively uniform, varying only fivefold compared to a threefold variation in healthy subjects. Intensive care patients are typically unstable. This instability expresses itself in a fluctuating hexobarbitone clearance. At the start of therapy, hexobarbitone metabolism can be lower than normal (Group I). During the 1st week there is usually a rapid rise (+87%, Group II), which can reach even higher values over the subsequent 2−3 weeks (+143%, Group III). These alterations are so great that 19-fold variations in hexobarbitone clearance can be measured in intensive care patients. This progressive increase in the rate of hexobarbitone metabolism is related to the extent of multiple drug therapy. The induction effects on enzyme ac-

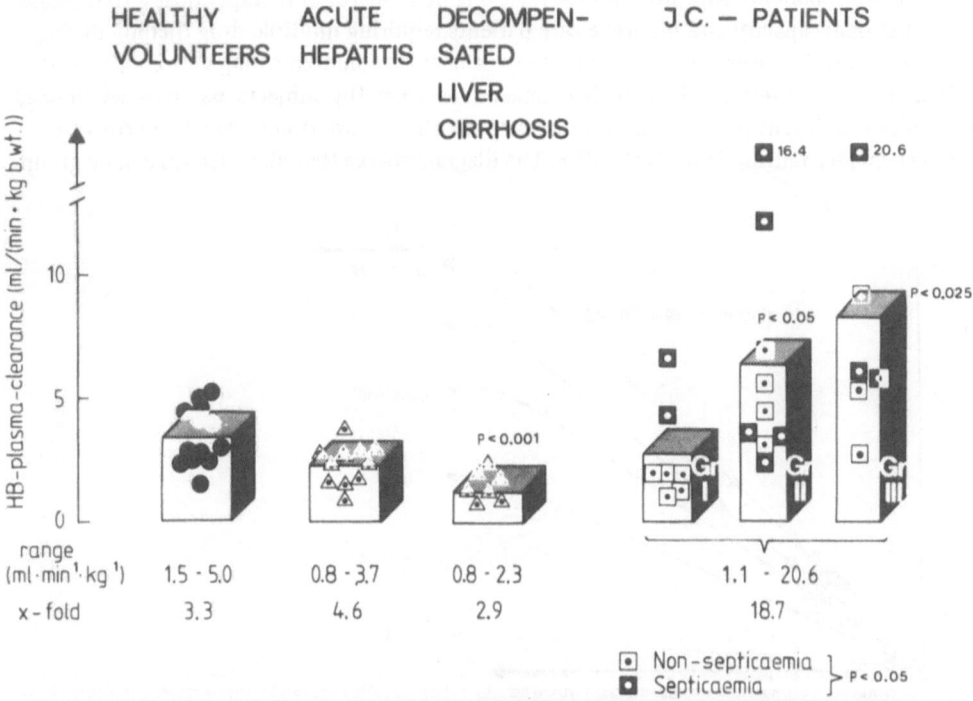

Fig. 2. Hexobarbitone plasma clearances in healthy volunteers, patients with acute hepatitis, decompensated liver cirrhosis and I.C. patients. The latter were divided into three groups. In group I patients were tested on the 3rd and 4th days, in group II between the 5th and 8th days and in group III between the 13th and 29th days after initiation of intensive care therapy. [Adapted from Breimer et al. [2], Keller [14], Rietbrock et al. [27], Zilly et al. [48]]

tivity appear gradually. The presence of septicaemia is usually associated with an elevated hexobarbitone clearance. This is surprising, since the addition of endotoxins to isolated liver mono-oxygenase preparations inhibits catalytic activity [24]. In patients with septicaemia, drug treatment leads to in vivo alterations in the liver cell membranes so that even a capacity limited drug like hexobarbitone can easily penetrate cells. When the plasma clearance in such patients exceeds 8 ml per min per kg b.wt. hexobarbitone must be regarded as a high clearance drug like lidocaine and propranolol. In these patients the hexobarbitone elimination is dependent on liver blood flow [27].

More insight into the influence of severe and complicated diseases requiring intensive care treatment and multiple drug therapy can be obtained by examining parameters of intrinsic drug metabolizing activity. Hepatic intrinsic activity is equivalent to the metabolic enzyme capacity of the entire liver and is related to the in vitro activity of microsomal enzyme preparations [7]. We have measured the hepatic extraction ratio for methohexitone. The hepatic extraction was determined directly by insertion of a catheter into the femoral artery and the hepatic vein or was measured indirectly from the area under the concentration time curves (AUC) following oral and intravenous doses in the same patient. This indirect method requires the use of the equation for a perfusion-limited model derived by Gibaldi et al. [12] and Rowland [29].

Figure 3 demonstrates the relationship between plasma clearance, hepatic extraction ratio and the apparent plasma flow for methohexitone [28]. The probands included healthy volunteers, patients with liver disease receiving phenobarbital therapeutically to increase liver functional capacity and intensive care patients requiring multiple drug therapy during artificial respiration. Hepatic extraction values in healthy volunteers ranged from 47%–90%. This large variation reflects the fact that some of these healthy subjects may have an induced metabolism. In intensive care and liver disease patients the variation in hepatic extraction was even greater ranging from 18%–99%. The diagram shows that all probands can be group-

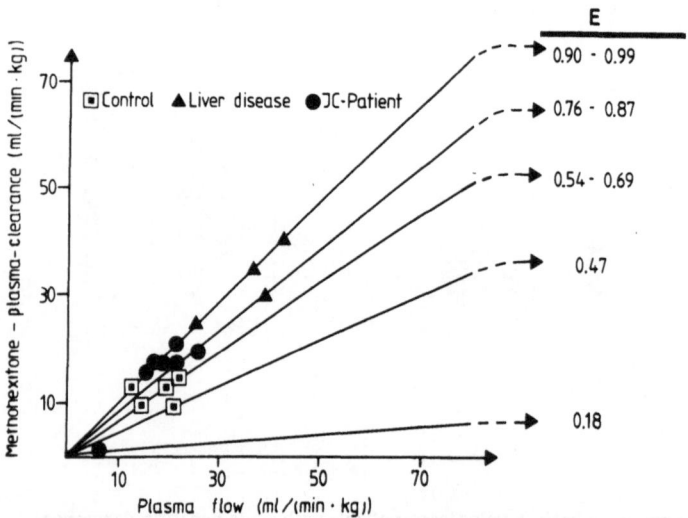

Fig. 3. The relationship between plasma clearance and apparent plasma flow within the given range of hepatic extraction ratios for methohexitone in healthy volunteers, patients with liver disease receiving phenobarbital therapeutically and I.C. patients requiring multiple drug therapy. [Adapted from Rietbrock et al. [28]]

ed according to their extraction ratio. The solid curves represent an approximation of the theoretical relationship between plasma clearance and plasma flow for the given ranges of hepatic extraction. The plasma clearance of methohexitone in the liver disease patients given phenobarbital was substantially higher than the control subjects and even higher than the intensive care patients. Since we know that liver disease patients without phenobarbital treatment have a limited metabolic capacity for drugs, these results with phenobarbital suggest that phenobarbital increases not only the extraction ratio but also the plasma flow.

Differences in the Oxidative and Reductive Pathways of Inhalation Anaesthetic Metabolism

The therapeutic importance of drug metabolism lies not only in the kinetics of drug elimination but also in the pharmacological activity and quantity of each metabolite produced. The main function of the mono-oxygenase system in the biotransformation process is the activation of molecular oxygen according to the following equation [16] (Fig. 4). In order to understand better the toxic side effects at the cellular and molecular level, which are controlled and regulated in vivo by cytochrome P_{450}, we have to study the details of these mechanisms. Cytochrome P_{450} is actually a family of similar but functionally different terminal oxidases, which differ slightly in their substrate binding spectrum [9, 13, 40, 44]. These differences in binding reflect the broad specificity of this enzyme system.

The mechanisms of action seem to be identical for all cytochrome P_{450} species [35, 36]. The ferrous iron in cytochrome P_{450} is the "catalytic site" for O_2 binding and the site of a reverse inhibition of the mono-oxygenases by carbon monoxide [21]. Cytochrome P_{450} contains one molecule of heme per polypeptide chain. P_{450} and polypeptides are linked together by the thiolate group of a cysteinyl residue. This bond is essential for hydroxylation. The "active site" of the enzyme, where the substrate binding occurs, is near the catalytic site at the sixth ligand opposite the thiolate ligand. In the first step of drug degradation, the cytochrome P_{450} binds the substrate in the oxidized form, causing the displacement of an unknown endogenous ligand, possibly a water molecule [20, 36] (Fig. 5).

The second step is the reduction of this enzyme substrate complex by an electron derived mainly from NADPH with the aid of a flavoprotein known as P_{450} reductase. The reduced heme rapidly reacts with molecular oxygen to form a dioxy-complex. A second electron from the reductase then forms a peroxo-complex. After addition of a proton water is released and we are left with the reactive intermediate complex [FeO]. This can either oxidize the substrate by hydroxylation or form epoxides [11, 35, 36, 39] (Fig. 6).

The most common metabolic pathway for inhalation anaesthetics is oxidation. During this process they are dehalogenated and/or O-dealkylated at the ether bridge [8]. Halothane is only dehalogenated leading to bromide, chloride and trifluoroacetic acid. The metabolism of a halogenated ether like enflurane and methoxyflurane includes both reactions. In contrast to methoxyflurane, with enflurane the metabolism is restricted due to its higher fluor-

$$RH + O_2 + DH_2 \rightarrow R\text{-}OH + H_2O + D$$

Fig. 4. Activation of molecular oxygen. *RH*, substrate; *DH₂*, reduced electron donor. [Adapted from Mason [16]]

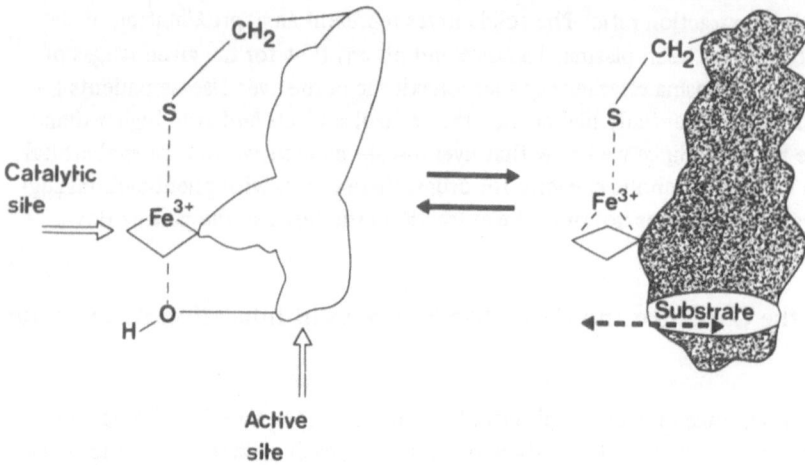

Fig. 5. Outline of the transition state of cytochrome P 450-catalyzed mono-oxygenation. [Adapted from Nebert et al. [20] and Ullrich [36]]

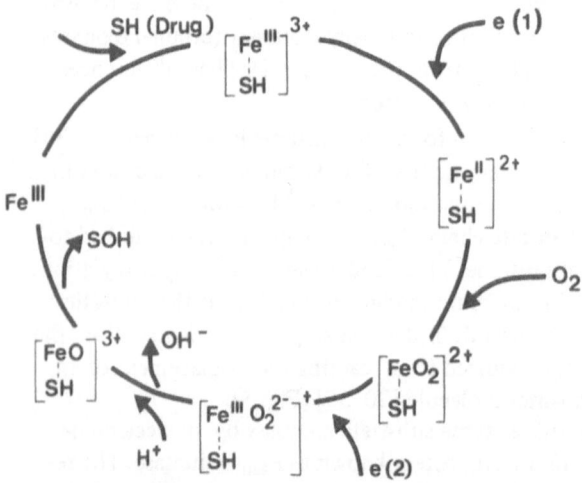

Fig. 6. Illustrates the electron transfer in drug oxidation. [Adapted from Estabrook et al. [11], Ullrich [35, 36], Ullrich and Staudinger [39]]

ide content. This is of clinical significance since a decreased fluoride release results in a lesser degree of renal damage with enflurane than with methoxyflurane.

We know that the formation of active radicals and intermediates precedes the formation of the final products of a reaction. Active radicals and some active intermediates have clinical importance since they can, under certain conditions, bind to cellular components and cause cellular damage such as liver necrosis. Such reactions have long been known to occur with chloroform [22, 23, 47]. They can also appear with halothane [33, 41], particularly during reductive metabolism [5, 6, 10, 17, 31, 34, 45]. During oxidative metabolism of halothane, when the O_2 supply is adequate, these active intermediates and active radicals readily combine with oxygen in preference to cell components and are thereby detoxified (Fig. 7).

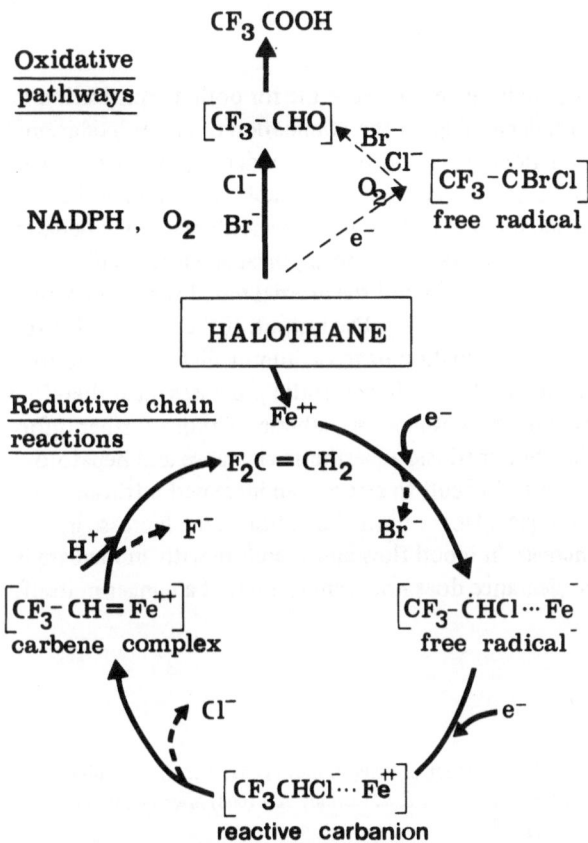

Fig. 7. Metabolic pathways of halothane. [Adapted from Mansuy et al. [15], Nastainczyk et al. [19], Stier [33], Ullrich and Schnabel [38], Van Dyke and Chenoweth [41], Van Dyke and Gandolfi [42]]

The oxidative pathway must therefore be regarded as a true detoxification pathway [25]. This has been verified by covalent binding studies using tissue components and ^{14}C-labelled halothane [43].

The reductive pathways of polyhalogenated hydrocarbons such as halothane are also catalysed by cytochrome P_{450} (Fig. 7). The electrons are used for the reductive elimination of chloride and bromide. During this process, the halogenated hydrocarbons can accept electrons from the ferrous iron of cytochrome P_{450} [38]. In the first step of the reductive pathway of halothane an electron from P_{450} leads to the formation of a debrominated radical. This represents a key step in the reductive metabolism of halothane. During hypoxia the covalent binding of this debrominated radical is very high, resulting in lipid peroxidation [4]. This is evident from the increased exhalation of 2-chloro-1,1,1-trifluoroethane and 2-chloro-1,1-difluoroethylene [18, 30]. The transfer of a second electron from cytochrome P_{450} may occur to form a carbanion [15, 19]. Following the reductive elimination of chloride, a carbene complex is formed at the ferrous iron of cytochrome P_{450}. β-elimination of fluoride and the acceptance of a proton gives rise to a 1,1-difluoroethane [15, 19, 38, 42]. In this manner these events constitute a cycle. This chain reaction process of halothane metabolism during hypoxia can lead to progressive liver damage (Fig. 7).

Regulatory Mechanisms of Hepatic Blood Flow

I have shown that the drug metabolism of halothane is responsible for both detoxification and the formation of toxic intermediates, depending on the domination of either oxidation or reduction pathways in the individual patient. This is in turn dependent upon the degree of hypoxia. The liver has more than one homeostatic mechanism available to overcome the hypoxia that could arise due to decreased hepatic blood flow during anaesthesia. When hepatic blood flow is reduced the oxygen extraction is increased in both portal and arterial blood. Furthermore, when the portal blood flow is compromised the arterial blood supply may increase. This phenomenon is coupled with an enhanced cardiac output. If the body is able to maintain these homeostatic processes, the accumulation of toxic intermediates of reductive metabolism will be prevented. The breakdown of these homeostatic processes must therefore be regarded as the cause of liver damage during halothane anaesthesia. Without further information on the relationship between inhalation intrinsic anaesthetic clearance and hepatotoxic reactive intermediate concentrations, it is difficult to assess if an increased intrinsic clearance causes or contributes to liver damage. Under normal conditions the increase in intrinsic clearance is coupled with an increase in blood flow and therefore with an increase in the oxygen availability. A high intrinsic clearance does not seem to present a danger in itself.

References

1. Breckenridge A, Bending MR, Brunner G (1977) Impact of drug monoxygenases in clinical pharmacology. In: Ullrich V, Roots I, Hildebrandt A, Estabrook RW, Conney AH (eds) Microsomes and drug oxidations. Pergamon Press, Frankfurt, p 385
2. Breimer DD, Zilly W, Richter E (1975) Pharmacokinetics of hexobarbital in acute hepatitis and after apparent recovery. Clin Pharmacol Ther 18:433
3. Brodie BB, Gillette JR (1971) Concepts in biochemical pharmacology. 2. In: Handbook of experimental pharmacology. Springer, Berlin Heidelberg New York, pp
4. Brown BR (1972) Hepatic microsomal lipoperoxidation and inhalation anesthetics: a biochemical and morphologic study on the rat. Anesthesiology 36:458
5. Brown BR, Sipes IG (1977) Biotransformation and hepatotoxicity of halothane. Biochem Pharmacol 26:2091–2094
6. Brown BR Jr, Sipes IG, Baker RK (1977) Halothane hepatotoxicity and the reduced derivative, 1,1,1-trifluoro-2-chloroethane. Environ Health Perspect 21:185–188
7. Cobby J, Makoid MC (1980) The use of marker drugs to measure organ function: a theoretical interpretation. Eur J Clin Pharmacol 18:511–516
8. Cohen EN, Van Dyke RA (1977) Metabolism of volatile anesthetics. Implications for toxicity. Addison-Wesley, Reading, Massachusetts; Menlo Park, California; London; Amsterdam, Don Mills, Ontario; Sydney
9. Coon MJ, Ballou DP, Haugen DA, Krezoski SO, Nordblom GD, White RE (1977) Purification of membrane-bound oxygenases: isolation of two electrophoretically homogeneous forms of liver microsomal cytochrome P 450. In: Ullrich V, Roots I, Hildebrandt A, Estabrook RW, Conney AH (eds) Microsomes and drug oxidations. Pergamon Press, Frankfurt, p 82
10. Cousins MJ, Sharp JH, Gourlay GK, Adams JF, Haynes WD, Whitehead R (1979) Hepatotoxicity and halothane metabolism in an animal model with application for human toxicity. Anaesth Intensive Care 7:9–24
11. Estabrook RW, Hildebrandt A, Ullrich V (1968) Oxygen interaction with reduced cytochrome P 450. Hoppe Seylers Z Physiol Chem 349:1605
12. Gibaldi M, Boyes RN, Feldman S (1971) Influence of first pass effect on availability of drugs on oral administration. J Pharm Sci 60:1338–1340

13. Haugen DA, Van der Hoeven TA, Coon MJ (1975) Purified liver microsomal cytochrome P 450. Separation and characterization of multiple forms. J Biol Chem 250:3567
14. Keller B (1976) Pharmakokinetische Untersuchungen zur Beurteilung der Hexobarbital-Toleranz bei Lebergesunden vor und nach einer Behandlung mit Prednison oder Rifampicin sowie bei Patienten mit akuter Hepatitis und Leberzirrhose. Inaugural Dissertation, Universität Würzburg
15. Mansuy D, Nastainczyk W, Ullrich V (1979) The mechanism of halothane binding to microsomal cytochrome P 450. Naunyn Schmiedebergs Arch Pharmacol 285:315–324
16. Mason HS (1957) Mechanisms of oxygen metabolism. Adv Enzymol 19:79
17. McLain GE, Sipes IG, Brown BR (1979) An animal model of halothane hepatotoxicity: roles of enzyme induction and hypoxia. Anesthesiology 51:321–326
18. Mukai S, Morio M, Fujii K, Hanaki C (1977) Volatile metabolites of halothane in the rabbit. Anesthesiology 47:248–251
19. Nastainczyk W, Ullrich V, Sies H (1978) Effect of oxygen concentration on the reaction of halothane with cytochrom P 450 in liver microsomes and isolated perfused rat liver. Biochem Pharmacol 27:387–392
20. Nebert DW, Kumaki K, Sato M, Kon H (1977) Association on type I, type II, and reverse type I difference spectra with absolute spin state of cytochrome P 450 iron. In: Ullrich V, Roots I, Hildebrandt A, Estabrook RW, Conney AH (eds) Microsomes and drug oxidations. Pergamon Press, Frankfurt, pp 224–231
21. Omura T, Sato R (1964) The carbon monoxide-binding pigment of liver microsomes. J Biol Chem 239:2370-2378
22. Paul BP, Rubinstein D (1963) Metabolism of carbon tetrachlorid and chloroform by the rat. J Pharmacol Exp Ther 141:141
23. Recknagel R, Glende E (1973) Carbon tetrachloride hepatotoxicity, an example of lethal cleavage. Crit Rev Toxicol 2:263-297
24. Renton KW, Mannering GJ (1977) Depression of hepatic cytochrome P 450-dependent mono-oxygenase systems with administered interferon inducing agents. In: Ullrich V, Roots I, Hildebrandt A, Estabrook RW, Conney AH (eds) Microsomes and drug oxidations. Pergamon Press, Frankfurt, p 484
25. Rietbrock I (1978) Zur Frage der Hepatotoxizität von Halothan. In: Kirchner E (ed) 20 Jahre Fluothane. Anaesthesiol Intensivmed Prax 109:25
26. Rietbrock I, Richter E (1978) Veränderungen der Pharmakokinetik unter der Intensivtherapie. In: Lawin P, Morr-Strathman U (eds) Aktuelle Probleme der Intensivbehandlung. Thieme, Stuttgart, p 207
27. Rietbrock I, Lazarus G, Richter E, Breimer DD (1981) Hexobarbital disposition at different stages of intensive-care treatment. Br J Anaesth 53:283
28. Rietbrock I, Richter E, Heusler H, Breimer DD (to be published) Methohexitone disposition in healthy subjects liver disease and intensive-care patients. Kinetics and clearance-apparent blood flow relationships. Br J Anaesthesiol
29. Rowland M (1972) Influence of route of administration on drug availability. J Pharm Sci 61:70–74
30. Sharp JH, Trudell JR, Cohen EN (1979) Volatile metabolites and decomposition products of halothane in man. Anesthesiology 50:2
31. Sipes IG, Podolsky TL, Brown BR (1977) Bioactivation and covalent binding of halothane to liver macromolecules. Environ Health Perspect 21:171–178
32. Sotaniemi EA, Ylostalo PR, Kauppila AJ (1974) Factors affecting drug administration in hospital. Eur J Clin Pharmacol 7:473
33. Stier A (1965) Der Stoffwechsel des Halothane und seine pharmakologisch-toxikologische Bedeutung. Habilitationsschrift, Universität Würzburg
34. Uehleke H, Hellmer KH, Taberelli-Poplawski S (1973) Metabolic activation of halothane and its covalent binding to liver endoplasmic proteins in vitro. Naunyn Schmiedebergs Arch Exp Pathol Pharmakol 279:39
35. Ullrich V (1972) Enzymatische Hydroxylierungen mit molekularem Sauerstoff. Angew Chem [Engl] 84:689
36. Ullrich V (1977) The mechanism of cytochrome P 450 action. In: Ullrich V, Roots I, Hildebrandt A, Estabrook RW, Conney AH (eds) Microsomes and drug oxidations. Pergamon Press, Frankfurt, pp 192–201

37. Ullrich V, Kremers P (1977) Multiple forms of cytochrome P 450 in the microsomal mono-oxyge-
     nase system. Arch Toxicol 39:41–50
38. Ullrich V, Schnabel KH (1973) Formation and binding of carbanions by cytochrome P 450 of liver
     microsomes. Drug Metab Dispos 1:176–183
39. Ullrich V, Staudinger HJ (1969) Aktivierung von Sauerstoff in Modellsystemen. In: Hess B, Staudin-
     ger HJ (eds) Biochemie des Sauerstoffs. Springer, Berlin Heidelberg New York, p 229
40. Ullrich V, Frommer U, Weber P (1973) Characterization of cytochrome P 450 species in rat liver
     microsomes. I. Differences in the 0-dealkylation of 7-ethoxycoumarin after pretreatment with phe-
     nobarbital and 3-methylcholanthrene. Hoppe Seylers Z Physiol Chem 354:514
41. Van Dyke RA, Chenoweth MB (1965) Metabolism of volatile anesthetics. Anesthesiology 26:348
42. Van Dyke RA, Gandolfi AJ (1976) Anaerobic release of fluoride from halothane. Relationship to
     the binding of halothane metabolites to hepatic cellular constituents. Drug Metab Dispos 4:40–44
43. Van Dyke RA, Wood CL (1975) In vitro studies on irreversible binding of halothane metabolite to
     microsomes. Drug Metab Dispos 3:51–57
44. Welton AF, O'Neal O, Chaney LC, Aust SD (1975) Multiplicity of cytochrome P 450 hemopro-
     teins in rat liver microsomes. J Biol Chem 250:5631
45. Widger LA, Gandolfi AJ, Van Dyke RA (1976) Hypoxia and halothane metabolism in vivo. Release
     of inorganic fluoride and halothane metabolite binding to cellular constituents. Anesthesiology 44:
     197
46. Wilkinson GR, Shand DG (1975) A physiological approach to hepatic drug clearance. Clin Pharmacol
     Ther 18:377
47. Wislow SG, Gerstner HB (1978) Health aspects of chloroform, a review. Drug Chem Toxicol 1:259–
     275
48. Zilly W, Breimer DD, Richter E (1978) Hexobarbital disposition in compensated and decompensated
     cirrhosis of the liver. Clin Pharmacol Ther 23:525

Hepatic Oxygenation and Fluoride Release During Halothane Anesthesia

L. Irestedt

Hepatic release of inorganic fluoride during halothane anaesthesia has been shown to indicate a reductive metabolic pathway resulting in the formation of other, potentially hepatotoxic halothane metabolites [Widger et al. 1976]. This knowledge is mainly based on experimental studies and obviously raises the question: "Does hepatic reductive halothane metabolism occur during clinical halothane anaesthesia in man"?

Most clinical studies have shown small or insignificant increases in F^--levels during halothane anaesthesia, except in very obese patients, where marked increases were found [Young et al. 1975]. Since low hepatic oxygen tissue pressure is a prerequisite for reductive halothane metabolism, it is essential to consider factors influencing hepatic oxygenation during halothane anaesthesia. Halothane seems to decrease hepatic blood flow and oxygenation to a greater extent than enflurane [Irestedt 1978; Hughes et al. 1980]. Upper abdominal surgery may further impair hepatic blood flow [Gelman 1976]. Another important factor may be an increase of hepatic oxygen uptake resulting from enzyme induction, which causes imbalance between oxygen supply and consumption during anaesthesia [Irestedt and Andreen 1978]. To find out whether or not clinical normoxic halothane anaesthesia is associated with hepatic fluoride release, we are performing a study from which preliminary results are given. Women undergoing hysterectomy under halothane anaesthesia preoperatively receive an arterial and a hepatic venous catheter from which blood is regularly sampled. Results from eight women during normoxic, normocapnic anaesthesia with 1% halothane show that hepatic fluoride release occurs in all patients throughout the operations. Arterial F^- concentration rose from 0.9 to 1.8 μmol and hepatic venous F^- concentration from 1 to 2.2 μmol during the operations. Hepatic venous oxygen tension decreased from 5.7 to 4.7 kPa.

The reason why hepatic fluoride release occurs during nonhypoxic halothane anaesthesia is probably the uneven distribution of hepatic tissue oxygen tensions, as demonstrated by Görnandt and Kessler [1973], resulting in low oxygen pressure areas within the liver, in spite of adequate hepatic oxygenation. In conclusion it seems as though halothane, to a small but certain extent, undergoes reductive metabolism under normoxic halothane anaesthesia in healthy patients. Factors such as obesity, enzyme induction, hyperventilation, hypovolemia, and upper abdominal surgery will probably increase this tendency.

References

1. Gelman SJ (1976) Disturbances in hepatic blood flow during anesthesia and surgery. Arch Surg 111: 881
2. Görnandt L, Kessler M (1973) PO_2 histograms in regenerating liver tissue. In: Kessler M, Bruley DF, Clark LC, Lübbers DW, Silver JA, Strauss J (eds) Oxygen in tissue. Urban & Schwarzenberg, München Berlin Wien, p 288
3. Hughes RL, Cambell D, Fitch W (1980) Effects of enflurane and halothane on liver blood flow and oxygen consumption in the greyhound. Br J Anaesth 52:1079
4. Irestedt L (1978) Haemodynamics and oxygen consumption during halothane, enflurane and neurolept anaesthesia. An experimental study in the dog with special reference to the liver and preportal tissues. Thesis, Karolinska institute, Stockholm
5. Irestedt L, Andreen M (1978) The effect of enzyme induction on hepatic oxygenation during enflurane anesthesia in the dog (Abstract). In: V European congress of anaesthesiology. Excerpta Medica, Amsterdam Princeton London Geneva New York (International congress series No. 452)
6. Widger LA, Gandolfi AJ, Van Dyke RA (1976) Hypoxia and halothane metabolism in vivo: Release of inorganic fluoride and halothane metabolite binding to cellular constituents. Anaesthesiology 44: 197
7. Young SR, Stoelting RK, Peterson C, Madura JA (1975) Anesthetic biotransformation and renal function in obese patients during and after methoxyflurane or halothane anesthesia. Anesthesiology 42:451

Current Status of Hepatotoxicity of the Halogenated Inhalation Anesthetics

B.R. Brown Jr.

The introduction of halothane to the clinical practice of anaesthesia was a milestone in its development. Here was an anaesthetic which was easily controllable, potent, pleasant for the patient, and with a minimum of deleterious side effects. Although there were individuals who voiced the opinion that the drug might have some of the potential hepatotoxic drawbacks of chloroform, Raventos' [1] early observations indicated that no direct liver toxicity was seen following anaesthesia with halothane in experimental animals. However, within a number of years following the release of halothane, there was a plethora of articles reporting unexplained and unanticipated jaundice and massive hepatic necrosis following anaesthesia with this drug [2, 3, 4]. These cases created considerable controversy, primarily more heat than light. The cases of jaundice were rare and sporadic. However, sufficient numbers were reached to spur the National Halothane Study [5], one of the largest epidemiologic works ever performed. Unfortunately, this study was inconclusive. There appeared to be a non-statistically significant hint of a problem involving halothane, but it was certainly not proven by this large nonrandomized and retrospective epidemiologic study.

Continuing case reports stimulated the search for a mechanism, however. Some means had to be postulated by which halothane could produce hepatic damage. Three possibilities were available: (a) that halothane was a hepatotoxin similar in nature to carbon tetrachloride; (b) that the hepatic reaction was immunologically mediated; or, (c) that the actual disease observed was viral hepatis. Since the lesion could not be demonstrated in experimental animals with normal anaesthetizing concentrations of halothane, the first speculation was received with little enthusiasm. The third possibility was widely entertained, particularly by advocates of the anaesthetic, for several years. Recent advances in serologic tests for hepatitis A and B have effectively ruled out these entities in many reported cases, however. Since many hepatologists were by virtue of training immunologists, the belief arose that the entity of so-called halothane hepatitis might be an allergenic phenomenon. This speculation was supported by the fact that there seemed to be a higher incidence following a second or multiple administration of the anaesthetic, and by the report that certain individuals believed to be susceptible to this process, when challenged with halothane, had alterations in liver enzymes and other hepatic variables indicating toxic damage [6, 7]. Predicated on this belief, several dogmas concerning halothane use were promulgated. These included restraint on use for a second administration for a variable period of time, from 3 months to 12 months, depending on the author. The fact of unexplained jaundice attending repeated administrations of halothane seemed to be fairly well confirmed. Little [8] reported that 49% of patients in his series of postsurgical jaundice had received two or more administrations of halothane prior to developing hepatic damage, and Klatskin [7] noted that 68% of the patients in his series had had more than one anaesthetic with the drug. Recent reports have confirmed that there seems to be a higher attack rate following more than one closely spaced administration. For example, a recent report by Trowell [9] and associates demonstrated that British women given halothane anaesthesia during radium therapy for carcinoma of the cervix had gross elevations of serum glutamic pyruvate transaminase plasma levels following multiple administrations of the anaesthetic, although none of the 39 patients in this series developed overt liver necrosis. Substantiation of the allergenic theory of the mechanism of halothane necrosis was reinforced by the findings of Paronetto and Popper [10]. These investigators found that there was increased incorporation of tritiated thymidine into lymphocytes harvested from supposed halothane hepatitis patients. Reports of eosinophilia, skin rashes, and arthralgia coincident with halothane hepatitis appeared confirmatory. A recent study by Vergani and co-workers [11] demonstrates that circulating antibodies reacting specifically with cell membranes of hepatocytes isolated from halothane-anaesthetized rabbits were detected in nine out of 11 patients with fulminant hepatic failure following halothane anaesthesia.

However, to detract from this thesis several phenomena were noted. The first, and most significant, was that many of the cases of halothane hepatitis represented first administrations. It is certainly difficult to understand how a patient could be made allergic to a drug during the first encounter. Also, there is a noticeable paucity of published case reports in infants and children, implying, at least in a negative sense, that the young are not susceptible to this disease. Yet individuals in this age-group do have a rather high frequency of allergically mediated diseases. There has been at least one published series [12] in which patients with multiple administrations of halothane had no liver problems whatsoever. The work of Trowell et al. [9] was repeated in a genetically dissimilar but pathologically similar group in South Africa, with no deleterious hepatic effects noted [13]. The lymphocyte transformation test has been repeated by several groups with negative results [14]. Resolution of these conflicting reports seems difficult.

It was only as recently as 1964 that it was recognized that halothane and other halogenated anaesthetics of similar genre are biotransformed [15, 16]. Previously, it had been taught categorically that anaesthetics were metabolically inert. During approximately the same era, parallel studies were looking at the cause of hepatic necrosis due to classic hepatotoxins such as carbon tetrachloride. It was observed that it is the biotransformation and bioactivation of carbon tetrachloride that is a vector in the hepatic damage produced by this halogenated alkyl, halide, and not the parent molecule [17]. Through the process of metabolic breakdown, carbon tetrachloride is converted to free radicals and/or reactive intermediates, which are capable of damaging hepatic molecular structures. If carbon tetrachloride is given to animals and the metabolism of the compound blocked, very little in the way of hepatic damage results. By the same token, the dosage of carbon tetrachloride required to produce hepatic damage in newborn animals (those with immature biotransformation systems) is much higher than in adults [18].

There are three known mechanisms by which halogenated compounds produce hepatic damage. These are: (a) lipoperoxidation, (b) decrease of intrinsic antioxidants, and (c) covalent binding. Lipoperoxidation is defined as a breakdown of long-chain fatty acids such as arachidonic, linoleic, and linolenic acids by an oxidative process. This consists primarily of abstraction of a hydrogen adjacent to a double-bonded carbon atom, followed by the attachment of oxygen which forms a peroxy radical. The peroxy radical then abstracts hydrogen from adjacent fatty acid molecules, with concomitant autocatalytic breakdown of the molecules to aldehydes. Thus lipoperoxidation is tantamount to destructive cleavage of integral phospholipids, proteins, and cellular membrane components. The net result is necrosis. Lipoperoxidation has been demonstrated during the biotransformation of halothane [19]. Not only has this effect been seen in animals, but it is also present in humans. Human patients anaesthetized with halothane show a variable degree of lipoperoxidation, as demonstrated by expired pentane. However, the dose-response relationships of lipoperoxidation are quite poor. Nevertheless, this destructive process does occur with each and every halothane anaesthetic, indicating that a certain degree of liver alteration occurs, even though this is clinically insignificant.

Antioxidant depletion seems unlikely to be one of the factors involved in halothane hepatotoxicity. One of the principal antioxidants in the liver is reduced glutathione. It serves as an antioxidant by virtue of its sulfhydryl group. Depletion of glutathione is integral in the hepatotoxicity of carbon tetrachloride and chloroform. Experimental research in animals indicates that in the case of halothane, even with the advent of necrosis there is no drop in glutathione concentration [20].

Let us now consider the third possibility, covalent bonding. When alkyl halides are metabolized to reactive intermediates, those intermediates with an unpaired, unstable covalent electron are capable of combining and binding with contiguous lipoprotein and protein molecules. Such binding alters the tertiary structure of these proteins and lipids, and hence alters functional integrity. Thus covalent bonding has been compared to liver damage. Several years ago, Uehleke and his co-workers [21] showed that the biotransformation of halothane will result in covalent bonding under very special circumstances. These circumstances are in the presence of nitrogen, or rather in the absence of oxygen. Stier and co-workers [15] in Germany, who first demonstrated biotransformation of halothane, indicated that this was primarily an oxidative destruction of the anaesthetic. This metabolism was mediated through cytochrome P_{450}, and resulted in the formation of the metabolites trifluoroacetic acid, chloride ion, and bromide ion. For years it was thought that this was the only pathway available for the biotransformation of halothane. However, if one looks at reductive or non-oxygen-dependent breakdown, the metabolic by-products are trifluoroethane and difluorochloroethylene. These metabolites are found in very small quantities in both animals and man when halothane is given. This implies that although halothane is metabolized mostly via the innocuous oxidative pathway, a small amount is metabolized via the reductive or non-oxygen pathway [22].

It the non-oxygen-dependent or reductive pathway is the one that produces a considerable quantity of free radicals, then increasing the amount of halothane being shunted down this pathway could result in liver damage. This has now been shown to be correct, and is the basis for the hypoxia animal model of halothane toxicity [23]. In this model animals are pretreated with the inducing drug, phenobarbital, so as to stimulate biotransformation of halothane. The animals are then anaesthetized in a slightly hypoxic environment, $FIO_2 = 0.14$, such that there is an obligatory non-oxygen-dependent opening of this pathway. Under these circumstances extensive hepatocellular damage occurs, with rises in transaminases and other features of hepatic destruction. The validity of this animal experiment has now been proven in several laboratories throughout the world. With this model there is also found a large increase in covalent bonding of fluorine-containing organic metabolites of halothane to liver tissue.

Thus the final vector of hepatotoxicity in the case of halothane may be altered biotransformation, particularly down the reductive or non-oxygen-dependent pathway. How can these experimental animal findings relate to the problem of hepatotoxicity in man? From epidemiologic studies it is known that there are certain variables which may increase the risk of a patient developing hepatic necrosis following the administration of halothane: age, degree of obesity, and genetics. Each of these will now be surveyed.

The disease seems to be primarily one of middle age. A recent review from Sweden [24] indicates that the peak of susceptibility to halothane hepatitis is at a later age than that to viral hepatitis, again pinpointing the drug interaction as one which is predominantly of middle age. The middle-aged group comprises those individuals with the highest-developed drug-metabolizing systems. Also during middle age, in the current drug-oriented society, the largest number of microsomal inducing agents are taken. On the other hand, attack rates for the very young and the very old for halothane hepatitis appear to be very low. This is consistent with the metabolic activation theory of halothane hepatitis, since the very young and the very old are at the tail-end of the spectrum of drug biotransformation. This may account for the safety of halothane for repeat anaesthetics in the very young.

There have been reports since soon after the introduction of halothane that obese patients are more susceptible to halothane hepatitis than are patients of normal weight [25]. Investigators have demonstrated that, for the same number of MAC hours, the obese patient metabolizes more halogenated volatile anaesthetic than his normal-weight counterpart. The reason for this is the highly lipophilic nature of the inhalation anaesthetics, which are stored in fat and slowly released back to the liver for biotransformation over a period of hours at the termination of the anaesthetic. Thus obesity fits well into the metabolic activation theory, from a quantitative aspect at least. Second administrations which seem to support an allergenic theory may actually give considerable weight to the bioactivation theory of halothane hepatitis. Many cases of second administration which this author has reviewed have been in patients who have been in hospital and received various inducing drugs, such as barbiturates, sedatives, etc., between anaesthetics. Obviously, these patients are in quite a different condition from that when they received the drug on the first occasion. During periods of hospitalization there is frequently some starvation, which enhances microsomal cytochrome P_{450}. These patients have undergone essential changes since they received their first administration.

There does seem to be a genetic predisposition to the disease. It has been noted in the United States that the Mexican/American female has a relatively very high incidence of attacks of halothane hepatitis [26]. Genetic links could imply activation of a certain metabolic pathway, which would be the reductive or non-oxygen-dependent pathway. This qualitative change, coupled with the quantitative change of obesity, could lead to enhanced reductive metabolism, generation of free radicals, covalent bonding of sufficient magnitude to progress to functional alteration, and eventual necrosis of the liver.

Is there any basis for the allergenic theory? Recent evidence indicates that there are certain haptenes formed by the interaction of halothane metabolites and cell membranes [11]. Even in the case of the classic hepatotoxin carbon tetrachloride, antigenic compounds similar to these are formed [27]. The antibodies demonstrated by the Vergani group [11] arose rather late to give strong sway to any primary antigenic effect of halothane or its metabolites. Perpetuation of liver disease in the human may in many cases be due to an antigenic component. For example, in viral hepatitis, chronic passive hepatitis can result even when there is no virus demonstrable. It is entirely plausible that the virus initiates a destructive process, producing hepatocytic antigens which perpetuate the liver destruction. In a parallel fashion halothane metabolites may produce antigenic material which will perpetuate and intensify the lesion. Therefore the metabolic activation theory could still have an allergic component for the long-term disease syndrome.

The newer halogenated anaesthetics, enflurane and isoflurane, seem to be metabolized at a far slower rate than halothane. It is also theoretically possible that metabolism of isoflurane produces less in the way of reactive intermediates than halothane, such that there are both qualitative and quantitative differences. It is interesting that after some 35 million administrations of enflurane, there are very few well-documented cases of subsequent hepatic necrosis. This phenomenon is seen in animals, where a sequence of halogenated anaesthetics can be graded according to quantitative hepatic injuries. Chloroform is far more injurious than fluroxene, and this compound more than halothane, and halothane more than enflurane, and enflurane more than isoflurane. In fact, animal studies with isoflurane even under stressful conditions of biotransformation indicate that there is no liver damage. With enflurane very mild liver damage is seen under those identical conditions which produce rather extensive lobular necrosis with halothane (personal observations). Thus the feature of low blood air partition coefficient, which means basically that the anaesthetic will not remain in the body very long, and a molecular structure such that there is impediment to biotransformation, can theoretically result in a lower incidence of hepatic necrosis. It is quite possible that the introduction of enflurane and isoflurane means that there is a decrease in the number of case reports of unexplained hepatic necrosis following anaesthesia, since both these anaesthetics have a decreased propensity for biotransformation.

In summary it may be concluded that the halogenated anaesthetics may have a propensity to produce hepatic damage under certain circumstances. Although it is unproven clinically, there is strong supporting experimental evidence to indicate that the initial cause of such damage may lie in metabolic activation of the compounds. Degree of metabolic activation to reactive intermediates is a multifactorial phenomenon involving qualitative and quantitative alterations of biotransformation, genetic predisposition, obesity, hepatic blood flow, partition coefficient, and structural configuration of the compound.

References

1. Raventos J (1956) The action of Fluothane – a new volatile anaesthetic. Br J Pharmacol Chemother 11:394
2. Virtue RW, Payne KW (1958) Post-operative death after Fluothane: Anesthesiology 19:562
3. Brody GL, Sweet RB (1963) Halothane anesthesia as a possible cause of massive hepatic necrosis. Anesthesiology 24:29
4. Lindenbauer J, Leifer E (1963) Hepatic necrosis associated with halothane anesthesia. N. Engl J Med 268:525
5. Bunker JP, Forest WH Jr, Mostell F et al. (eds) (1965) The national halothane study. A study of the possible association between halothane anesthesia and postoperative hepatic necrosis. NIGMS, Bethesda
6. Belfrage S, Ahlgren I, Axelson S (1966) Halothane hepatitis in an anesthetist. Lancet 2:1466
7. Klatskin G, Kimberg DV (1969) Recurrent hepatitis attributable to halothane sensitization in an anesthetist. N Engl J Med 280:515
8. Little DM (1968) Effects of halothane on hepatic function. In: Greene NM (ed) Halothane. F.A. Davis, Philadelphia
9. Trowell J, Peto R, Crampton-Smith A (1975) Controlled trial of repeated halothane anesthetics in patients with carcinoma of the uterine cervix treated with radium. Lancet 1:821
10. Paronetto F, Popper H (1970) Lymphocyte stimulation induced by halothane in patients with hepatitis following exposure to halothane. N Engl J Med 283:277

11. Vergani D, Mieli-Vergani G, Alberti A, et al. (1980) Antibodies to the surface of halothane-altered rabbit hepatocytes in patients with severe halothane-associated hepatitis. N Engl J Med 303:66
12. Gronert GA, Schaner PJ, Gunther RC (1968) Multiple halothane anesthesia in the burn patient. JAMA 205:878
13. Allen PJ, Downing JW (1977) A prospective study of hepatocellular function after repeated exposures to halothane or enflurane in women undergoing radium therapy for cervical cancer. Br J Anaesth 49:1035
14. Walton B, Dumond DC, Williams C, et al. (1973) Lymphocyte transformation: Absence of increased responses in alleged halothane jaundice. JAMA 225:494
15. Stier A, Alter H, Hessler O, et al. (1964) Urinary excretion of bromide in halothane anesthesia. Anesth Analg 43:723
16. Van Dyke RA, Chenoweth MB, Van Poznak A (1964) Metabolism of volatile anesthetics. I. Conversion in vivo of several anesthetics to $^{14}CO_2$ and chloride. Biochem Pharmacol 13:1239
17. Recknagel R, Ghoshal A (1966) Lipoperoxidation as a vector in carbon tetrachloride hepatotoxicity. Lab Invest 15:132
18. Castro JA, Sasame HA, Sussman H, et al. (1968) Diverse effects of SKF 525-A and antioxidants on carbon tetrachloride induced changes in liver P–450 content and ethylmorphine metabolism. Life Sci 1:129
19. Brown BR Jr (1972) Hepatic microsomal lipoperoxidation and inhalation anesthetics: A biochemical and morphologic study in the rat. Anesthesiology 36:458
20. Brown BR Jr, Sipes IG, Sagalyn AM (1974) Mechanisms of acute hepatic toxicity: Chloroform, halothane, and glutathione. Anesthesiology 41:454
21. Uehleke H, Hellmer KH, Tabarelli-Poplawski S (1973) Metabolic activation of halothane and its covalent binding in liver endoplasmic proteins in vitro. Arch Pharmacol 279:39
22. Widger LA, Gandolfi AJ, Van Dyke RA (1976) Hypoxia and halothane metabolism in vivo: Release of inorganic fluoride and halothane metabolites binding to cellular constituents. Anesthesiology 44:197
23. Brown BR Jr, Sipes IG (1977) Biotransformation and hepatotoxicity of halothane. Biochem Pharmacol 26:2019
24. Bottinger LE, Dalen E, Halten B (1976) Halothane induced liver damage: An analysis of the material reported to the Swedish adverse drug reaction committee, 1966–1973. Acta Anaesth Scand 20:40
25. Peters RL, Edmonson HA, Reynolds TA, et al. (1969) Hepatic necrosis associated with halothane anesthesia. Am J Med 47:748
26. Hoft RH, Bunker JP, Goodman HJ, et al. (1981) Halothane hepatitis in three pairs of closely related women. N Engl J Med 304:1023
27. Dienstag JL (1980) Halothane hepatitis: Allergy or idiosyncrasy? N Engl J Med 303:102

Present Status of Chronic Exposure to Trace Concentrations of Volatile Anaesthetics

H.O. Stoeckel and P.M. Lauven

Since Vaisman [28] reported in 1967 for the first time an increasing occurrence of miscarriages in female anaesthesists who had performed mainly ether anaesthesias, more and more attention has been paid to the putative detrimental effects caused by chronic exposure to trace concentrations of volatile anaesthetics.

According to a survey of anaesthetic procedures practised in the university clinics and large municipal hospitals in the Federal Republic of Germany, about 60% of the anaesthesias have been performed with volatile agents, 30% by means of intravenously administered anaesthetics plus nitrous oxide and about 10% as regional anaesthesias during recent years. In other countries the percentage of inhalation anaesthesia is presumably even higher.

The still evident importance of inhalation anaesthesia and the possibly toxic potency of volatile anaesthetics discussed in numerous publications since 1967 call again and again for a critical evaluation of the risk, together with a demand for protective measures.

Moreover, uncritical comments in newspapers, TV and radio as well as the law for protection of motherhood disconcert the public (and personnel), and there are already suits for damages pending.

The relevant literature comprises in vitro studies on cellular toxicity, animal experiments in laboratories, epidemiological investigations with the affected groups of persons as well as — with regard to one special problem, namely psychomotor performance — experiments with test subjects.

Furthermore, investigations concerning the efficiency of protective measures against contamination of the room air have been carried out. So far, the following putative lesions in man have been described. Influences on:

1. Fertility (rates of abortions, premature deliveries and anomalies)
2. Possible cancerogenity
3. Impairment of psychomotor activity

The studies carried out with in vitro models — such as cell cultures of different kinds, preparations of rat liver mitochondria and so on — can be neglected in this review, since they do not deal with long-term exposure to trace concentrations, but with clinically relevant dosages of inhalation anaesthetics. The same applies to studies on the suppressive effects of cellular immunity and on haematopoiesis.

Controlled animal experimental studies constitute the only alternative for applying results to man. For well-known reasons, including, for example, frequently missing or inadequate statistical methods, these results call, however, for sceptical evaluation. It should also be noted that the majority of these studies, too, are related to clinically relevant dosages. These doses are 100- to 10 000-fold higher than the room air concentrations and will therefore also not be considered here. Investigations with gnawers, which with respect to time of exposure and room air concentrations corresponded to clinical conditions, led to contradictory results for halothane, N_2O and chloroform as well as methoxyflurane and enflurane.

In analogy to clinical conditions, exposure times of 4-8 h/day for 5 days/week were used in such investigations. Total examination period ranged from 4 up to a maximum of 32 weeks. After an exposure time of 4 h without special protective measures, as for instance exhaust system or gas-absorbing coal filter, the following room air concentrations in operating rooms were determined within a distance of 1 metre from the anaesthesist's workplace:

N_2O: 5600 ppm (Lauven and Stoeckel, 1981)

Halothane: 57 ppm (Nikki et al., 1972)

Enflurane: 130 ppm (Lauven and Stoeckel, 1981)

In a poorly ventilated room these concentrations may be even higher.

Studies in animal experiments on hepatotoxic effects showed that halothane did not exhibit toxic effects under the conditions mentioned. The same is true for histologically detectable lesions of the kidneys.

With regard to fertility, investigations of Bruce [3] as well as of Wharton and co-workers [2, 30] showed that in experiments with mice under halothane influence there were no differences concerning frequency of pregnancies, miscarriages, premature births and anomalies as compared to control animals.

According to a study of Corbett et al. [9], a significant decrease in pregnancy frequency and a marked increase in the rate of miscarriages was to be observed in rats exposed to trace doses of N_2O (15 000 ppm). Fink [8] found an influence on rat fetuses only after long-term exposure plus clinically relevant dosages of at least 25% N_2O.

In the reports quoted so far only a single agent per se, namely N_2O or halothane, was administered. A study of Coate [6], however, demonstrated that, in rats, dose-dependent cytogenetic alterations in the medulla and in the spermatogones were found following a combined administration of both drugs, as is usual in clinical practice. The applied concentrations were 1 ppm halothane with 50 ppm N_2O and 10 ppm halothane with 500 ppm N_2O. Moreover, rate of ovulation decreased as did implantation of the ovum; furthermore, a retardation of fetal development was observed. Garro and Phillips [15] recently reported on a mutagenic effect of the BCD (bromine-chlorine-difluoroethylene) metabolite, while the Standford group [11] found that this BCD metabolite may be generated outside the organism in anaesthetic apparatuses working with CO_2-absorption chalk.

The question of a possible carcinogenity was investigated by Linde and Bruce [20] in rats under exposure to halothane. The authors could not detect pathological alterations in any of the organs examined; this could have indicated the growth of fresh tumours.

Epidemiological studies in groups of persons exposed to trace concentrations were performed several times and constituted the starting point for the discussion of the problem; this discussion has been going on now for 14 years.

To come to the point, the results in the available literature are extremely contradictory and have repeatedly led to critical comments. The difficulties of performing epidemiological studies will be mentioned here cursorily and at the same time as criticism of the studies in the literature [12]: too small groups, no control groups or only ones that cannot be compared to each other, wrong methodological procedures or misleading interpretations of statistical date. The well-known disadvantages of restrospective studies and last but not least the disregard of other variables has led to wrong conclusions.

The present studies primarily deal with questions of fertility and cancerogenity.

Apart from the early reports of Vaisman in 1967 [28] and Askrog and Harvald in 1970 [1], above all the working groups around Ellis N. Cohen [7] in the United States as well as those around Knill-Jones [18] and Spence [27] in Great Britain should be mentioned here. The most extensive and best known investigation is the American publication in 1974 entitled *Occupational disease among operating room personnel. A national study* [7].

Without being able to enter here into the numerous details of the American *National study* [7], which comprises about 7600 persons exposed to trace concentrations and without being able to consider the many details of the international analysis of the independent data compiled in the United States and Great Britain by Spence, E. Cohen, Knill-Jones and other authors [27] from 2200 exposed persons, the essential points are summarized as follows:

1. The rate of miscarriages in female doctors exposed to trace concentrations is raised
2. The rate of anomalies in children of exposed female doctors is raised
3. Male anaesthetists exhibit a higher incidence of hepatic diseases
4. The children of male anaesthetists exhibit an increased rate of anomalies
5. In the wives of the anaesthetists exposed to trace concentrations the incidence of miscarriages is not raised
6. In male anaesthetists the rate of cancer is not increased

Despite emphasizing that there was no evidence for a cause-effect relationship, it follows from these statements that the mere possibility of a causal relationship justifies the application of all measures for diminishing the room contamination. As a possible serious cause for a cause-effect relationship one has to discuss, however, at least one other variable — and that is stress.

It is true that the existence of other causes than the trace dosages of inhalation anaesthetics cannot be proved exactly at the time being; these causes, however, cannot be precluded either. So, for instance, it is still absolutely impossible at the moment to appropriately judge and evaluate permanent stress by environmental factors such as foreign substances of an industrialized surrounding, living habits (foodstuff additives, stimulants like alcohol, etc., smoking) or genetic factors.

Walts et al. [29], Fink and Cullen [14] as well as Ferstandig [12] extensively criticize the epidemiological studies — in particular the American National Study [7] and the British-American study of Spence and co-workers [27]. The harshest criticism is expressed with regard to the methods of data gathering, statistical shortcomings and the logic of conclusions. These critics conclude that none of the previous epidemiological studies provide a clear proof that trace doses of volatile and gaseous anaesthetics are injurious to health.

Based on an extensive epidemiological survey on American dentists and their personnel, Cohen and co-workers recently established, however, that subsequent to use of N_2O an elevated rate of spontaneous abortions was to be observed in both female dentists and wives of dentists exposed to trace doses and that the teratogenicity of the fetuses of exposed women increased, as did the incidence of cancer with these women. This study, in which dental personnel not involved with the use of N_2O served as the control group, makes it reasonable to assume a relationship between exposure to N_2O and the injuries to health described above.

The third complex of possible injuries caused by exposure to trace dosages under discussion comprises psychomotor disorders. Investigations on impairments of the power of concentration under defined conditions have led to contradictory results. Thus, Bruce et al. [4] found in test subjects that 500 ppm N_2O strongly affected the power of concentration, while 500 ppm N_2O plus 15 ppm enflurane (or 10 ppm halothane) did not cause impairments as compared to control groups. Strangely enough, the same authors also observed an increase in vigilance at 50 ppm N_2O plus 1 ppm halothane in comparison to control experiments [5]. On the other hand, Smith and Shirley [26] did not find any changes in the psychomotor behaviour of test subjects who were exposed to 50 000 ppm N_2O plus 100 ppm halothane or 500 ppm N_2O plus 10 ppm halothane. Alterations in psychomotor behaviour were observed only upon administration of subtherapeutical concentrations, i.e. after 10 Vol% (100 000 ppm) N_2O and 0.1 Vol% (1000 ppm halothane).

Thus, at the moment it appears more likely that trace doses of inhalation anaesthetics in concentrations which usually are to be found in operating rooms without special exhaust devices do not cause an impairment of the psychomotor behaviour and that there is no reason to expect the contrary.

If one tries to summarize the findings of all the investigations mentioned and to venture from this an evaluation of the risk for the personnel in an operating room, one can say — under consideration of all aforementioned reservations concerning the vailidity of the data reported in literature — the following:

1. Neither the animal experiments nor the epidemiological studies can establish with certainty a cause-effect relationship with regard to trace doses of inhalation anaesthetics — the more so as the importance of other variables and co-variables, respectively, cannot be excluded. In the present state of knowledge a multifactorial aetiology has to be considered.

2. At present, however, the possibility of a causal relation cannot be excluded with certainty.

3. Thus, for the time being, the question of an indication for the introduction of protective measures, particularly of exhaust devices, cannot be clearly substantiated or rejected from the scientific point of view.

4. As long as the situation is unclear, most authors recommend a reduction of room air concentrations, above all the authors of the extensive British-American epidemiological study as well as the most important critics of these studies [14, 29].

The majority of the authors, including above all those who have published this year the report of the ASA ad hoc Committee on Effects of Trace Anaesthetic Agents on Health of Operating Room Personnel, call for a reduction to the absolutely possible minimum. In this connection conclusions drawn from animal experiments in the past years have played a role. These conclusions imply a possible importance of the BCD metabolite of halothane and interactive effects of halothane in combination with N_2O.

Finally, the necessity for elimination of anaesthetic gases and vapours was clearly defined in 1979 by legislature in the Federal Republic of Germany (law for Protection of Motherhood, article 4, paragraph 1). In 1977 the Trade Cooperative Association of Health Service and Welfare Work issued a corresponding recommendation.

What requirements must be met by an elimination of trace doses from the room air? The basis for the calculation of permissible maximum concentrations at workplaces (MAK values) is the rule that one-tenth to one-twelfth [22] of the toxic threshold concentrations ought to prevent injuries to health. The difficulty, however, is the determination of the threshold values on the basis of exact experimental data. In 1977, the National Institute of Security and Health (NIOSH) in the United States recommended limit concentrations which were particularly low, i.e. 0.5 ppm for halothane and enflurane. If N_2O is administered simultaneously, the MAK values, however, decrease to 0.2 ppm, with the N_2O value of 25 ppm remaining unchanged. Similar recommendations with values of 0.5 ppm for halothane and 30 ppm for N_2O also exist in Great Britain.

The only recommendation hitherto in the Federal Republic of Germany is 5 ppm for halothane; in the German Democratic Republic a limit of 6 ppm is recommended for chronic exposure and of 18 ppm for short-term exposure. In the Federal Republic of Germany recommendations for enflurane are in preparation, but non-corresponding ones for N_2O, since the competent board of experts at the "Deutsche Forschungsgemeinschaft" considers this agent as being unproblematical. This view is based on the consideration that trace doses of N_2O alone do not exhibit toxic effects up to subtherapeutical dosages of 20 Vol%. Right now it still remains open in how far a revision will be necessary here due to the most recent results of investigations in animals on the effects of combined administration of volatile anaesthetics and due to the so-called Dental Report [8], the most recent epidemiological study carried out in the United States in 1980. Air-conditioning, by the way, is under no circumstances a suitable means for achieving an adequate reduction to the low MAK values called for.

The efficiency of absorption filters and exhaust apparatuses manufactured by Dräger was tested by us [19] as well as by quite a number of other authors during anaesthesias via mask and intubation.

It could be seen that

1. N_2O — as expected — was not sufficiently absorbed by filters

2. Continuous exhaustion during mask anaesthesia lessens contamination considerably, but the recommended MAK values (United States and United Kingdom) cannot be achieved if the mask does not fit tightly enough

3. During endotracheal intubation and exhaustion from the circuit system the measured values are lower than the MAK data.

With halothane the measured values during mask anaesthesia with filter or exhaust device nearly reached or lay just above the limit of the MAK values, due to inappropriate tightness of the mask, while during intubation with filter or exhaustion the (German) MAK values were not exceeded. Even though we did not look for leakages in the circuit system during our studies, it is very doubtful whether the 0.5 ppm for ether and hydrocarbon called for in the United States and Great Britain can be achieved at all. Under identical experimental conditions we could achieve comparable results with enflurane.

The results confirm the reports about the efficiency of suitable exhaust devices for all anaesthetic gases and vapours usually administered today as well as the efficiency of the filters for volatile agents with the exception of N_2O.

In conclusion it can be stated that at present there is still quite a number of uncertainties with regard to possible health injuries for operating room personnel caused by long-term exposure to trace doses of inhalation anaesthetics, but that on the grounds of most recent reports in the literature the indications for damages are increasing. Protective measures such as exhaust devices turn out to be efficient as long as their capacity is sufficient and as long as they work perfectly and are properly serviced. Legal regulations force us to take adequate protective measures and most recent literature ought to help us to watchfully follow further developments.

References

1. Askrog V, Harvald B (1970) Teratogen effect of inhalation anaesthetica. Saerty k Nord Med 3:490–500
2. Baden JM, Brinkenhoff M, Whartons RS, et al. (1976) Mutagenicity of volatile anesthetics: halothane. Anesthesiology 45:311–318
3. Bruce DL (1973) Murine fertility uneffected by traces of halothane. Anesthesiology 38:473–477
4. Bruce DL, Bach MJ, Arbit J (1974) Trace anesthetic effects on perceptual, cognitive and motor skills. Anesthesiology 40:453–458
5. Bruce DL, Bach MJ (1976) Effects of trace anesthetic gases on behavioral performance of volunteers. Brit J Anesth 48:871–876
6. Coate WB, Kapp RW Jr, Ulland BM, et al. (1979) Toxicity of low concentration long term exposure to an airborne mixture of nitrous oxide and halothane.
7. Cohen EN, Brown BW, Bruce DL, et al (1974) Occupational disease among operating room personnel. A national study. Anesthesiology 41:321–340
8. Cohen EN, Brown BW, Wu MJ, et al. (1980) Occupational disease in dentistry and chronic exposure to trace anesthetic gases. J Am Dent Assoc 101:21
9. Corbett TH, Cornell RG, Enders JL, et al. (1973) Effects of low concentrations of N_2O on rat pregnancy. Anesthesiology 39:299–301
10. Corbett TH, Cornell RG, Enders JL, et al. (1974) Birth defects among children of nurse-anesthetists. Anesthesiology 41:341–344
11. Edmunds HN, Badden JM, Simmons VF (1979) Mutagenicity studies with volatile metabolites of halothane in man. Anesthesiology 51:424–429
12. Ferstandig LL (1978) Trace concentrations of anesthetic gases: A critical review of their disease potential. Anesth Analg 57:328–345
13. Fink BR, Shepard TH, Blandau RJ (1967) Teratogenic activity of nitrous oxide. Nature 214:146–148
14. Fink BR, Cullen BF (1976) Anesthetic pollution: what is happening to us? Anesthesiology 45:79–83 79-83
15. Garro AJ, Phillips RA (1978) Mutagenicity of the halogenated olefin, 2-bromo-2-chloro-1,1, difluoroethylene, a presumed metabolite of the inhalation anesthetic halothane. Mutation Res 54:17–22
16. Garro AJ, Phillips RA, Milliken RA, Leslie-Rendell-Baker (1979) Chronic Anesthetic Exposure – what is the margin of safety? Anesthesiology 50:77–78
17. Garstka G, Wagner K-L, Hamacher M (1975) Schwangerschaftskomplikationen bei Anästhesistinnen. Geburtshilfe Frauenheilkd 35:826–833
18. Knill-Jones RP, Mewman BJ, Spence AA (1975) Anaesthetic practice and pregnancy. Controlled survey of male anaesthetists in the United Kingdom. Lancet 2:807–808
19. Lauven PM, Stoeckel HO (1981) Raumluftkonzentrationen der Inhalationsanästhetika im Operationssaal unter Berücksichtigung von Schutzmaßnahmen. Anästh Intensivther Notfallmed 16: (im Druck)
20. Linde AW, Bruce DL (1969) Effects of chronic exposure of rats to traces of halothane. Proc IV. World Congr of Anesthesiologists London. Excerpta Medica Amsterdam, S. 923
21. Mazze R, Cascorbi H, Jones T, et al. (1981) Waste anesthetic gases in operating room air: A suggested program to reduce personnel exposure. ASA-Ad hoc committee of effects of trace anesthetic agents on health of operating room personel
22. McGowan JC (1972) Effects of anaesthetics and related substances on the division of living cells. Lancet 2:279–280
23. Michenfelder JD (1980) Editorial: Exposure to anesthetic gases and health problems in dental workers. Anesthesiology 53:1–2
24. Nikki P, Pfäffli P, Ahlmann K, Ralli R (1972) Chronic exposure to anaesthetic gases in the operating theatre and recovery room. Ann Clin Res 4:266–272
25. Sharp H, Trudell JR, Cohen EN (1979) Volatile metabolites and decomposition products of halothane. Anesthesiology 50:2–8

26. Smith G, Shirley WA (1976) Failure to demonstrate effects of low concentrations of nitrous oxide and halothane on psychomotor performance. Br J Anaesth 48:274
27. Spence AA, Cohen EN, Brown BW Jr, Knill-Jones RP, Himmelberger DU (1977) Occupation hazards for operating roombased physicians. JAMA 238:955–959
28. Vaisman AH (1967) Arbeitsbedingungen in den Operationsräumen und ihr Einfluß auf die Gesundheit der Anästhesiologen. Eksp Khir Anestheziol 3:44
29. Walts LF, Forsythe AB, Moore JG (1975) Critique: occupational disease among operating room personnel. Anesthesiology 42:608–611
30. Wharton RS, Mazze RJ, Baden JM, et al. (1978) Fertility, reproduction and postnatal survival in mice chronically exposed to halothane. Anesthesiology 48:167–174

Aspects of Possible Health Hazards from Traces of Waste Anaesthetic Vapours and Gases

K. Taeger

The atmosphere of induction-, operating-, and recovery-rooms is polluted by traces of waste anaesthetic vapours and gases such as halothane, enflurane, and nitrous oxide [1, 2, 3]. Can an atmosphere polluted by these agents cause acute or chronic illness in operating-room personnel? In my opinion this question cannot be answered with certainty, though epidemiological surveys [4-13] have suggested that persons working in operating-rooms experience an unusually high incidence of spontaneous abortions, congenital malformations in offspring, underweight newborn, cancer, and diseases of the liver and kidneys. Is there really a cause-effect relationship? What is the contribution of other factors, such as stress, work overload, abuse of alcohol, cigarette smoking, and vapours from disinfectants? Could it be that the observed health hazards are, at least in part, random events? First, we would like to point out that the authors of the epidemiological studies did not state, but only supposed, pollution of the atmosphere in operating-rooms to be responsible for acute or chronic illness in operating-room personnel.

In the mean time, Lecky [14], Fink and Cullen [15], Vessey [16], and Ferstandig [17] have criticized the performance and interpretation of the available epidemiological studies. Is it justified, then, to dispense with measures to reduce the pollution? Not at all! In that respect the critics agree with the criticized. An unproven harmfulness does not prove harmlessness. Therefore it is generally thought desirable, as formulated in 1974 by the "Deutsche Gesellschaft für Anaesthesie und Wiederbelebung" (German Society for Anaesthesia and Resuscitation), together with the "Berufsverband deutscher Anaesthesisten" (Professional Association of German Anaesthetists) [18], to ". . . oblige hospital authorities to install effective scavenging systems", while ". . . in the mean time the use of charcoal filters ought to be prescribed".

The use of charcoal filters instead of scavenging systems seems to me to be acceptable only as a temporary measure. As early as 1972, Eichler [19] demonstrated that even small amounts of halothane, adsorbed by charcoal filters, diffused through the whole charcoal layer and were continuously released into the atmosphere after a period of hours to days. The release of halothane from filters might not be perceived, since the olfactory threshold lies at around 80-100 ppm. Charcoal filters have to be replaced every 8 h. Nitrous oxide is not absorbed by charcoal filters, though it too is a potential health hazard.

In 1977, the National Institute of Occupational Safety and Health (NIOSH) proposed upper limits for the concentrations of inhalation anaesthetics in the atmosphere of operating-rooms, e.g. 0.5 ppm for halothane and 25 ppm for nitrous oxide. According to Smith and Shirley [20] and Mazze [21], these limits are essentially based upon the results of an epidemiological survey performed by Cohen et al. in 1974 [8]. Performance and interpretation of the results were seriously doubted by some, including Ferstandig [17]. The NIOSH limits are further based upon the results of a survey, performed by Bruce and Bach [22]. They reported an impairment of cognitive and motor skills of healthy volunteers resulting from exposure to 50 ppm nitrous oxide and 1 ppm halothane. Their results, however, could not be confirmed by the work of Frankhuisen [23], Smith and Shirley [24], and Cook [25]. The NIOSH limits, therefore, seem not to be based upon convincing experimental results.

What measures should now be taken to eliminate any possible health hazards for the personnel brought about by pollution of the atmosphere of operating-rooms? Anaesthetic gases should be scavenged by means of vacuum systems and exhausted outside the building. Operating-rooms should be ventilated by fresh air. Polluting the operating-room air by anaesthetic gases should be avoided by proper anaesthetic techniques, e.g. no addition of anaesthetic gases to the gas mixture in the anaesthetic circuit before intubation or before gastight position of the face-mask. At least 5 min before the end of anaesthesia, the addition of anaesthetic gases and vapours ought to be stopped. Leaks should be hunted for at regular intervals by means of proper methods, and should be eliminated. In operating-rooms ventilated with fresh air and equipped with an effective scavenging device, where proper anaesthetic techniques are used, health hazards for the personnel caused by traces of waste anaesthetic gases and vapours largely cease to exist.

References

1. Linde HW, Bruce DL (1969) Occupational exposure of anesthetists to halothane, nitrous oxide and radiation. Anesthesiology 30:363–368
2. Whitcher CE, Cohen EN, Trudell JR (1971) Chronic exposure to anesthetic gases in the operating room. Anesthesiology 35:348–353
3. Piziali RL, Whitcher C, Sher R, Moffat RJ (1976) Distribution of waste anesthetic gases in the operating room air. Anesthesiology 45:487–494
4. Askrog V, Harvald B (1970) Teratogen effekt af inhalationsanaestetika. Saertryk Nord Med 83: 498–500
5. Cohen EN, Bellville JW, Brown BW (1971) Anesthesia, pregnancy, and miscarriage. A study of operating room nurses and anesthetists. Anesthesiology 35:343–347
6. Knill-Jones RP, Moir DD, Rodrigues LV, Spence AA (1972) Anaesthetic practice and pregnancy. Controlled survey of women anaesthetists in the United Kingdom. Lancet 2:1326–1328
7. Corbett TH, Cornell RG, Lieding K, Endres JL (1973) Incidence of cancer among Michigan nurse-anesthetists. Anesthesiology 38:260–263
8. American Society of Anesthesiologists (1974) Occupational disease among operating room personnel: A national study. Report of an ad hoc committee on the effect of trace anesthetics on the health of operating room personnel. Anesthesiology 41:321–340
9. Corbett TH, Cornell RG, Endres JL, Lieding K (1974) Birth defects among children of nurse-anesthetists. Anesthesiology 41:341–344
10. Knill-Jones RP, Newmann BJ, Spence AA (1975) Anaesthetic practice and pregnancy. Controlled survey of male anaesthetists in the United Kingdom. Lancet 2:807–809
11. Cohen EN, Brown BW, Bruce DL, Cascorbi HF, Corbett TH, Jones TW, Whitcher CE (1975) A survey of anesthetic health hazards among dentists. J Am Dent Assoc (JADA) 90:1291–1296
12. Pharoah POD, Alberman E, Doyle P (1977) Outcome of pregnancy among women in anaesthetic practice. Lancet 1:34–36
13. Tomlin PJ (1979) Health problems of anaesthetists and their families in the West Midlands. Br Med J 1:779–784
14. Lecky JH (1980) Anesthetic pollution in the operating room. A notice to operating room personnel. Anesthesiology 52:157–159

15. Fink BR, Cullen BF (1976) Anesthetic pollution: What is happening to us? Anesthesiology 45: 79–83
16. Vessey MP (1978) Epidemiological studies of the occupational hazards of anaesthesia – a review. Anaesthesia 33:430–438
17. Ferstandig LL (1978) Trace concentrations of anesthetic gases: a critical review of their disease potential. Anesth Analg 57:328–345
18. Empfehlung der deutschen Gesellschaft für Anaesthesie und Wiederbelebung und des Berufsverbandes deutschen Anaesthesisten (1974) Anaesth Inform 15:292–294
19. Eichler J, Kukulinus K, Naumann P (1972) Über das Aufnahmevermögen von Halothanfiltern. Anaesth Inform 4:123–128
20. Smith G, Shirley AW (1976) Failure to demonstrate effects of low concentrations of nitrous oxide and halothane on psychomotor performance. Br J Anaesth 48:274
21. Mazze RJ (1980) Waste anesthetic gases and the regulatory agencies. Anesthesiology 52:248–256
22. Bruce DL, Bach MJ (1976) Effects of trace anaesthetic gases on behavioural performance of volunteers. Br J Anaesth 48:871–876
23. Frankhuizen JL, Vlek CAJ, Burm AGL, Rejger V (1978) Failure to replicate negative effects of trace anaesthetics on mental performance. Br J Anaesth 50:229–234
24. Smith G, Shirley AW (1978) A review of the effects of trace concentrations of anaesthetics on performance. Br J Anaesth 50:701–712
25. Cook TL, Smith M, Starkweather JA, Winter PM, Eger EI II (1978) Behavioral effects of trace and subanesthetic halothane and nitrous oxide in man. Anesthesiology 49:419-424

The Kinetics of the Uptake and Elimination of Halothane and Enflurane

H. Schmidt and R. Dudziak

The general presentation of the pharmacokinetics of halothane and enflurane, using numerous mathematical models [2, 6, 9, 12, 13, 24, 25, 30, 34], like the corresponding clinical experimental investigations is based upon measurements of the inspiratory and/or end-expiratory concentration of the anaesthetic in question [8, 14, 23, 29, 31, 33], and upon determinations of the solubility of the individual inhalation anaesthetics in the various body fluids and tissues [18, 21, 22, 32]. On the other hand, measurements of the halothane or enflurane concentration in the arterial or venous blood of humans are used almost exclusively for the determination of partial pharmacokinetic or pharmacodynamic aspects [1, 3, 7, 10, 11, 16, 17, 19, 20, 26]. Only the serum half-lives calculated for halothane by Duncan and Raventos [11], which fluctuate between 3 and 45 min, are based upon nephelometric determinations of the halothane level in the venous blood.

The object of our own investigations was to determine, quantitatively as far as possible, the behaviour of the central venous blood levels of halothane and enflurane under the conditions of a largely standardized anaesthetic procedure on a fairly large number of patients, and to deduce pharmacokinetic parameters from this. There were two separate investigation series, in each case involving 32 patients aged between 20 and 70 years with a healthy circulation, who had to undergo surgical operations lasting 2–3 h. The venous blood concentrations were determined during the administration of halothane with an inspiratory concentration of 1 Vol%, or of enflurane with an inspiratory concentration of 2 Vol%, for a period of 60 min; and for a measurement period of 240 min after interruption of the administration of the anaesthetic measurements were made by means of head-space gas chromatography. For this, after the intravenous induction of anaesthesia, relaxation, and intubation, the patients were put on controlled ventilation with a nitrous oxide and oxygen mixture (FIO_2 = 32–34 Vol%). A semi-open system was used in 16 patients from one investigation series, and a semi-closed anaesthetic circuit system in the remaining 16 patients. Three to 5 min after the induction of anaesthesia, 1 Vol% halothane or 2 Vol% enflurane was added to the fresh gas mixture, via a specially calibrated vaporizer, for a period of 60 min. After this period of exposure the patients received 0.1–0.2 mg fentanyl intravenously at intervals of between 20 and 30 min for the remaining duration of the anaesthesia. Pancuronium bromide was administered to maintain the muscle relaxation. Throughout the whole of the period of observation, in addition to the usual surveillance during anaesthesia (measurement of the pulse-rate and of the peripheral arterial blood-pressure, ECG monitoring), following a precisely laid down time schedule, the cardiac minute volume, respiratory minute volume, and oesophageal temperature were also measured; arterial blood samples were taken to determine the blood gas values, the acid-base status, the haemoglobin and haematocrit values, and

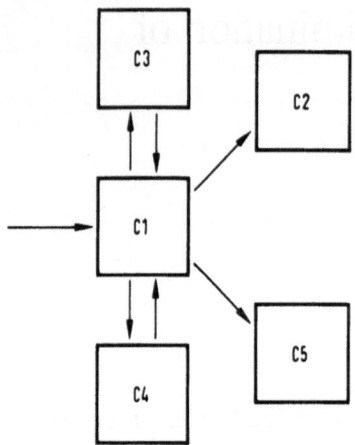

Fig. 1. Multi-compartment model of the computer program BIC 261/Model 44, used to calculate the pharmacokinetic parameters of halothane and enflurane. *C1*, central compartment (blood); *C2*, O; *C3* and *C4*, hypothetical side-compartments; *C5*, elimination via the lungs

the triglyceride level; and central venous blood samples from a venous catheter placed close to the right atrium were taken for the measurement of the blood levels of the inhalation anaesthetic.

The gas-chromatographic analysis procedure, like the methods of measurements used to determine the other parameters, has been described in detail elsewhere [28]. The evaluation of the results obtained from the determination of the blood concentrations of halothane and enflurane was carried out using the computer calculating programme BIC 261/Model 44. The calculations were based upon a multi-compartment model, which is shown diagrammatically in Fig. 1. Here C1 corresponds to the central compartment of the blood, and C3 and C4 to hypothetical side-compartments. The correlation coefficient (r) as a measure of the fit between the experimentally determined measurements and the calculated data amounted, for the two halothane groups, to 0.9987 and 0.9981, and for the enflurane groups to 0.9968 and 0.9963 (Tables 1 and 2).

Since the uptake, distribution, and elimination of an inhalation anaesthetic depend upon the inspiratory concentration, the exposure time, and the solubility of the anaesthetic agent in the blood and individual tissues, just as much as upon the alveolar ventilation and the cardiac output of the patient, the administration of the anaesthetic and the alveolar ven-

Table 1. Pharmacokinetic parameters of halothane

		$t_{0.5}(\alpha)$ (min)	$t_{0.5}(\beta)$ (min)	$t_{0.5}(\gamma)$ (min)	Clearance totalis (l/kg/h)	r^a
Halothane, semi-open	x̄	2.237	16.31	134.02	2.259	0.9987
system (n = 16)	SD	2.064	7.78	61.63	0.33	0.0011
Halothane, semi-closed	x̄	2.813	18.75	99.81	2.456	0.9981
system (n = 15)	SD	2.482	10.02	31.84	0.54	0.0016

[a] Correlation coefficient

Table 2. Pharmacokinetic parameters of enflurane

		$t_{0.5}(\alpha)$ (min)	$t_{0.5}(\beta)$ (min)	$t_{0.5}(\gamma)$ (min)	Clearance totalis (l/kg/h)	r^a
Enflurane, semi-open	$\bar{x}$	1.607	13.48	111.26	3.468	0.9968
system (n = 15)	SD	1.483	8.8	42.59	0.333	0.0027
Enflurane, semi-closed	$\bar{x}$	2.743	16.89	100.25	3.284	0.9963
system (n = 16)	SD	1.991	7.14	23.66	0.49	0.0028

[a] Correlation coefficient

tilation were kept constant in the individual patients in both investigation series. The slight fall in oesophageal temperature of between 0.5 and 1.5 °C is not expected to have any lasting significance for the pharmacokinetics of the investigated anaesthetics. And since, under the experimental conditions described, no statistically significant fall could be demonstrated in the cardiac index and the stroke volume during the administration of halothane or enflurane for the four groups of patients, the influence of this parameter upon the elimination of the investigated anaesthetics can be excluded (Figs. 2–5).

The changes in the solubility of halothane in the blood with high triglyceride levels, demonstrated in vitro by Saraiva et al. [27], also have no adverse effect upon the uptake and elimination of the anaesthetic. Although triglyceride levels of 1031 mg/dl and 554.2 mg/dl were measured in two patients of the halothane series, the venous halothane concentrations did not deviate from the measurements obtained in the other patients.

Additional influence upon the kinetics of halothane and enflurane, through the concentration effect described by Eger [12] or "the second gas effect" found by Epstein et al. [14] with the simultaneous administration of volatile anaesthetics and nitrous oxide, could largely be excluded for the present investigations, because these phenomena are only of clinical significance if halothane or enflurane are administered in a higher inspiratory concentration than that used by us. From our personal results it is seen that the venous blood concentrations of halothane and enflurane, regardless of the anaesthetic circuit system used, exhibit a steep rise in the first 30 min, which slows down distinctly in the next 30 min, and that they do not reach any steady state at the end of the period of exposure (Figs. 9–13). Under comparable experimental conditions Grothe et al. [17] obtained similar results. By contrast with this, Gostomzyk [16] reported that, regardless of the amount of halothane administered, a concentration plateau supervenes in the blood 15 min after the start of halothane anaesthesia. According to present-day findings, this claim can no longer be maintained.

Taking into account the semi-saturation times, which were calculated, not measured, by Cowles et al. [9] for the inspiratory halothane concentration of 1 Vol%, and which on average amount to 20.4 min for the well-perfused organs, to 206 min for the skeletal musculature, and to 2330 min for the fat, the possibility must be excluded that the steady state can be reached with a clinically relevant dosage of halothane. By analogy with this, similar results are to be expected for enflurane anaesthesia. After interruption of the administration of the anaesthetic, one must rather reckon with redistribution processes, which, as regards their duration and intensity, are determined solely by the partial pressure difference between the arterial blood and the tissues [13]. From this it may be deduced that after the end

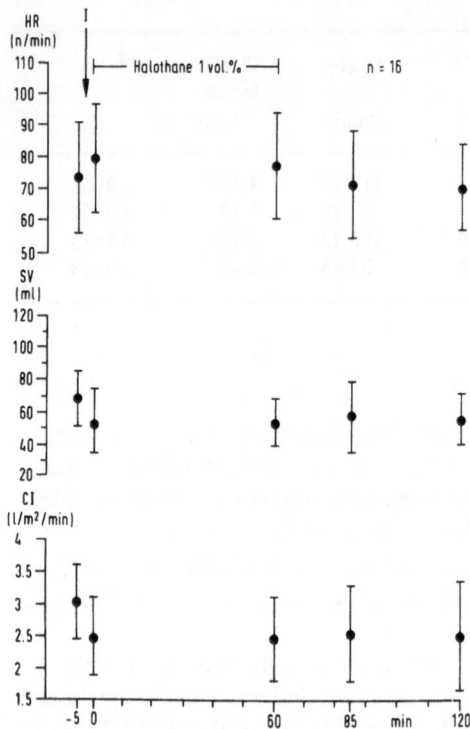

Fig. 2. Mean changes in heart rate (*HR*), stroke volume (*SV*), and cardiac index (*CI*) after intravenous induction (*I*) of anaesthesia and during and after administration of halothane in 16 patients ventilated by a semi-open system. $\bar{x} \pm SD$

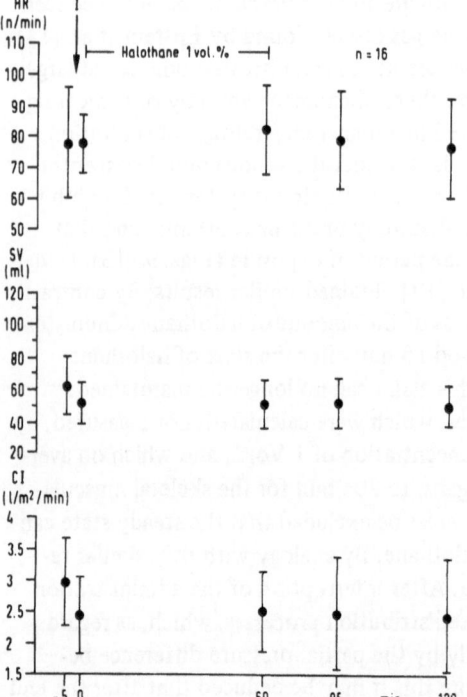

Fig. 3. Mean changes in heart rate (*HR*), stroke volume (*SV*), and cardiac index (*CI*) after intravenous induction (*I*) of anaesthesia and during and after administration of halothane in 16 patients ventilated by a semi-closed system. $\bar{x} \pm SD$

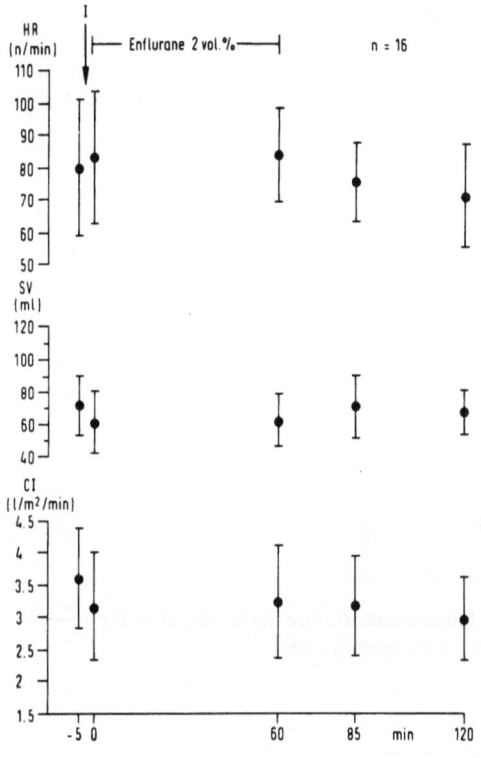

Fig. 4. Mean changes in heart rate (*HR*), stroke volume (*SV*), and cardiac index (*CI*) after intravenous induction (*I*) of anaesthesia and during and after administration of enflurane in patients ventilated by a semi-open system. x̄ ± SD

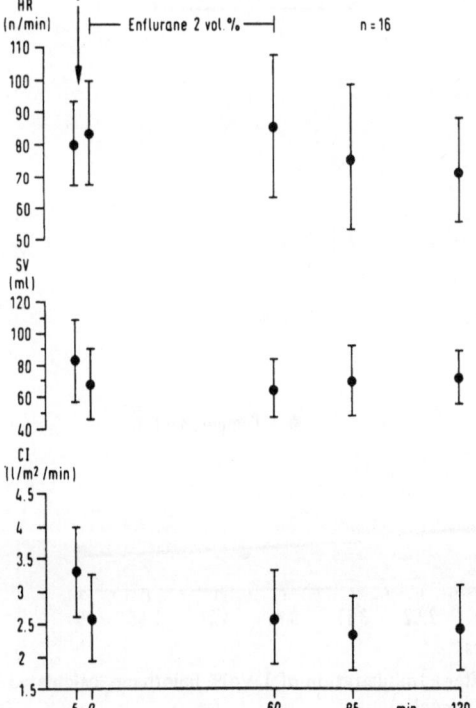

Fig. 5. Mean changes in heart rate (*HR*), stroke volume (*SV*), and cardiac index (*CI*) after intravenous induction (*I*) of anaesthesia and during and after administration of enflurane in 16 patients ventilated by a semi-closed system. x̄ ± SD

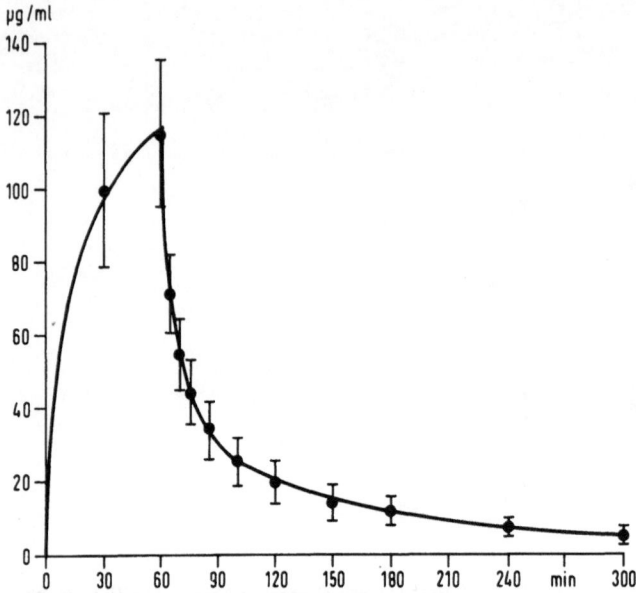

Fig. 6. Calculated mean values of the halothane venous blood concentration during and after the administration of 1 Vol% halothane in 16 patients ventilated by a semi-open system

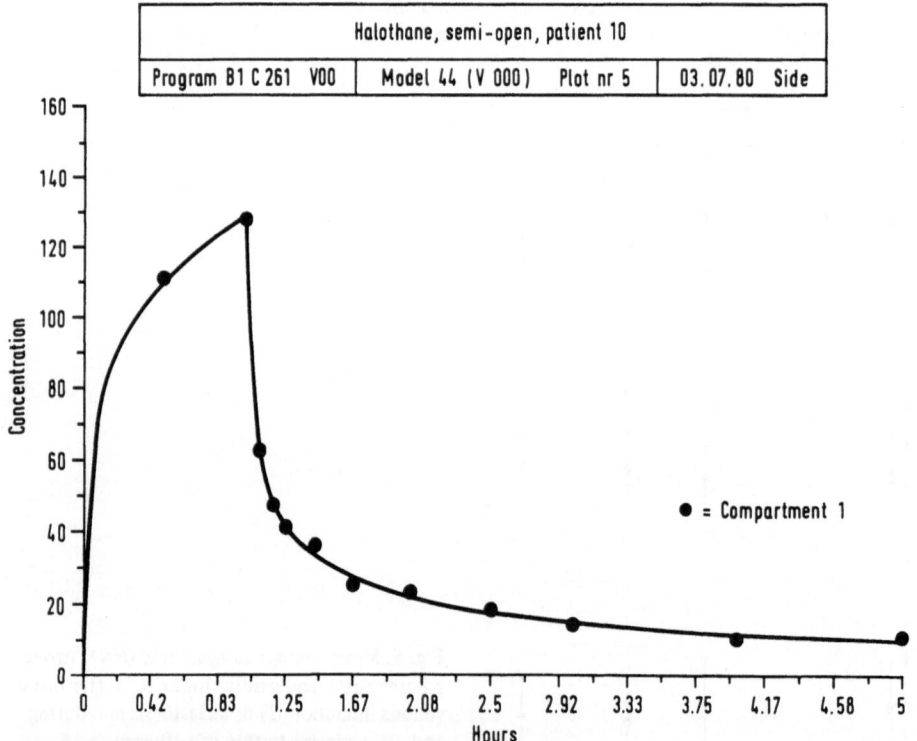

Fig. 7. Venous blood concentration curve during and after administration of 1 Vol% halothane, calculated by the computer program from the experimental data (*triangles*)

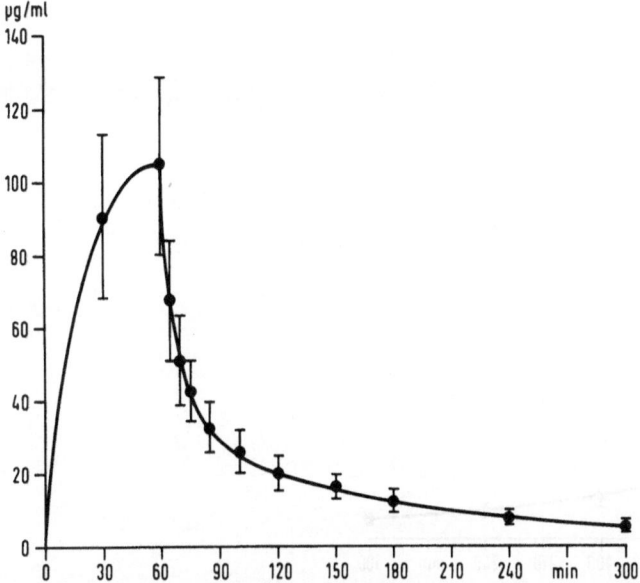

Fig. 8. Calculated mean values of the halothane venous blood concentration during and after administration of 1 Vol% halothane in 15 patients ventilated by a semi-closed system

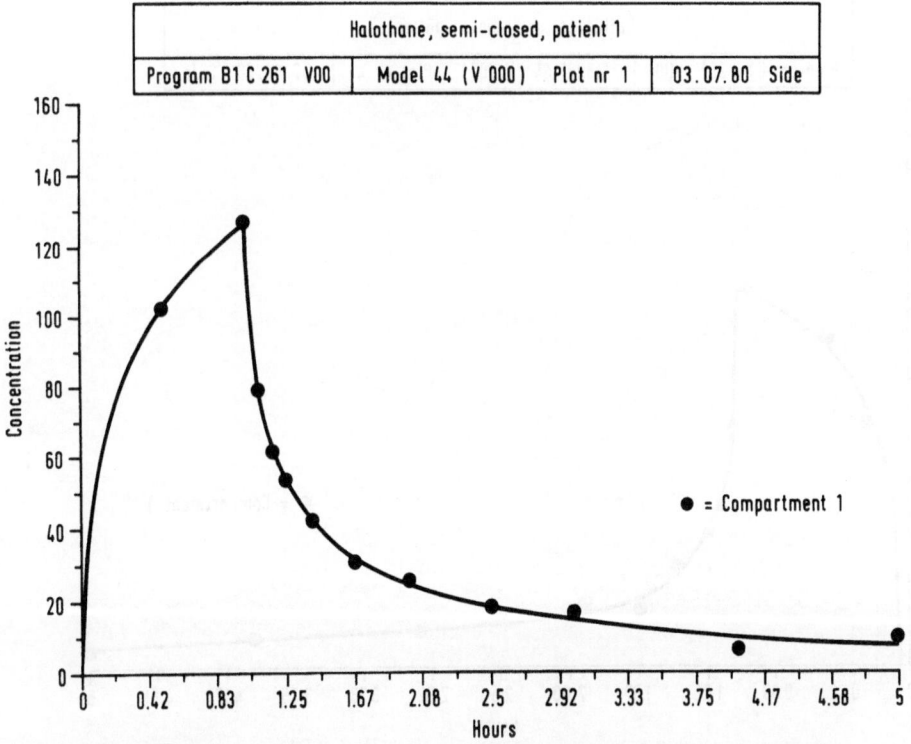

Fig. 9. Venous blood concentration curve during and after administration of 1 Vol% halothane, calculated by the computer program from the experimental data (*triangles*)

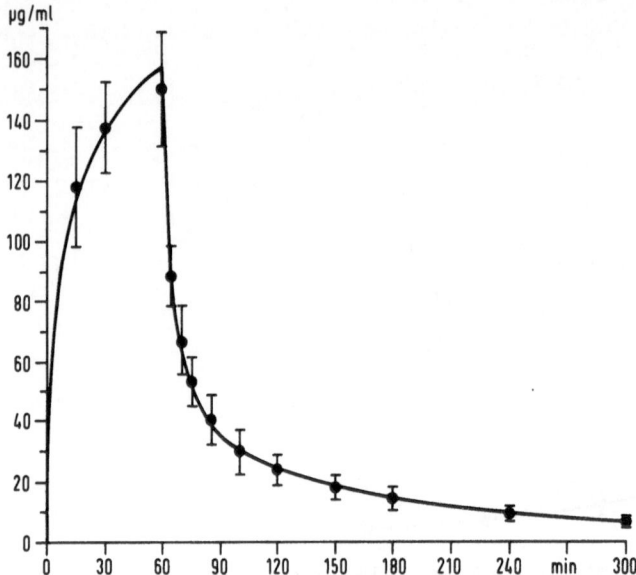

Fig. 10. Calculated mean values of the enflurane venous blood concentration during and after administration of 2 Vol% enflurane in 15 patients ventilated by a semi-open system

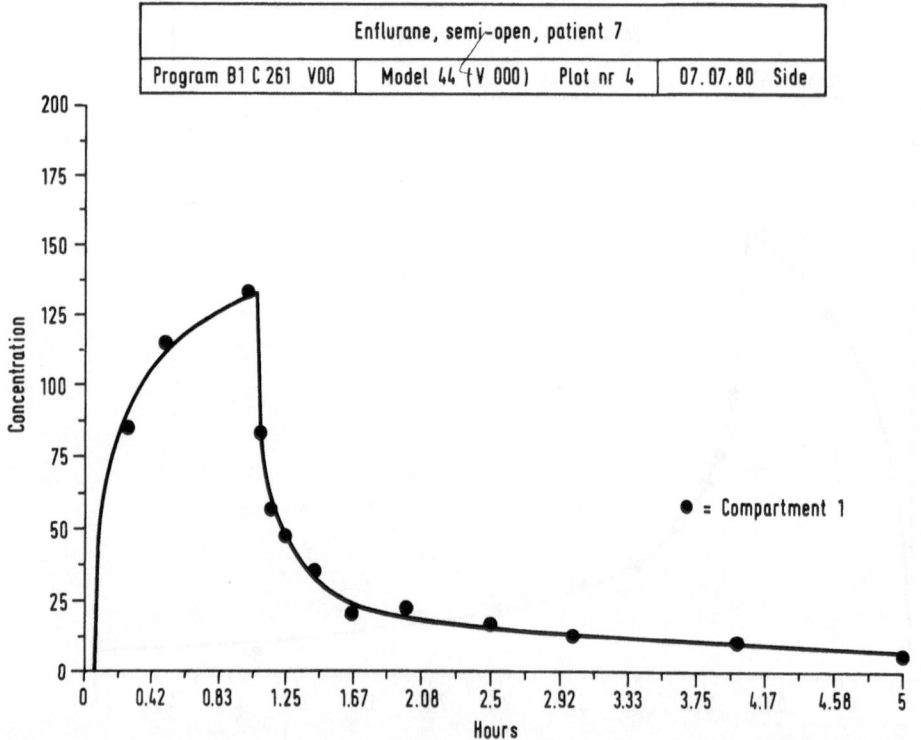

Fig. 11. Venous blood concentration curve during and after administration of 2 Vol% enflurane, calculated by the computer program from the experimental data (*triangles*)

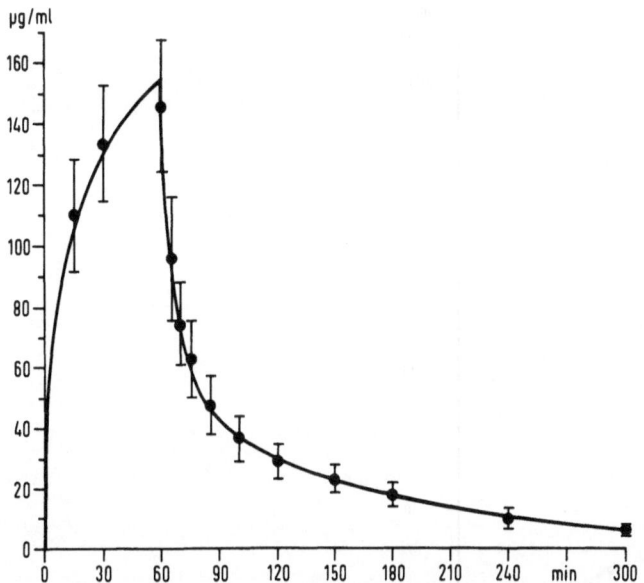

Fig. 12. Calculated mean values of the enflurane venous blood concentration during and after administration of 2 Vol% enflurane in 16 patients ventilated by a semi-closed system

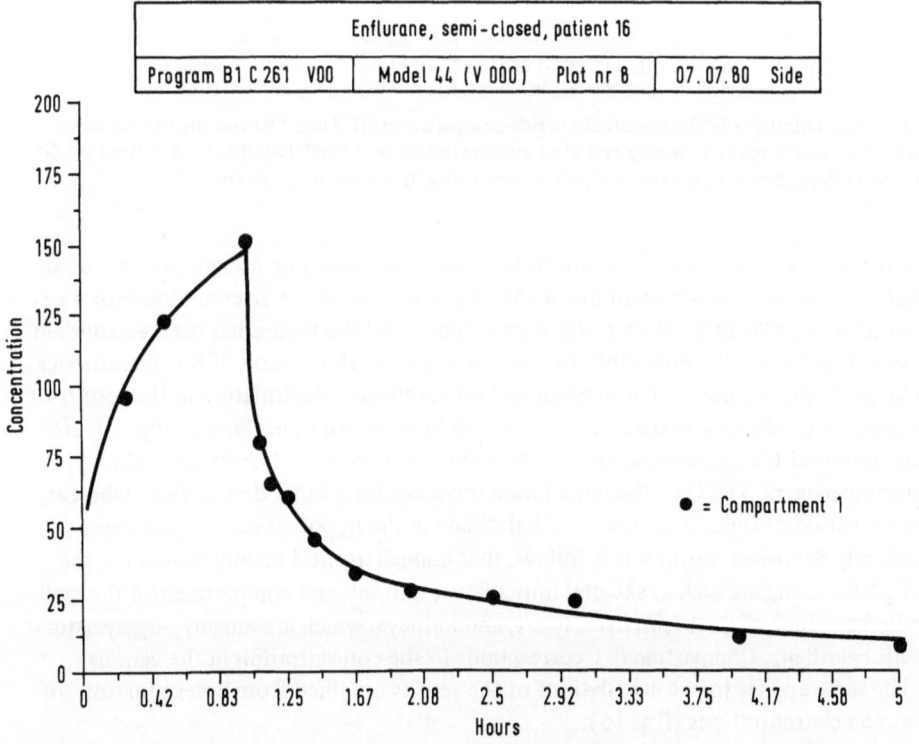

Fig. 13. Venous blood concentration curve during and after administration of 2 Vol% enflurane, calculated by the computer program from the experimental data (*triangles*)

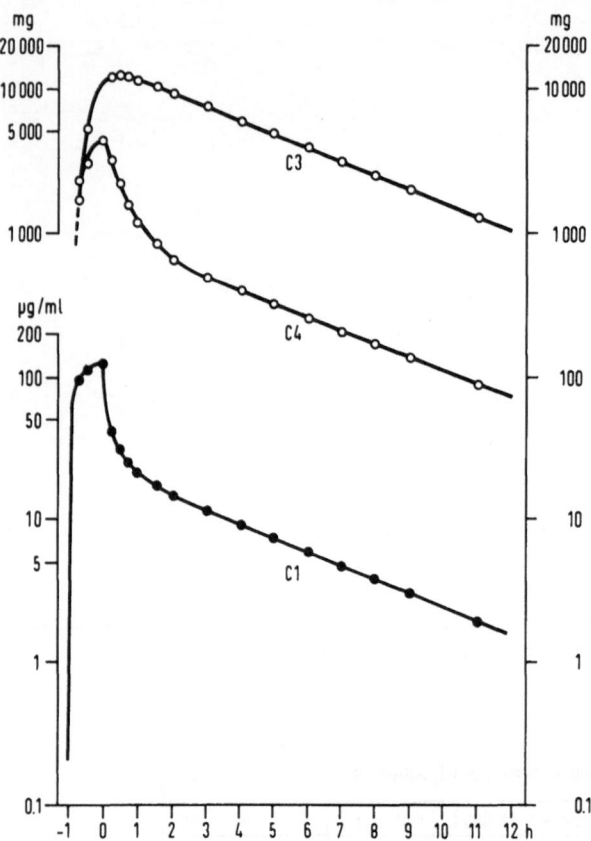

Fig. 14. Levels of halothane in the hypothetical side-compartments (*C3* and *C4*) and the venous blood concentration of halothane (*C1*) during and after administration of 1 Vol% halothane, calculated by the computer from the experimental data on a patient ventilated by a semi-open system

of anaesthesia, organs which at this point in time have only taken up a slight amount of an anaesthetic can extract certain amounts of the anaesthetic from the arterial blood for a period up until an equilibrium between the arterial blood and the tissues has been established. The process is influenced considerably by the simultaneous elimination of the anaesthetics via the lungs. These theoretical considerations find additional confirmation in the results of the calculations of our own measurements. As may be seen from the graph in Fig. 14, after the interruption of the administration of halothane, the amount of halothane in the hypothetical compartment 3 (C3) of the model used increases for a short time at first, whereas, in the same period of time, the amount of halothane in the hypothetical compartment 4 (C4) distinctly decreases. From this it follows that compartment 3 mainly represents the less well perfused organs such as skeletal musculature and fat, and compartment 4 the well-perfused organs such as the brain, liver, heart, and kidneys, which are already largely saturated with halothane. Compartment 1 corresponds to the concentration in the venous blood. The same applies to the calculations of the results obtained from determinations of the enflurane concentrations (Fig. 15).

Consequently, in measurements of the venous blood levels of halothane and enflurane after the end of anaesthesia, redistribution processes are picked up, as is also the simulta-

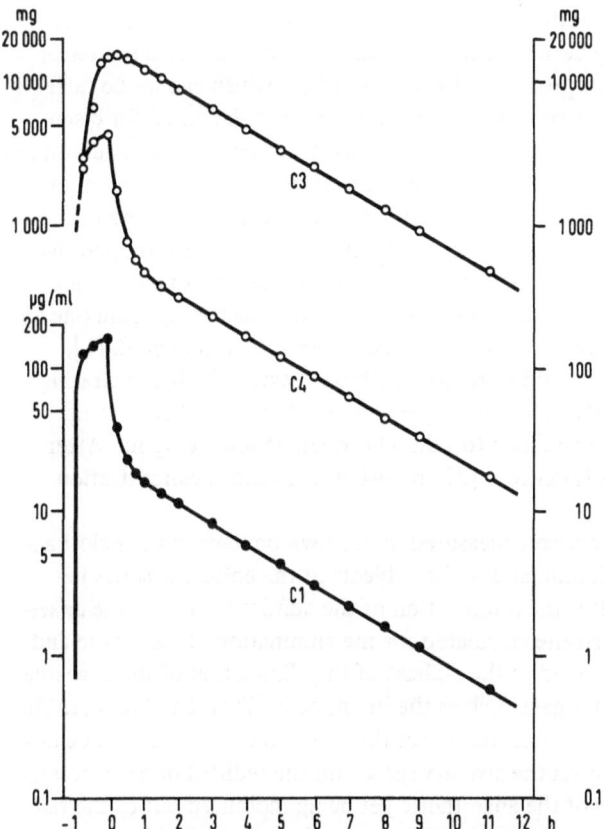

Fig. 15. Levels of enflurane in the hypothetical side-compartments (*C3* and *C4*) and the venous blood concentration of enflurane (*C1*) during and after administration of 2 Vol% enflurane, calculated by the computer from the experimental data on a patient ventilated by a semi-closed system

neous elimination of the anaesthetics via the lungs. In detail, for the elimination of halo-thane from the blood we determined three successive phases with half-lives of 2.237±2.004 min for the α-phase, 16.31±7.78 min for the β-phase, and 134.02±61.31 min for the γ-phase with anaesthesia in a semi-open system, and of 2.813±2.428 min for the α-phase, 18.75± 10.02 min for the β-phase, and 99.81±31.84 min for the γ-phase with anaesthesia in the semi-closed system (Table 1). The difference between the data calculated for the two differ-ent anaesthetic circuit systems is not statistically significant. This also applies to the para-meters determined under enflurane anaesthesia. This finding is in agreement with the results obtained by Goldman et al. [15] in comparative investigations. For the elimination of enflur-ane from the blood the detailed half-lives amounted to 1.607 ± 1.483 min for the α-phase, 13.48±8.80 min for the β-phase, and 111.25±42.59 min for the γ-phase with anaesthesia in the semi-open system, and 2.743±1.991 min for the α-phase, 16.89±7.24 min for the β-pha-se, and 100.25 ± 23.66 min for the γ-phase with anaesthesia in the semi-closed system (Table 2).

The range of scatter of the individual results, which taken as a whole is very large, per-mits the conclusion that mean values only allow very general statements about the uptake and elimination of halothane and enflurane. For precise data it is necessary to determine the concentration of the anaesthetic in question in the individual patient. The question as to whether there is a causal relationship between the very great range of individual scatter of the reported data and the distribution processes already described, which cannot be differentiated in detail and which possibly vary very considerably, can only be raised for discussion here. Reliable conclusions about this can only be obtained from simultaneous determinations of the concentration of an inhalation anaesthetic in the blood and the individual organs. For the allocation of the elimination phases determined from our own results to the different body compartments, use can be made, above all, of the results from comparative investigations between halothane or enflurane concentrations and the time of awakening after anaesthesia. Despite experimental conditions which differed considerably from one another, and despite the use of very different methods of measurement, Ardoin et al. [1], Duncan and Raventos [11], and Kessler and Haferkorn [20] were agreed in demonstrating that after halothane anaesthesia patients obeyed simple commands such as "Open your eyes", if the venous halothane levels had fallen to values between 25 and 50 μg/ml. After enflurane anaesthesia, as Kessler and Haferkorn [20] reported, the venous concentration had fallen to 60 μg/ml by this time.

Corresponding venous blood levels were measured in our own patients in the halothane series between the 15th and the 40th min, and in the subjects of the enflurane series between the 10th and the 25th min, after the interruption of the administration of the anaesthetic. In agreement with this, the half-life calculated for the elimination of halothane and enflurane from the blood can be allocated to the β-phase of the elimination of the anaesthetic in question from the well-perfused organs such as the brain, heart, liver, and kidneys. The α-phase of the fall in the venous blood concentration of the anaesthetics would then be determined above all by the elimination via the alveolar space and the redistribution processes described, without essential amounts of the anaesthetic yet being mobilized out of the tissues, whereas the γ-phase would correspond to the elimination from the musculature and the fat. This interpretation of the phases of elimination agrees in principle with the allocation of the elimination phases carried out by Eger from model calculations for the fall in the alveolar concentration [13]. The conclusions drawn by Torri et al. [33] from the results of comparative measurements of the end-tidal concentration after halothane and enflurane anaesthesia contradict this. The investigators interpret the initial fall in the wash-out curve as elimination from the well-perfused organs, the following flattening of the course of the curve as elimination from the musculature, and the subsequent very flat course of the curve as the elimination from the adipose tissues. It is not apparent from the reports of Torri et al. [33], however, whether the elimination curves upon which their calculations are based represent individual observations or have been derived from mean values. Nor are the half-lives, which are generally given for the description of the elimination, reported. From measurements of the alveolar enflurane concentration after the end of anaesthesia, Chase et al. [8] calculated elimination half-lives which exhibited a very broad scatter of the individual values. The data obtained by these authors deviate considerably from the parameters calculated from our personal investigations. From the animal experiments of Beneken Kolmer et al. [4, 5] it is apparent that the end-expiratory halothane concentration initially falls more rapidly in the elimination phase than the concentration in the mixed venous blood. So far corresponding investigations have not been carried out in humans.

From the consideration of our personal results as a whole, it can be observed that determinations of the venous blood concentrations of volatile anaesthetics are more suitable than measurements of the end-expiratory concentration for answering clinically important questions such as the minimum duration of post-anaesthetic surveillance, possible interactions with other drugs given in the elimination phase, suitable anaesthetic procedures for repeated anaesthetics to be given within a short period of time, or time of discharge of out-patients. In addition it would also first have to be demonstrated that the measured end-expiratory concentrations are in fact identical with the alveolar concentrations. This particularly applies when the measurements are carried out under spontaneous respiration. The pharmacokinetic parameters reported here for the first time for halothane and enflurane have a mainly theoretical importance for the clinical questions.

References

1. Ardoin D, Hingson RA, Tomaro AJ, Fike WW (1966) Chromatographic blood-gas studies of halothane in ambulatory oral surgical anesthesia. Anesth Analg 45:275–281
2. Ashman MN, Blesser WB, Epstein RM (1970) A nonlinear model for the uptake and distribution of halothane in man. Anesthesiology 33:419–429
3. Bencsath FA, Drysch K, List D, Weichardt H (1978) Analysis of volatile air pollutants by charcoal adsorption with subsequent gas chromatographic head space analysis by desorption with benzylalcohol. Angewandte Chromatographie No. 32 E, Bodenseewerk. Perkin-Elmer & Co, Überlingen
4. Beneken Kolmer HH, Burm AG, Cramers CA, Ramakers JM, Vader HL (1975) The uptake and elimination of halothane in dogs: a two or multicompartment-system? I: Gaschromatographic determination of halothane in blood and in inspiratory and end-tidal gases. Br J Anaesth 47:1049–1052
5. Beneken Kolmer HH, Burm AG, Cramers CA, Ramakers JM, Vader HL (1975) The uptake and elimination of halothane in dogs: a two or multicompartment-system? II: Evaluation of wash-in and wash-out curves. Br J Anaesth 47:1169–1175
6. Bourne JG (1964) Uptake, elimination and potency of inhalational anaesthetics. Anaesthesia 19: 12–32
7. Butler RA (1963) Halothane. In: Papper EM, Kitz RJ (eds) Uptake and distribution of anesthetic agents. McGraw-Hill, New York Toronto London, pp 274–283
8. Chase RE, Holaday DA, Fiserova-Bergerova V, Saidman LJ (1971) The biotransformation of Ethane in man. Anesthesiology 35:262–267
9. Cowles AL, Borgstedt HH, Gillies AJ (1968) Uptake and distribution of inhalation anesthetic agents in clinical practice. Curr Res Anesth Analg 47:404–414
10. Dick W, Knoche E, Traub E, Eckstein K-L (1975) Ethrane in der Geburtshilfe. In: Kreuscher H (ed) Ethrane, neue Ergebnisse aus Forschung und Klinik. Schattauer, Stuttgart New York, pp 73–85
11. Duncan WAM, Raventos J (1959) The pharmacokinetics of halothane (Fluothane) anaesthesia. Br J Anaesth 31:302–315
12. Eger EI II (1963) Applications of a mathematical model of gas uptake. In: Papper EM, Kitz RJ (eds) Uptake and distribution of anesthetic agents. McGraw-Hill, New York Toronto London, pp 88–103
13. Eger EI II (1976) Anesthetic uptake and action. William & Wilkins, Baltimore
14. Epstein RM, Rackow H, Salanitre E, Wolf GL (1964) Influence of the concentration effect on the uptake of anesthetic mixtures: The second gas effect. Anesthesiology 25:364–371
15. Goldman E, De Campo T, Aldrete JA (1979) Enflurane concentration: influence of semi-closed system (Abstr). Anesthesiology 51:23
16. Gostomzyk JG (1971) Bestimmung der Narkosegas-Konzentration im Blut mit der Dampfraum-Gaschromatographie. Anaesthesist 20:212–215
17. Grothe B, Doenicke A, Hauck G, Lindström D, Bauer T, Kugler J (1976) Untersuchungen zur Metabolisierung von Halothan und Ethrane am Menschen mit und ohne Vorbehandlung von Phenobarbital. Anaesthesiol Wiederbeleb 99:31–41
18. Han YH, Helrich MH (1966) Effect of temperature on solubility of halothane in human blood and brain tissue homogenate. Anesth Analg 45:775–780
19. Hennes HH (1975) Ethrane in der Kinderanaesthesie. In: Kreuscher H (ed) Ethrane, neue Ergebnisse aus Forschung und Klinik. Schattauer, Stuttgart New York, pp 87–99

20. Kessler G, Haferkorn D (1977) Vergleichende Untersuchungen über die postnarkotische Phase nach Kurznarkosen mit Halothan und Ethrane. Z Prakt Anaesth 12:269–274
21. Larson CP Jr, Eger EI II, Severinghaus JW (1962) The solubility of halothane in blood and tissue homogenates. Anesthesiology 23:349–355
22. Lowe HJ, Hagler K (1969) Determination of volatile organic anesthetics in blood, gases, tissues and lipids: partition coefficients. In: Porter R (ed) Gas chromatography in biology and medicine. A Ciba Foundation symposium. Churchill, London, pp 86–112
23. Mapleson WW (1962) Rate of uptake of halothane vapour in man. Br J Anaesth 34:11–18
24. Mapleson WW (1963) An electric analogue for uptake and exchange of inert gases and other agents. J Appl Physiol 18:197–204
25. Mapleson WW (1972) Kinetics. In: Chenoweth MB (ed) Modern inhalation anesthetics. Springer, Berlin Heidelberg New York, pp 326–344
26. Miller MS, Gandolfi AJ (1979) A rapid, sensitive method for quantifying enflurane in whole blood. Anesthesiology 51:542–544
27. Saraiva RA, Willis BA, Steward A, Nunn JN, Mapleson WW (1977) Halothane solubility in human blood. Br J Anaesth 49:115–119
28. Schmidt H (1981) Das Verhalten der venösen Blutspiegel von Halothan und Enfluran unter den Bedingungen einer weitgehend standardisierten Narkose. Habilitationsschrift, Frankfurt/M
29. Sechzer PH, Linde HW, Dripps RD (1962) Uptake of halothane by the human body. Anesthesiology 23:161–162
30. Smith NT, Zwart A, Beneken JEW (1972) Interaction between circulatory effects and the uptake and distribution of halothane: use of a multiple model. Anesthesiology 37:47–58
31. Stoelting RK, Eger EI II (1969) The effect of ventilation and anesthetic solubility on recovery from anesthesia. Anesthesiology 30:290–296
32. Stoelting RK, Longshore RK (1972) Effect of temperature on the solubility of fluoxene, halothane and methoxyflurane blood/gas and cerebrospinal fluid/gas partition coefficients. Anesthesiology 36:503–505
33. Torri G, Damia G, Fabiani ML, Frova G (1972) Uptake and elimination of enflurane in man. A comparative study between enflurane and halothane. Br J Anaesth 44:789–794
34. Zwart A, Smith NT, Beneken JEW (1972) Multiple model approach to uptake and distribution of halothane: use of analog computer. Comp Biol Med Res 5:228–238

Molecular Basis for Unitary Theories of Inhalation Anaesthesia

J.R. Trudell

Introduction

Recent knowledge of the molecular structure of nerve cell membranes provides a basis for understanding and discussing unitary mechanisms of anaesthesia. A unitary mechanism is a general mechanism by which any of the many forms of inhalation anaesthetic may alter many of the functions of the nervous system. The wide variety of molecular shapes and sizes of anaesthetics that produce general anaesthesia at equimolar membrane concentrations, and the diversity of nervous, muscular, respiratory, and cardiovascular effects, argue for a unitary mechanism of anaesthesia. My discussion of theories of anaesthesia will be in three parts. First, I will review the current knowledge of the molecular structure of the phospholipid bilayer membranes that surround the function-controlling proteins of the nerve cell. Secondly, I will describe research on molecular mechanisms of anaesthesia performed during the last 10 years. I will concentrate my discussion on theories that involve perturbations of phospholipid-protein interactions by inhalation anaesthetics. Finally, I will present a new model system developed by Galla and myself for studying the effect of inhalation anaesthetics on a protein-induced lateral phase separation.

Molecular Structures of Membranes

A discussion of unitary theories of anaesthesia must begin with a review of current knowledge of the molecular structure of the phospholipid bilayer membranes that surround function-controlling proteins of the nerve cell. Protein-containing phospholipid bilayers are a ubiquitous structure in all cells. Of particular importance to anaesthesia, these phospholipid bilayers make up the thin, insulating nerve cell membrane that allows control of transmembrane potentials, fluxes of ions, and permeability by water, as well as the exocytosis and reception of transmitter molecules. Because I have attempted to formulate a unitary mechanism of anaesthesia that would attempt to explain how inhalation anaesthetic drugs may exert all of their many effects on synaptic transmission, axonal conduction, cardiac contractility, and vascular tone, I have sought a model system that would have properties common to the membranes in all cellular tissues.

An excellent illustration of the general properties of a phospholipid bilayer is included in a paper by Singer and Nicholson [1]. There is an insulating layer in the center of a bilayer formed by the opposing fatty acid chains of phospholipid molecules. Highly polar phosphate head-groups form an interface with either the extracellular or intracellular aqueous phases.

This phospholipid bilayer is so thermodynamically stable that it will form spontaneously when purified synthetic phospholipids are simply added to a water system and shaken by hand. This bilayer membrane may contain many forms of proteins, some of which are able to span the membrane and protrude into both the intra- and extracellular spaces. This class of proteins includes the ion channels and active transport pumps. Other proteins either rest on the top of the membrane, where they may form multiprotein complexes, or intracollate halfway into the membrane, where part of the protein is exposed to a hydrophobic region and the other part is available to either the intra- or extracellular aqueous phase.

Cory-Pauling-Koltrum (CPK) models are an excellent way to visualize the motions possible in phospholipid bilayer membranes, as well as the possible interactions between intrinsic membrane proteins and the phospholipids that make up the surrounding bilayer membrane. In Fig 1, the possibilities of rotation of the phosphate head-group of a phosphatidylcholine molecule is shown in the upper left model; the wag and flexing motion possible in the fatty acid chains of the phospholipid are shown in the lower left model; and on the right side of the figure are shown the anaesthetics chloroform, diethyl ether, methoxyflurane, and halothane, with a molecule of water at the bottom for comparison of size.

Phospholipid Perturbation Theories

Much of our early work on the theories of inhalation anaesthesia centered around the increase in molecular motion in the head-group and fatty acid chain region of the phospholipids in pure synthetic bilayers. We were able to add synthetically prepared spin labels to phospholipid bilayers and make quantitative measurements of the increase in fluidity as a function of anaesthetic concentration. The change in the fluidity of these bilayers was measured by electron paramagnetic resonance. We observed that as inhalation anaesthetics were added to the bilayer, they expanded the surface layer of the bilayer and increased the motional freedom or fluidity of the fatty acid chains [2]. However, it was not easy to develop a theory to explain how these small changes in fluidity of a nerve cell membrane could result in loss of activity of the proteins that control nerve function.

As a consequence, several laboratories began studying the effect of inhalation anaesthetics on a special property of mixtures of phospholipids known as a lateral phase separation [3, 4, 5]. A lateral phase separation in a phospholipid bilayer occurs when the temperature of a two-component system is maintained such that the lower melting component is in a fluid phase and the higher melting component segregates itself into small islands or domains of gel phase that essentially float in the fluid phospholipid phase. The size of these domains may be from 10 to several hundred phospholipids. An important property of lateral phase separations with regard to protein function is that, at the boundary between the fluid and the gel phase, there exists a defect in the packing and long-range order of the bilayer. This defect region has very high lateral compressibility. We have pointed out that lateral phase separations may be very important to the function of intrinsic membrane proteins if these proteins must increase in volume during some phase of their function [6]. For example, in the case of a pore protein, the entire protein may expand when the pore opens. Other proteins may simply have to go from a low-volume state, through a larger-volume transition state, before recoiling into a second low-volume catalytic form. A lateral phase separation makes such volume changes in proteins much easier thermodynamically. The phospholipids that are near a lateral phase separation exist in two forms; the gel phase is tightly packed in

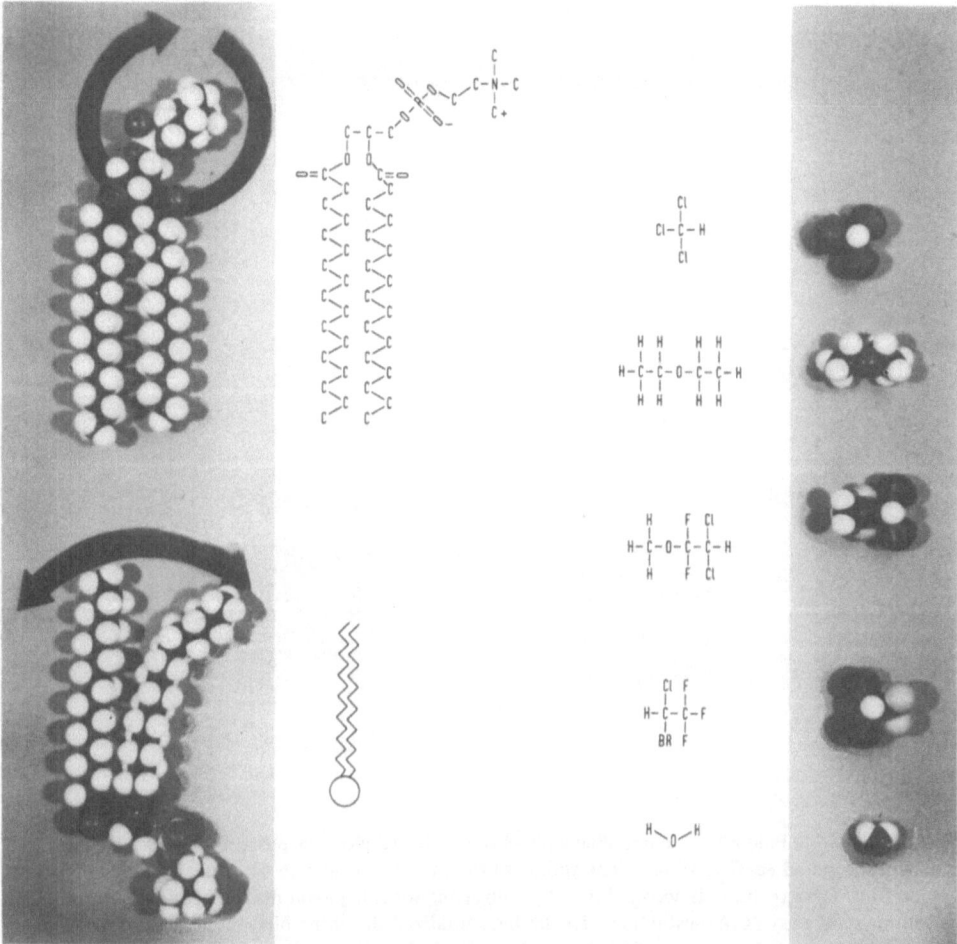

Fig. 1. In the *first vertical column to the left* are two exact-scale space-filling molecular models of phospholipid molecules arranged as they would be in a bilayer. In the *second vertical column from the left at the top* is an atomic structure of the corresponding phospholipid. *Below it in the same column* is the ball-and-wavy-line representation of a phospholipid. In the *third vertical column* are the atomic structures of chloroform, diethyl ether, methoxyflurane, halothane, and water. In the *fourth column* are the corresponding molecular models on the same scale as the phospholipids on the left. In the molecular models the *white balls* are hydrogen (*H*), the *black balls* are carbon (*C*), the *dark gray balls* are oxygen (*O*), the *medium gray balls* are phosphorus (*P*), and the *light gray balls* are nitrogen (*N*)

an ordered configuration that has low volume per phospholipid. The fluid phase is much less ordered and occupies considerably more volume per phospholipid molecule. Thus, whenever a lateral phase separation exists, room may be made for the lateral expansion of proteins by some of the fluid phase phospholipids being rapidly converted into the ordered gel phase. This has the effect of allowing lateral expansion of proteins without creating long-range dislocations in the membrane. In a series of experiments, we have shown that inhalation anaesthetics destroy these lateral phase separations.

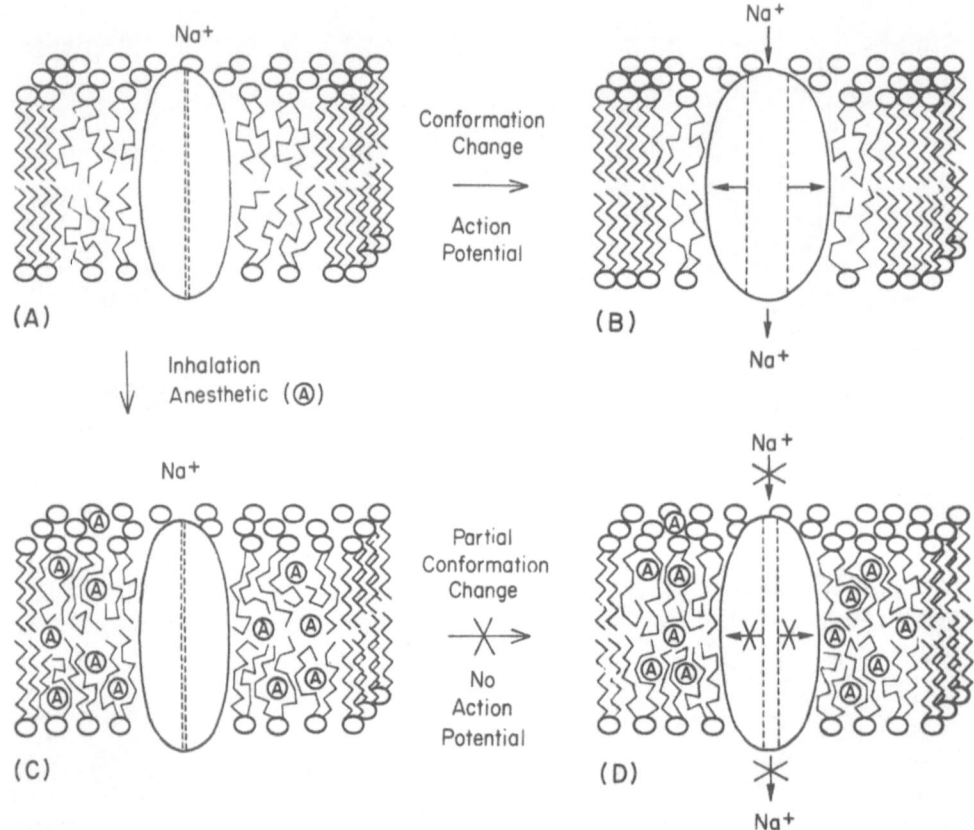

Fig. 2. A A phospholipid bilayer containing a membrane-solvated globular protein that has a sodium channel in the closed configuration. B The globular protein has expanded in conformation to allow a sodiumion flux. The expansion is accomplished by converting some high-volume fluid-phase lipids into the low-volume solid phase. C Anaesthetic molecules have fluidized the entire bilayer and destroyed the regions of solid phase. D Conversion of the high-volume fluid-phase lipids into the low-volume solid phase is a high-energy process. Therefore, the protein is unable to expand or change conformation, and the excitation process does not occur. Trudell JR [6]

In Fig. 2, the basic idea of a theory based on these experiments is described. In the upper left-hand drawing, a sodium channel protein is shown in its closed configuration; it is surrounded by fluid phase lipids which are themselves surrounded by the highly ordered gel phase lipids. In the transition to the drawing in the upper right, it is seen that as the pore protein expands, some of the fluid phase phospholipids have converted to the lower-volume gel phase lipids and allowed the expansion of the protein with very little activation energy. In contrast, in the lower left drawing, the lateral phase separation is shown destroyed by an inhalation anaesthetic. All of the phospholipids are essentially in a fluid phase. It is seen that the transition to the open configuration in the drawing at the lower right is now not aided by low lateral compressibility and either does not open, or opens with a much greater activation energy.

I would like to emphasize that although the protein shown in Fig. 2 is depicted as a sodium channel, this same sort of theory is meant to apply to any protein that exists in a phospholipid bilayer membrane, and must change its volume during its function. Therefore the perturbation of these lateral phase separations in the bilayer of cardiac tissue, nerve axons, synapses, and the many membranes of the brain may all simultaneously produce effects on their respective functional proteins.

Peptide-Induced Lateral Phase Separation Model

Although theories based on perturbations of membrane properties are very attractive, it has been difficult to test them in nerve membranes because of the enormous complexity of the many kinds of phospholipids and proteins that are always present. Galla has developed a model system in which a positively charged polypeptide antibiotic named polymyxin was bound to a negatively charged phosphatidic acid vesicle [7]. This model has the unique property that the peptide not only binds to the surface of the phosphatidic acid vesicle, but it clusters together after binding to make domains of a tight peptide-phospholipid complex. The phospholipids in this peptide-phospholipid domain have properties that are very distinct from those in the remainder of the bilayer. The properties of the two different phases are measurable by electron paramagnetic resonance techniques that determine the partition coefficient of the small spinprobe "Tempo". It is seen that as the peptide binds to the surface of the phospholipid vesicle, it forms a lateral phase separation in the phospholipids below it. This is exactly the kind of model system that is appropriate for a study of the effect of inhalation anaesthetics on lateral phase separations. Galla and I have performed a series of experiments on these lateral peptide-induced phase separations to determine the effect of inhalation anaesthetics.

In Fig. 3, the melting transition of pure phosphatidic acid (solid circles) is shown as measured by the electron paramagnetic resonance technique that uses the value of the parti-

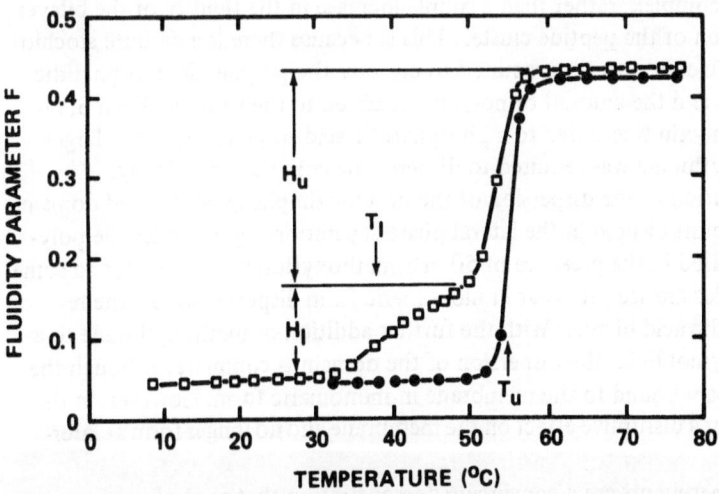

Fig. 3. Phase transition curves of dipalmitoylphosphatidic acid bilayers at pH 9 and a sodium concentration of 0.05 M without (black dots) and after incorporation of polymyxin, 4 mole % (white squares). A second phase transition step with a lowered phase transition temperature, T_1, as compared with that of mixed phosphatidic acid bilayers, appears at T_u. The step height of each of these phase transitions is designated by H_1 or H_u respectively. Galla HJ and Trudell JR [9]

tion coefficient of "Tempo" between gel and fluid phases expressed as fluidity parameter (F).
The effect of adding 4 mole % of polymyxin is depicted by the open squares. Each polymyxin peptide has four positive charges available for binding to phosphatidic acid. Therefore,
4 mole % of polymyxin can interact strongly with 16% of the total phospholipids at the bilayer surface. The amount of phosphatidic acid in this polymyxin-phosphatidic acid domain
is denoted by H_1. It may be seen that the phosphatidic acid that surrounds the polymyxin-
phosphatidic acid domain and melts between 50 ° and 55 ° exhibits a broader and lower
melting transition. It is clear that the effect of the addition of polymyxin has created two distinct phases of phospholipids with very different properties. A lateral phase separation must
exist between these two phases.

The famous Meyer-Overton rule states that clinical concentrations of any inhalation
anaesthetic produce anaesthesia when the nerve membranes contain a concentration of
30–60 mM anaesthetic/mol lipid [8]. In Fig. 4, the effect of a concentration of 75 mM metho-
xyflurane/mol phospholipid on the fluidity parameter of a polymyxin-phospholipid vesicle
system is seen. In the control measurement, the free phosphatidic acid phase melts at between 48° and 55°, while the phosphatidic acid in the polymyxin-phosphatidic acid domain
melts at between 30° and 48°. The effect of methoxyflurane is to increase the amount of
free phosphatidic acid, as well as to lower the midpoint of the melting transition of the free
phosphatidic acid phase. The melting transition of the phosphatidic acid in the polymyxin-
phosphatidic acid domain is lowered, and the amount of phospholipid in the domain is clearly reduced [9].

We have studied the concentration dependence of methoxyflurane on the dispersion of
the phosphatidic acid-polymyxin domain. The size of the domain decreases as a function of
inhalation anaesthetic concentration; at 100 mM anaesthetic/mol lipid, the phosphatidic
acid-polymyxin domain ceases to exist and the entire amount of phosphatidic acid in the bilayer begins to behave as though the polymyxin were not present. We have shown that there
is some direct molecular interaction between the methoxyflurane molecules and the polymyxin-phosphatidic acid complex, rather than a simple increase in the fluidity of the bilayer
causing a gradual disruption of the peptide cluster. This is because there is a definite stochio-
metry between anaesthetic concentration required to disperse the polymyxin-phosphatidic
acid complex completely, and the amount of polymyxin added to the vesicles. When 6, rather than 4, mole % polymyxin was added to a phosphatidic acid suspension, a 50% larger
concentration of methoxyflurane was required to disperse the complex completely.

A pictorial representation of the dispersion of the polymyxin-phosphatidic acid domain
is given in Fig. 5. The amount of lipid in the lateral phase separation region under the polymyxin is seen to be decreased in the presence of 50 mM methoxyflurane/mol lipid, and some
of the polymyxin molecules are seen to exist in monomeric form dispersed across the remainder of the phosphatidic acid bilayer. With the further addition of methoxyflurane to a
concentration of 100 mM/mol lipid, the dispersion of the domain is complete, although the
polymyxin molecules remain bound to the membrane in monomeric form. However, in this
form they have much less of a disruptive effect on the membrane and no longer form at lateral phase separation.

We feel that these experiments are a convincing demonstration that clinical concentrations of inhalation anaesthetics are able to disrupt lateral phase separations in membranes.
This simple model system is a long way from the complex lipid-protein interactions observed
in nerve membranes [10]. However, it is clear that those proteins that form channels by
existing as polymeric complexes, or that require the presence of nearby lateral phase separa-

tions for facile expansion during their activation, will be strongly affected by clinical concentrations of inhalation anaesthetics.

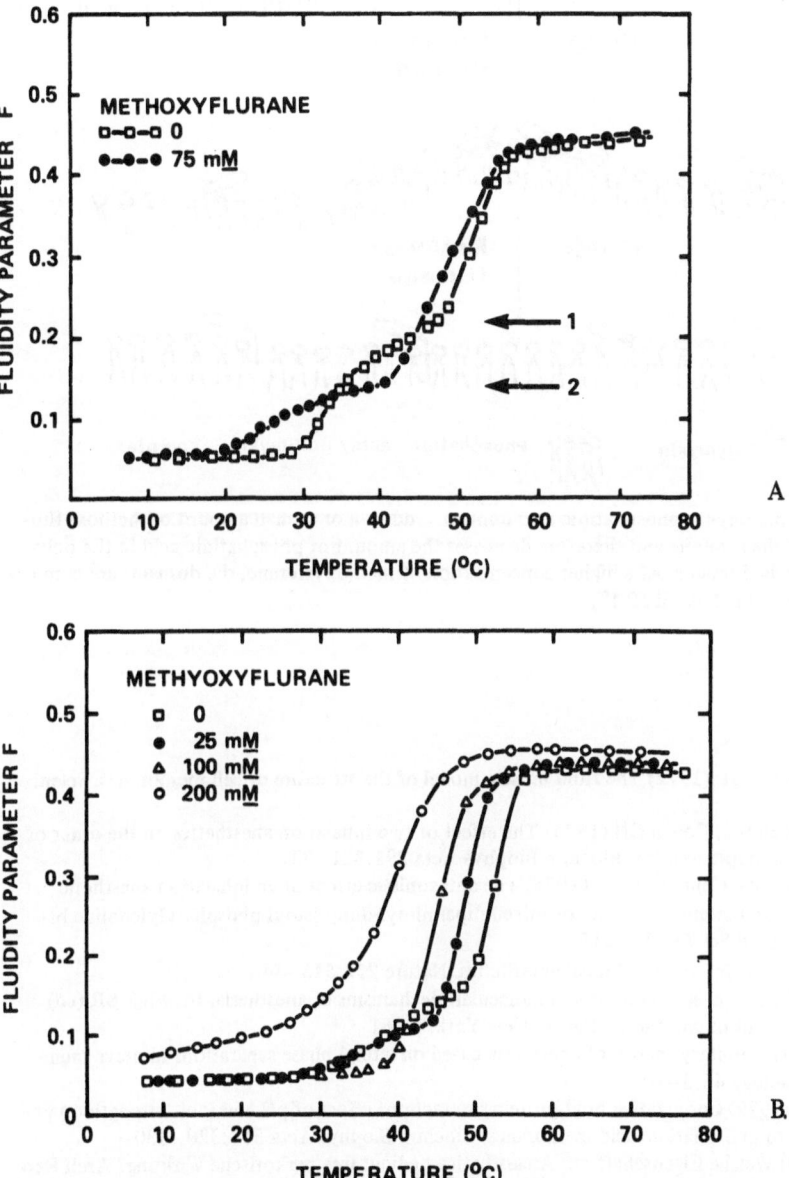

Fig. 4 A, B. Phase transition curve of dipalmitoylphosphatidic acid bilayers. A Polymyxin, 6 mole %, in the absence (white squares) and presence (black dots) of 75 mmol methoxyflurane per mol lipid. *Arrows 1 and 2* point out the step height of the lower phase transition step designated as H_1 in Fig. 3. B Equivalent bilayer preparations as in A but with polymyxin, 4 mole %. The phase transition curves are given for different amounts of anaesthetic between 25 and 200 mmol/mol lipid. *White squares* represent O; *black dots* represent 25 mM; *white triangles* represent 100 mM; and *white circles* represent 200 mM. The lower phase transition disappears at concentrations of methoxyflurane greater than 100 mmol/mol lipid. Galla HJ and Trudell JR [9]

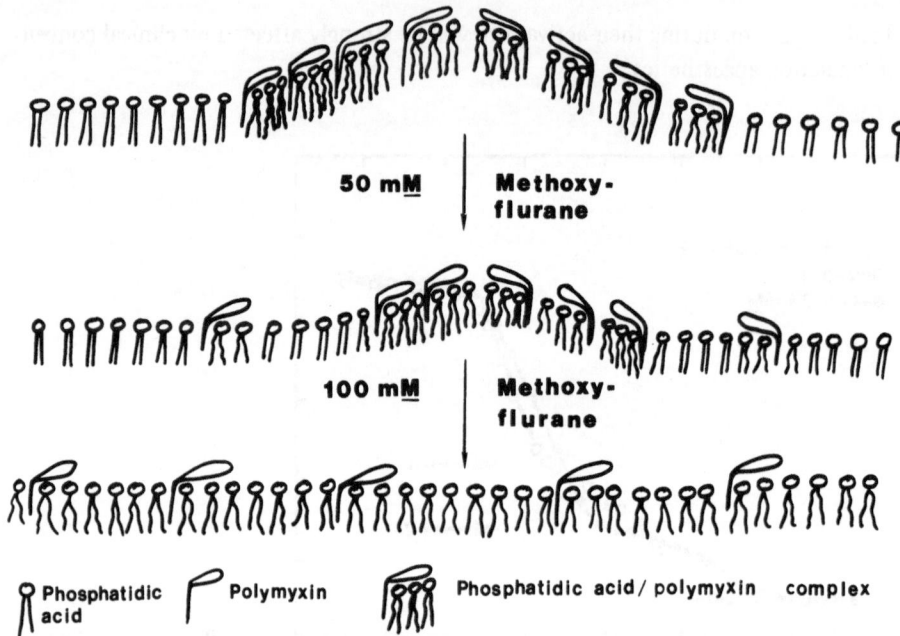

Fig. 5. Model for the polymyxin-phosphatidic acid domain. Addition of a small amount of methoxyflurane disperses some of the subunits and therefore decreases the amount of phosphatidic acid in the polymyxin-phosphatidic acid domains. At a higher concentration of methoxyflurane, the domains are completely dispersed. Galla HJ and Trudell JR [9]

References

1. Singer SJ, Nicholson GL (1972) The fluid mosaic model of the structure of cell membranes. Science 175:720–730
2. Trudell JR, Hubbell WL, Cohen EN (1973) The effect of two inhalation anesthetics on the order of spin-labeled phospholipid vesicles. Biochim Biophys Acta 291:321–327
3. Trudell JR, Payan DG, Chin JH, et al. (1975) The antagonistic effect of an inhalation anesthetic and high pressure on the phase diagram of mixed dipalmitoyl-dimyristoyl-phosphatidylcholine bilayers. Proc Natl Acad Sci 72:210–213
4. Lee AG (1976) Model for action of local anesthetics. Nature 262:545–548
5. Trudell JR (1980) Biophysical concepts in molecular mechanisms of anesthesia. In: Fink BR (ed) Molecular mechanisms of anesthesia. Raven, New York, p 261
6. Trudell JR (1977) A unitary theory of anesthesia based on lateral phase separations in nerve membranes. Anesthesiology 46:5–10
7. Sixl F, Galla HJ (1979) Cooperative lipid-protein interaction: effect of pH and ionic strength on polymyxin binding to phosphatidic acid membranes. Biochim Biophys Acta 557:320–330
8. Meyer HH (1899) Welche Eigenschaft der Anaesthetica bedingt ihre narkotische Wirkung? Arch Exp Pathol Pharmacol 42:109–118
9. Galla HJ, Trudell JR (1981) Perturbation of peptide-induced lateral phase separations in phosphatidic acid bilayers by the inhalation anesthetic methoxyflurane. Mol Pharmacol 19:432–437
10. Bosterling B, Trudell JR, Galla HJ (1981) Phospholipid interactions with cytochrome P-450 in reconstituted vesicles: Preference for negatively-charged phosphatidic acid. Biochim Biophys Acta 643:547–556

Clinical Implications of the Pharmacodynamics of Inhalation Anaesthetics

G. Torri, C. Martani und V. Perotti

An important and relatively new development in anaesthesiology is the increasing interest in learning about the body's uptake and distribution of anaesthetic agents to various organs and tissues. These studies are, in fact, fundamentally pharmacological, but the knowledge derived can be applied almost directly to improve patient care. Pharmacodynamic studies will support many data relevant to the three phases of anaesthesia: induction, maintenance, and recovery.

The induction of anaesthesia has always been correlated to the speed of equilibration between alveolar and inspired concentration. The progressive increase in alveolar concentration depends on many factors: alveolar ventilation, blood flow, blood solubility, body temperature, and pulmonary shunt; these have been reviewed by Eger [2]. When all physiological parameters are constant the only equilibration factor is represented by the solubility of the anaesthetic in blood and tissue, which is usually expressed by the blood/gas partition coefficient. The lower the blood solubility coefficient, the shorter the equilibration time between alveolar and inspired concentration, as shown by the following simplified formula:

$$\frac{F_A}{F_I} \propto \frac{1}{\text{blood solubility}}$$

This finding is supported by experimental data obtained from various sources [6, 9, 10], and is graphically represented in Fig. 1.

As shown in Fig. 1 the equilibration between inspired and alveolar concentration in normal subjects is faster with enflurane than with halothane [8]. However, the equilibration time alone cannot be used to predict the speed of induction of the anaesthesia. In clinical practice a very important factor which largely helps to determine the speed of anaesthesia induction is represented by the anaesthetic potency, but this parameter is rarely considered in pharmacodynamic studies. For normal values of the physiological parameters involved in the uptake and distribution of inhalation anaesthetics, the speed of induction is directly proportional to the anaesthetic potency and inversely proportional to the blood and tissue solubility, according to the following formula:

$$\text{Speed of induction} \propto \frac{\text{potency}}{\text{blood solubility}}$$

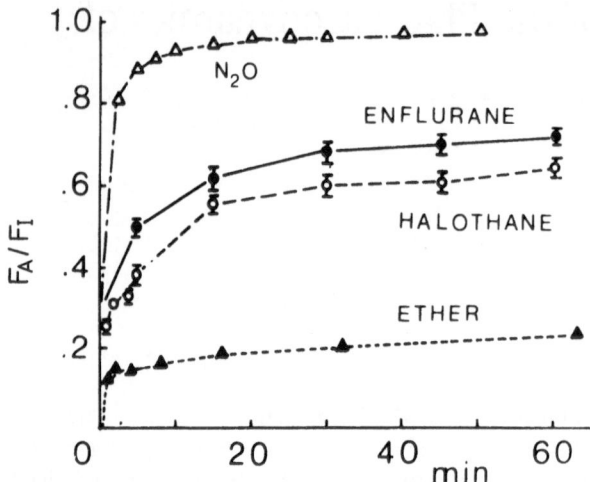

Fig. 1. Rate of rise of alveolar (F_A) anaesthetic concentration towards the inspired (F_I) concentration is most rapid with the least soluble agent (nitrous oxide) and least rapid with the most soluble agent (ether). All data are from studies in man by Salanitre et al. [6] (nitrous oxide), Torri et al. [8] (enflurane), and Wahrebrock et al. [10] (halothane and ether)

As a result, if two agents provide the same solubility the speed of induction will depend on their potency: the higher the potency the higher the speed of induction. On the other hand, should the potency be the same for the two agents, the higher speed of induction would be that of the less soluble anaesthetic.

The modern inhalation agents greatly differ in potency or in blood solubility. The minimum alveolar concentrations (MACs) of methoxyflurane, halothane, and enflurane are 0.16%, 0.76%, and 1.68% respectively [3, 5]. Consequently, the potency of enflurane is 50% that of halothane. Since the wash-in curves of these two agents do not greatly differ, in clinical practice it can be shown that, when the same inspired concentration is preset at the vaporizer, the speed of induction is higher with halothane than with enflurane. To obtain a rapid induction with enflurane the preset inspired concentration must be proportional to the potency of this anaesthetic. When equipotent inspired concentrations of enflurane and halothane are used, the induction of anaesthesia will be faster with enflurane than with halothane.

The induction of anaesthesia in a patient is never started with the same partial pressure of anaesthetic as that required for maintenance of anaesthesia, but with higher partial pressure. The anaesthesiologist knows intuitively that it takes time to achieve an equilibrium in the body with a given inspired concentration. Accordingly, he initially uses a higher concentration in order to establish the required anaesthetic partial pressure rapidly. If induction of halothane anaesthesia is achieved in a short time using 1.5%–2% of halothane in the inspired concentration, induction of enflurane anaesthesia will require 2.5%–3% in the inspired concentration.

As shown in Fig. 1, if inspired concentration is held constant, in a few minutes the alveolar concentration reaches a steady-state value which allows a constant level of anaesthesia to be maintained during surgical procedures. Nevertheless, many factors may affect the value of alveolar concentration: changes in alveolar ventilation or cardiac output, changes in ventilation/perfusion ratio or pulmonary shunt, or changes in blood solubility due to variations in body temperature. When the anaesthetic partial pressure at alveolar level is held constant for at least 15–20 min, its value is very similar to the partial pressure at brain level. [1, 8]. Consequently, the continuous monitoring of the end-tidal concentration by modern anaesthetic analysers represents a new scientific approach to the control of anaesthesia level. Furthermore, by this technique many problems concerning the reliability of the vaporizer may easily be overcome.

We turn next to a discussion of some differences in the recovery from anaesthesia that cannot accurately be analysed by the wash-out curves. Some years ago we applied to inhalation agents the Noerhen [4] concept of pulmonary clearance [7]. At the end of the anaesthesia, when the inspired concentration of anaesthetics is zero, the pulmonary clearance of anaesthetic agents ($\dot{C}1$) represents a useful index of their elimination from the lungs. Its value depends on pulmonary blood flow ($\dot{Q}$), alveolar ventilation ($\dot{V}_A$), and anaesthetic blood solubility (γ), according to the following equation:

$$\dot{C}1 = \frac{\dot{V}_A \quad \dot{Q}}{\dot{V}_A + \lambda \dot{Q}}$$

This equation is derived from: (a) alveolar ventilation equation; (b) Fick equation; and (c) partition coefficient (γ). The relation between pulmonary clearance values and anaesthetic blood solubility is graphically represented in Fig. 2.

The more soluble the anaesthetic in the blood, the lower the value of its pulmonary clearance and the longer the recovery time. Among the different halogenated compounds, enflurane has the highest value of pulmonary clearance, which may explain the rapid recovery observed in clinical application of this drug (see Table 1).

When different anaesthetics are considered, it can be found that a similar change in alveolar ventilation or in cardiac output determines a different change in pulmonary clearance,

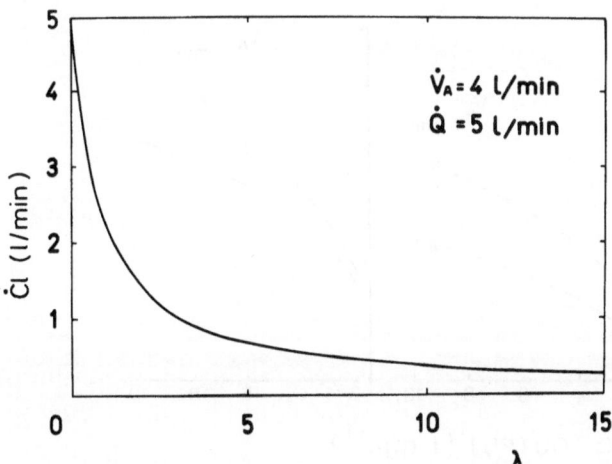

Fig. 2. Pulmonary clearance value ($\dot{C}1$) of anaesthetic agents plotted against anaesthetic blood solubility (λ). $\dot{Q}$, pulmonary blood flow

Table 1. Blood/gas partition coefficient and pulmonary clearance values at normal values of alveolar ventilation (4 l/min) and pulmonary blood (5 l/min)

Anaesthetic agent	Blood/gas partition coefficient	Pulmonary clearance (l/min)
Nitrous oxide	0.468	3.1
Enflurane	1.91	1.476
Halothane	2.36	1.2
Methoxyflurane	13	0.28

which depends on anaesthetic blood solubility (Fig. 3). The pulmonary clearance of highly soluble gases such as methoxyflurane is very low, and affected to little extent by changes in alveolar ventilation or in cardiac output. On the other hand, the pulmonary clearance of poorly soluble gases is very high, and greatly increased by an increase in alveolar ventilation. The present analysis being limited to the halogenated compounds, the largest increase in pulmonary clearance determined by an increase in alveolar ventilation demonstrated here is that of enflurane at every value of ventilation/perfusion ratio (Fig. 4).

Of the three factors governing the pulmonary clearance of inhalation anaesthetics (i.e. alveolar ventilation, cardiac output, and blood solubility), the alveolar ventilation represents the only parameter under the control of the anaesthetist. Consequently, all anaesthetics which may be defined as "ventilation-dependent" in their uptake and elimination represent, together with controlled ventilation, an improvement in modern anaesthesia.

In conclusion, pharmacodynamic studies point out two clinical advantages of enflurane:
1. The pulmonary clearance of enflurane is higher than that of the other halogenated anaesthetics.

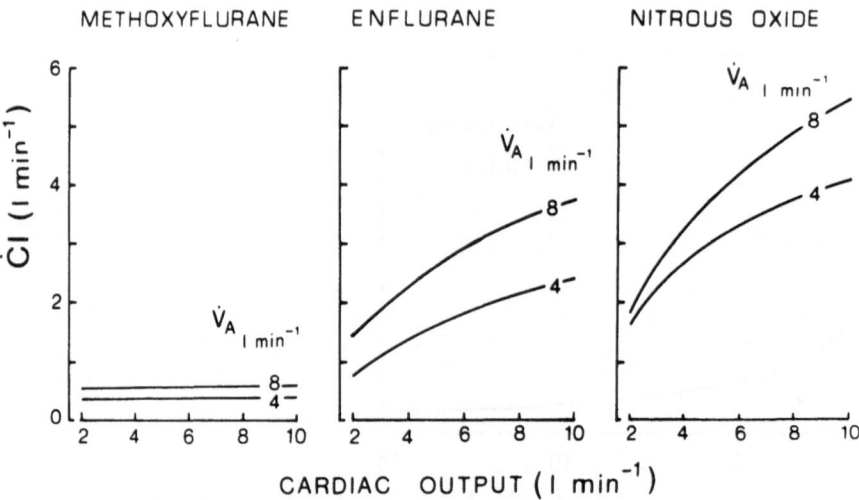

Fig. 3. Pulmonary clearance value ($\dot{C}I$) of three anaesthetics plotted against blood flow ($\dot{Q}$) at different alveolar ventilation values ($\dot{V}_A$)

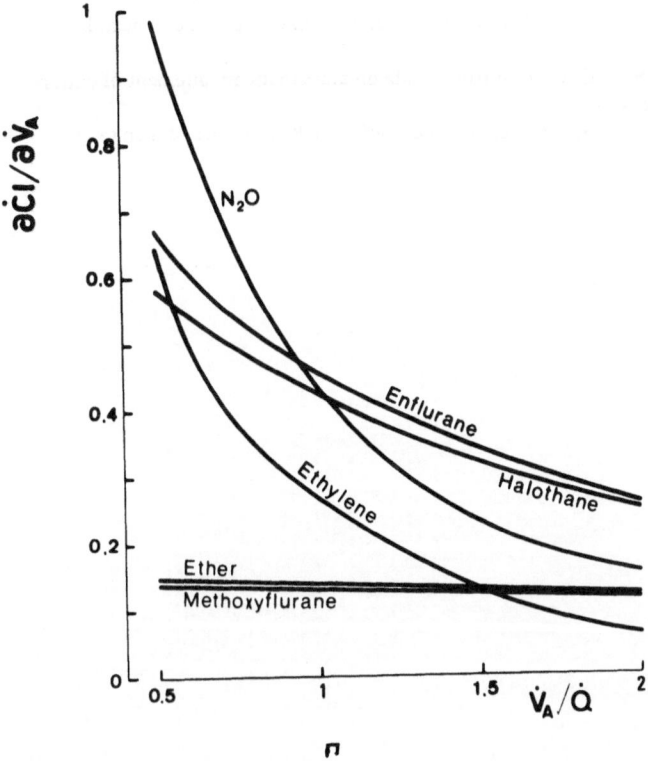

Fig. 4. Changes of pulmonary clearance determined by increase in alveolar ventilation $(a\dot{C}l/a\dot{V}_A)$ at different alveolar ventilation $(\dot{V}_A)$ blood flow (Q) values for different anaesthetic agents

2. By increasing alveolar ventilation the anaesthetist can to a large extent increase the pulmonary clearance of enflurane and easily control the recovery from anaesthesia.
These pharmacodynamic results may explain the clinical flexibility of enflurane, with particular reference to its uptake and elimination.

References

1. Eger EI II, Balhman SH (1971) Is the end-tidal anesthetic partial pressure an accurate measure of arterial partial pressure? Anesthesiology 35:301
2. Eger EI II (1974) Anesthetic uptake and action. Williams & Wilkins, Baltimore
3. Gion H, Saidman LPG (1971) The minimum alveolar concentration of enflurane in man. Anesthesiology 35:361
4. Noerhen TH (1962) Pulmonary clearance of inert gases with particular reference to ethyl ether J Appl Physiol 17:795
5. Saidman LPG, Munson ES, Babad AA, Muallen M (1967) Minimum alveolar concentration of methoxyflurane, halothane, ether and cyclopropane in man: correlation with theories of anesthesia. Anaesthesiology 28:994
6. Salanitre E, Rackow H, Greene LT, et al. (1962) Uptake and excretion of subanesthetic concentrations of nitrous oxide in man. Anesthesiology 23:814
7. Torri G, Damia G (1968) Pulmonary clearance of anaesthetic agents. A theoretical study. Br J Anaesth 40:757

8. Torri G, Damia G, Fabiani ML, Frova G (1972) Uptake and elimination of enflurane in man. Br J Anaesth 44:784
9. Torri G, Damia G, Fabiani ML (1974) Effect of nitrous oxide on anaesthetic requirement of enflurane. Appendix 2. Br J Anaesth 46:468
10. Wahrenbrock EA, Eger EI, Laravuso RB, et al. (1974) Anesthetic uptake of mice and man (and whales). Anesthesiology 40:19

Advances in Cardiovascular Pathophysiology

B.E. Strauer

Introduction

Chronic hypertrophic heart disease (hypertensive, non-hypertensive) is one of the most common cardiac diseases in man [1, 12, 17, 22–24]. Its aetiology may be outlined as follows (Table 1).

From the functional point of view, ventricular hypertrophy provides one of the basic mechanisms that permit the heart to maintain normal cardiac pump function despite abnormal pressure, or stress or volume load [4, 5]. On the other hand, cardiac hypertrophy is a significant precursor of cardiac enlargement and failure. The aetiology of cardiac failure may be schematized as follows (Table 2a, b).

With regard to the significance and influence of the type (abnormal pressure or volume load, heart rate changes, metabolic disorders, etc.), the duration (acute or chronic cardiac overload) and the degree of cardiac overload (appropriate or inappropriate), this presentation will focus some recent results on hypertrophic, congestive, and coronary heart disease. These may be considered under the following heads:

1. Ventricular and myocardial function
2. Contraction energetics and coronary blood flow
3. Pharmacological interventions
a) Analgesics; b) Digitalis glycosides; c) Vasodilating drugs (hydralazine)

Because of the abundance of data, facts, and concepts representing recent advances in cardiovascular pathophysiology, some basic results from the past few years will be discussed in this report which — from the point of view of the cardiologist — may be of pharmacotherapeutical relevance for diagnostics and management of the cardiac patient in anaesthesia.

Table 1. Etiology of cardiac hypertrophy

I.	Primary hypertrophic cardiomyopathy (hereditary cardiomyopathy, hypertrophic obstructive cardiomyopathy etc.)
II.	Secondary cardiac hypertrophy, due to
	— pressure overload (arterial hypertension, valvular heart disease etc.)
	— volume overload (valvular heart disease, cardiac and vascular shunts etc.)
	— high output (hypoxemia, anemia etc.)
	— metabolic disorders (coronary artery disease, hormonal disease etc.)

* Supported by Deutsche Forschungsgemeinschaft.

Table 2a. Etiology of cardiac failure

I.   Abnormal preload
     a) Cardiac valve incompetence (aortic regurgitation, mitral regurgitation etc.)
     b) Intra- and extracardial shunts (atrial septum defect, ventricular septal defect, ductus arteriosus Botalli apertus etc.)
     c) Hypervolemia (fluid excess, renal failure etc.)
     d) Hypovolemia (bleeding, blood-letting, exsiccosis etc.)
II. Abnormal afterload
     a) Intraventricular pressure overload (aortic stenosis, hypertrophic obstructive cardiomyopathy etc.)
     b) Extraventricular pressure overload (arterial hypertension, coarctation aortae, cor pulmonale etc.)
     c) Inappropriate ventricular hypertrophy (inadequate hypertrophy with high wall stress, decrease in mass-to-volume ratio etc.)
     d) Abnormal pressure decrease (blood-letting, excess vasodilatation etc.)
III. Abnormal contractility
     a) Alterations in myocardial contractility (primary cardiomyopathies, disturbances of contractile protein synthesis, abnormal contraction enzymes, changes of calcium transport etc.)
     b) Pharmacological interventions (negatively inotropic agents, intoxications etc.)
     c) Coronary circulation disorders (coronary insufficiency, myocardial infarction etc.)
     d) Extracardiac diseases (anemia, hypoxia, alterations in blood viscosity etc.)
IV. Abnormal heart rate
     a) abnormal increase in heart rate (ventricular, supraventricular tachycardia)
     b) abnormal decrease in heart rate (extreme bradycardia)

Table 2b. Extracardiac reasons for cardiac failure

Arterial hypertension
  − hypertensive heart disease (hypertensive hypertrophy and failure)
Secondary cardiomyopathies
  − thyreotoxicosis, hypothyroidism, oxalosis, amyloidosis, hemochromatosis, uremia, diabetes mellitus, anemia etc.
Ischemic heart disease (coronary artery disease)
  − hypoxidosis, polyglobulia, paraproteinemia, arteriitis (reduced oxygen availability to the myocardium)
  − abnormal pressure load, hypertensive emergency crisis, acute cor pulmonale, abnormal volume load, fever (increased oxygen demand of the myocardium)
Systemic immunopathies
  − Lupus erythematodes, progressive sclerodermia, periarteriitis nodosa, immune complex vasculitis with coronary involvement etc.
Pharmacologically induced cardiac failure (toxic)
  − Barbiturates, betareceptor blocking agents, analgesics, inhalation anesthetics, antiarrhythmic-drugs, adriamycin, glucocorticoids, ethanol etc.

Advances in cardiovascular pathophysiology

I.   Ventricular and myocardial function
II. Contraction energetics and coronary blood flow
III. Pharmacological interventions
       − analgesics
       − digitalis glycosides
       − vasodilating drugs (hydralazine)

Patient Population and Methods

The majority of data presented in this report are based on studies on more than 900 patients during diagnostic cardiac catheterizations 1968–1981 [16–20], including patients with hypertensive, coronary, congestive, valvular, septal, and myocardial heart disease. Methods have previously been described in detail. Quantitative ventriculography was performed in all patients [6–9]. Wall stress was calculated frame by frame from ventriculograms until the peak value of circumferential stress was obtained [6, 8, 9]. Left ventricular (LV) mass and LV mass to volume ratio were determined from end-diastolic chamber dimensions [22–24]. Coronary blood flow was measured by the argon method, with gas-chromatographic analysis of argon in the arterial and coronary sinus blood [3, 20, 27]. The experimental design for examination of isolated ventricular myocardium has been published elsewhere [15, 17–19].

Results

Pathophysiological Implications of Cardiac Hypertrophy

During the development of cardiac hypertrophy, ventricular wall mass increases. This may have at least three consequences with regard to intraventricular volume and wall thickness. First, in compensated pressure overload, as in arterial hypertension and in aortic stenosis, the ventricular wall becomes thickened and the mass is augmented, whereas end-diastolic volume remains normal or mildly increases. This leads to an increase in the mass to volume ratio, and is termed concentric hypertrophy [12]. Here the ventricular response is appropriate to the pressure load burdened upon the ventricular wall. Secondly, in both decompensated pressure and volume overload, ventricular mass and volume increase, whereas wall thickness may remain unchanged or only moderately increases. This leads to ventricular dilatation, with constancy or even decrease in the mass to volume ratio, and is termed excentric hypertrophy [12]. Here, ventricular response is inappropriate, since the heart dilates out of proportion to wall thickness changes. Thirdly, in chronic pressure overload, as well as in hypertrophic obstructive cardiomyopathy, excess increase in wall thickness and mass may occur, thereby narrowing the intraventricular hole. Consequently, the mass to volume ratio increases excessively. This type of excess hypertrophy is termed irregular inappropriate hypertrophy. Here, the ventricular response is inappropriate, because the wall thickens out of proportion to intraventricular volume changes.

These three types of hypertrophy occur in experimental and in clinical hypertrophic heart disease, and are associated with different cardiac dimensions and wall stress. Wall stress represents the force per unit cross-sectional area of the ventricular wall and is, according to the law of Laplace, expressed in dyn/cm^2 [14, 22–24]. Stress, in accordance with the Laplace equation, is directly related to pressure (p) and radius (r) and is inversely related to wall thickness (d).

There are at least three kinds of stress acting at the ventricular wall [8]: radial stress acts perpendicular to the endocardial surface; longitudinal stress acts within the wall parallel to the long axis of the heart, and circumferential wall stress, which in a quantitative sense is the most important one, acts within the wall parallel to the short axis of the ventricle. If wall hypertrophy is adequate with regard to the ventricular load (e.g. concentric hypertrophy), then the stress remains normal. If hypertrophy is inappropriate for the pressure and volume demand, then stress increases. If the wall thickens out of proportion to pressure and volume load, then stress is reduced.

Cardiac Dimensions in Chronic Pressure and Volume Overload

In the course of ventricular hypertrophy, heart size, ventricular mass, intraventricular volume, and stress may change. In a series of more than 400 patients we compared intraventricular volumes, as measured by quantitative cardiac ventriculography [25]. In cronic pressure overload, for example in arterial hypertension and in aortic stenosis, left ventricular end-diastolic volume is nearly normal, varying between 130 and 170 ml (normals 152 ± 2 ml) (Fig. 1) [25]. Accordingly there is normal filling volume, and stroke volume is also normal. On the other hand, chronic volume overload, for example in valvular or septal heart disease, involves large increase in heart size and in end-diastolic volume, varying from 200 to 360 ml (Fig. 2) [25]. This increased filling volume leads to considerable increase in total stroke volume, whereas the effective forward stroke volume, as a result of valvular regurgitation in these cases, does not change significantly.

Heart Size and Heart Function

Left ventricular (LV) size as determined by the end-diastolic volume shows an inverse relationship with LV function as evidenced by the ejection fraction (Fig. 3) [25]. With increase in end-diastolic volume the ejection fraction decreases for all patient groups with inborn or acquired heart disease. However, steepness of this characteristic is quite different: lowest de-

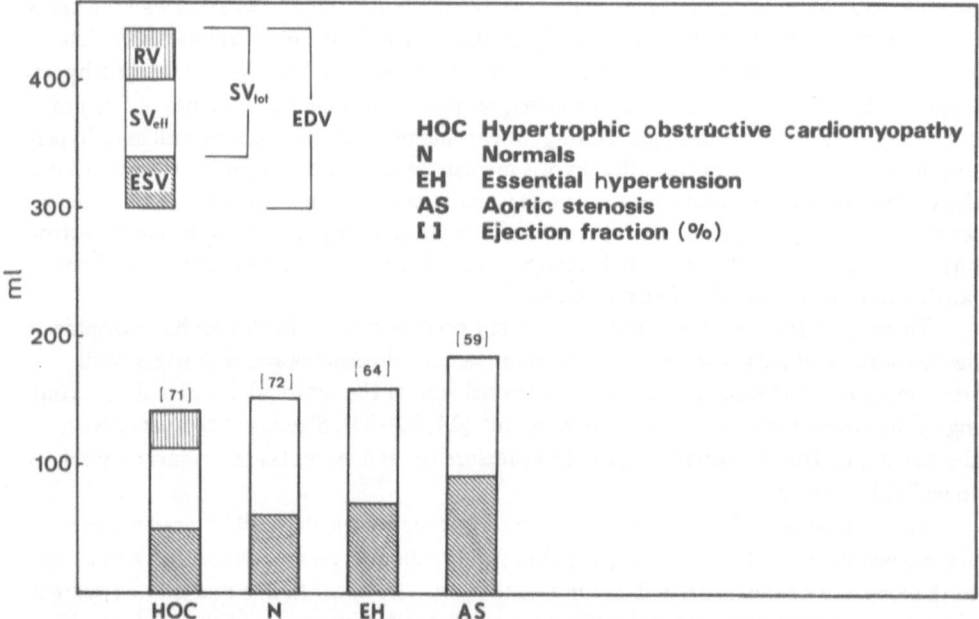

Fig. 1. Left ventricular volumes in chronic pressure overload (n = 112). *EDV*, end-diastolic volume; *ESV*, end-systolic volume; *SV*, stroke volume (*tot*, total; *eff*, effective; *RV*, regurgitation volume

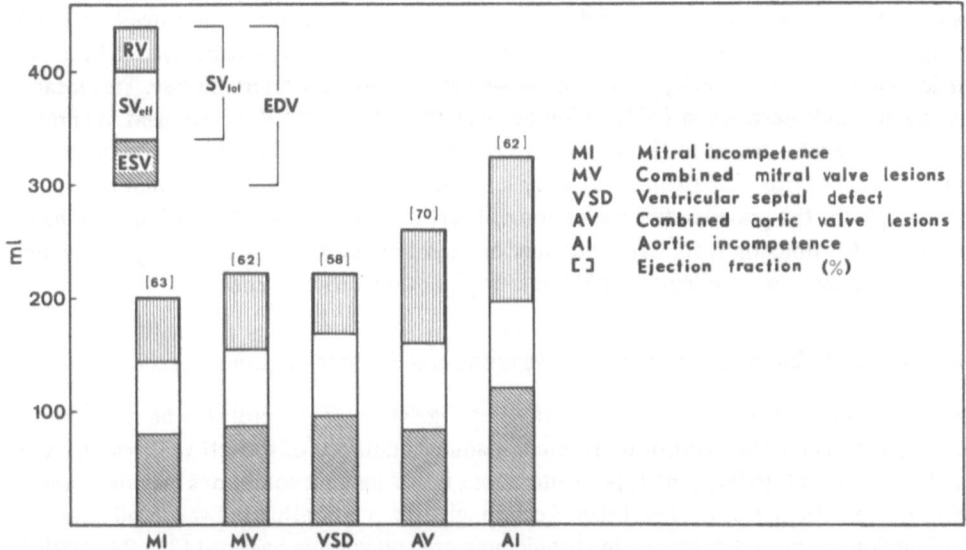

Fig. 2. Left ventricular volumes in chronic volume overload (n = 132). *EDV*, end-diastolic volume; *ESV*, end-systolic volume; *SV*, stroke volume (*tot*, total; *eff*, effective); *RV*, regurgitation volume

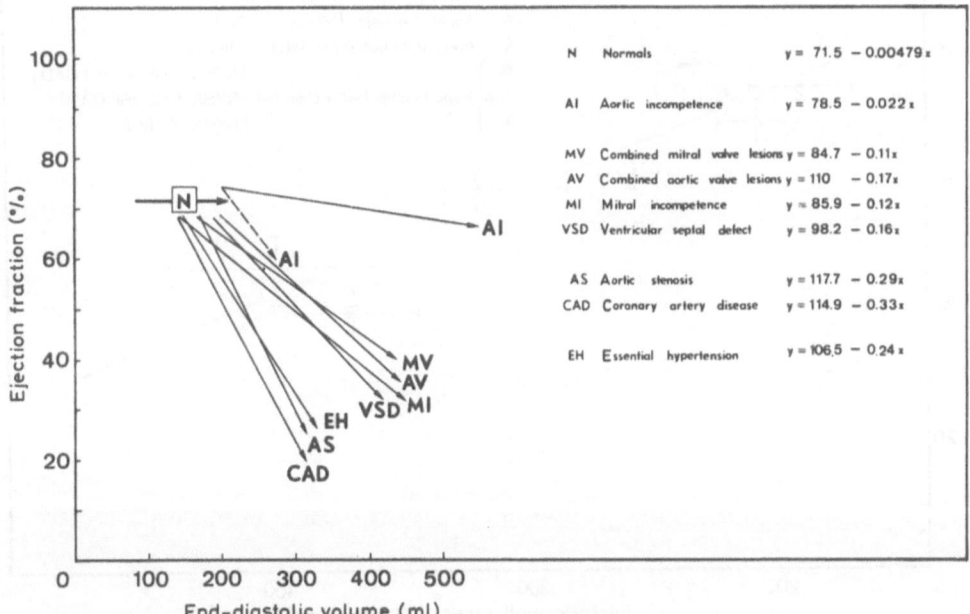

Fig. 3. Relationship between end-diastolic volume and the ejection fraction (EDV-ESV/EDV). *EDV*, end-diastolic volume; *ESV*, end-systolic volume

crease in function with increase in end-diastolic volume is present for volume overload (e.g.), aortic incompetence, whereas largest decrease is found for chronic pressure overload due to aortic stenosis and essential hypertension, as well as for coronary artery disease. This means that considerable decrease in LV function occurs with only small LV enlargement in chronic pressure overload, whereas in chronic volume overload normal LV function may exist even where there is a large increase in LV size [25]. From the practical diagnostic point of view, for example for the pre-operative evaluation of heart function, these relationships may help to evaluate LV function from left ventricular or heart size on routine chest X-rays, provided the clinical reason or a etiology for LV hypertrophy or dilatation is known.

Wall Stress and Ventricular Function – Diagnostic and Therapeutic Consequences

The different courses of these characteristics (see Fig. 3) may most probably be related to differing contractile state and/or to different loading conditions of the left ventricle. Except for changes in contractility, the typical alterations in LV loading conditions may decrease LV function with increase in heart size. Accordingly, the relationship between wall stress and function has been determined in chronic pressure and volume overload [22–24]. With increase in systolic wall stress, the left ventricular function, as evidenced by the ventricular ejection fraction, decreased (Fig. 4). Doubling of stress led to reduction in the ejection fraction by approximately 50% [22–24]. Since systolic wall stress results from systolic pressure and from the mass to volume ratio, it equals the ventricular after-load which is imposed on

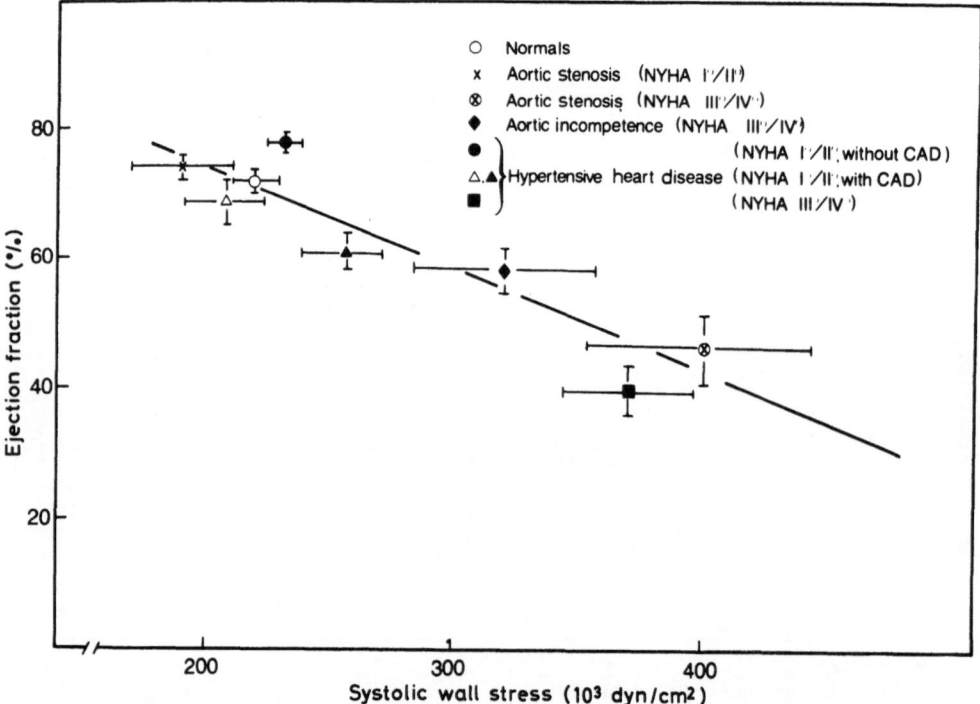

Fig. 4. Relationship between systolic wall stress (left ventricular overload) and the ejection fraction (n = 139). *CAD*, coronary artery disease; *NYHA I°* etc., (New York Heart Association, clinical degree I)

the left ventricular wall. It may therefore be concluded that heart size, i.e. end-diastolic volume, and systolic wall stress are primary determinants of ventricular performance [22–24].

The practical diagnostic consequences of the relationships imply that both heart and left ventricular size, as estimated from chest x-rays or from two-dimensional echocardiography, belong to the most practicable and relevant diagnostic parameters in the non-invasive assessment of ventricular function. If necessary, the ventricular after-load, that is systolic wall stress, can be derived from these non-invasive procedures by simultaneous determinations of pressure and ventricular geometry.

The therapeutic results which can be obtained by means of these diagnostic procedures therefore involve use of the whole spectrum of pharmacological and other therapeutic resources in order to reduce heart size and left ventricular size, thereby reducing systolic wall stress and improving left ventricular function.

Myocardial Oxygen Consumption in Chronic Heart Disease

Myocardial oxygen consumption (MVO_2) per unit weight is quite different in clinical heart disease (Fig. 5) [2, 23]. It is lowest in normotensive patients with coronary artery disease; it is normal in concentric and clinically compensated LV hypertrophy, even with extreme pressure load; and it is increased in dilated hearts with aortic valve disease.

There was no correlation between the oxygen consumption and ventricular function parameters, such as cardiac index, isovolumic contractility indices, and ejection phase parameters.

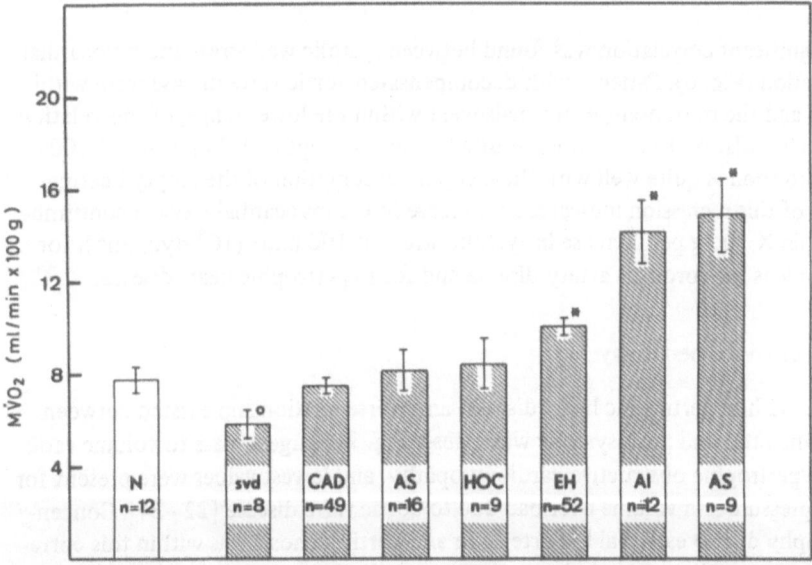

Fig. 5. Myocardial oxygen consumption ($M\dot{V}O_2$) in various hypertrophic and dilatative heart diseases. *N*, normals; *svd*, (= small vessel disease); *CAD*, coronary artery disease; *AS*, aortic stenosis (NYHA I°/ II°); *HOC*, hypertrophic obstructive cardiomyopathy; *EH*, essential hypertension; *AI*, aortic incompetence; AS* (NYHA III°/IV°); o indicates p 0.001 and * indicates p 0.01

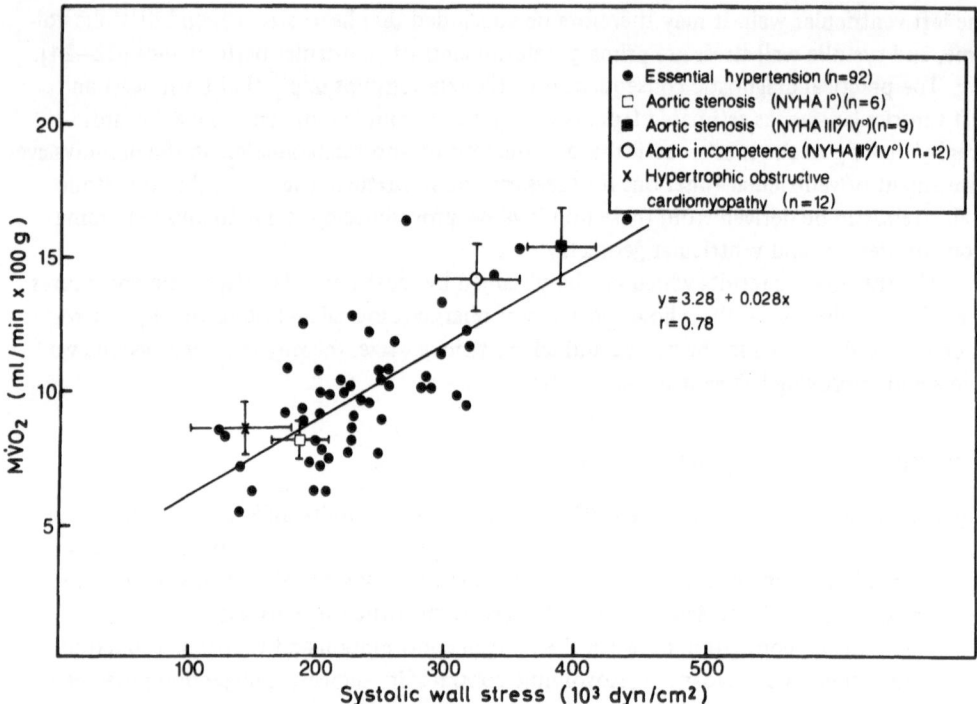

Fig. 6. Relationship between systolic wall stress per unit area and myocardial oxygen consumption ($M\dot{V}O_2$) per unit weight (n = 131). *NYHA I°* etc.

However, significant correlation was found between systolic wall stress and myocardial oxygen consumption (Fig. 6). Patients with decompensated aortic valve disease were within the upper range, and the normotensive normals were within the lower range, of this relationship [22–24]. Extrapolation to zero stress resulted in an intercept of 1.29 ml/min $\times$ 100 g, a value which corresponds quite well with the oxygen consumption of the empty beating heart. Steepness of this regression indicates an increase in the myocardial oxygen consumption by 3.4 ml/min $\times$ 100 g per increase in systolic stress of 100 units (10^3 dyn/cm^2), for the normals as well as for coronary artery disease and for hypertrophic heart disease.

Appropriateness of LV Hypertrophy

In patient groups with hypertrophic heart disease, an inverse relationship existed between the mass to volume ratio and peak systolic wall stress (Fig. 7). Largest mass to volume ratio was found for hypertrophic obstructive cardiomyopathy, and lowest values were present for decompensated pressure and volume overload due to aortic valve disease [22–24]. Concentric LV hypertrophy due to essential hypertension and aortic stenosis was within this correlation, whereas normotensives were shifted to lower systolic stress at equal mass to volume ratio, that is to a lower isobaric relationship.

With regard to this characteristic, at least three types of LV hypertrophy may be distinguished (Fig. 8) [22–24]:

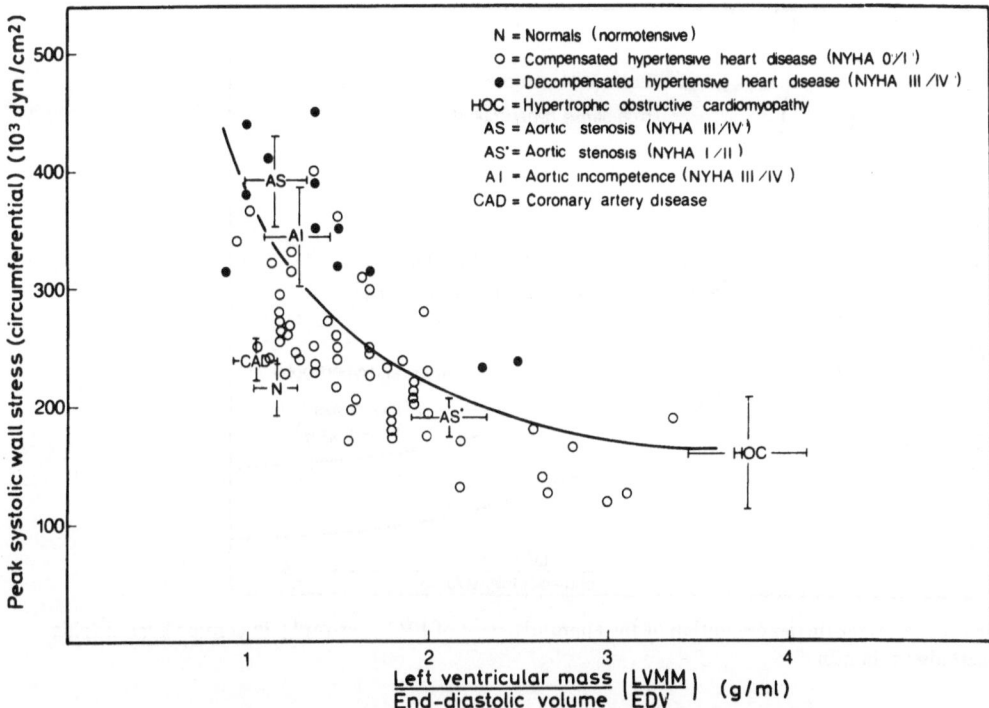

Fig. 7. Relation between left ventricular mass to volume ratio (LVMM/EDV) and peak systolic wall stress. A decrease in wall stress with an increase in mass to volume ratio is demonstrated. *The curve* (= isobar for all patients with essential hypertension) was calculated by polynome fitting ($Y = 31.2 + 371.2 \times 1/X$, where Y = wall stress, X = mass to volume ratio). Normotensive normal subjects (N) and normotensive subjects with coronary artery disease have shifts to lower wall stress at comparable mass to volume ratio (= lower isobar). The appropriateness of left ventricular hypertrophy in essential hypertension may be derived from the course of this curve: at a normal mass to volume ratio, an increased wall stress is present for decompensated hypertensive disease (NYHA class III or IV) (high stress hypertrophy), whereas an appropriate increase in mass to volume ratio despite an enhanced systolic pressure load may maintain normal systolic wall stress (normal stress hypertrophy). In contrast, excess augmentation of left ventricular mass out of proportion to volume may lead to a decrease in systolic wall stress (low stress hypertrophy). [3] Hypertrophic heart disease (AS, AI, HOC) may be situated within the isobaric characteristics of hypertensive heart disease, if systolic pressure is increased at comparable mass to volume ratio. [4] Left ventricular hypertrophy due to aortic stenosis may have increased wall stress (AS; NYHA class III or IV) (high stress hypertrophy) or normal wall stress (AS^x, NYHA class I or II) (normal stress hypertrophy), and wall stress may be even reduced, despite increased intraventricular systolic pressure load in hypertrophic obstructive cardiomyopathy (low stress hypertrophy). NYHA = New York Heart Association

1. Appropriate hypertrophy which keeps systolic wall stress normal even at extreme pressure load, as a result of an appropriate increase in the mass to volume ratio parallel to pressure load

2. Inappropriate, i.e. low-stress hypertrophy, which is associated with marked increase in LV mass out of proportion to intraventricular volume

3. Inappropriate, i.e. high-stress hypertrophy, which is characterized by excess dilatation out of proportion to ventricular mass development.

Thus at least two forms of inappropriate hypertrophy may occur in chronic hypertrophic heart disease.

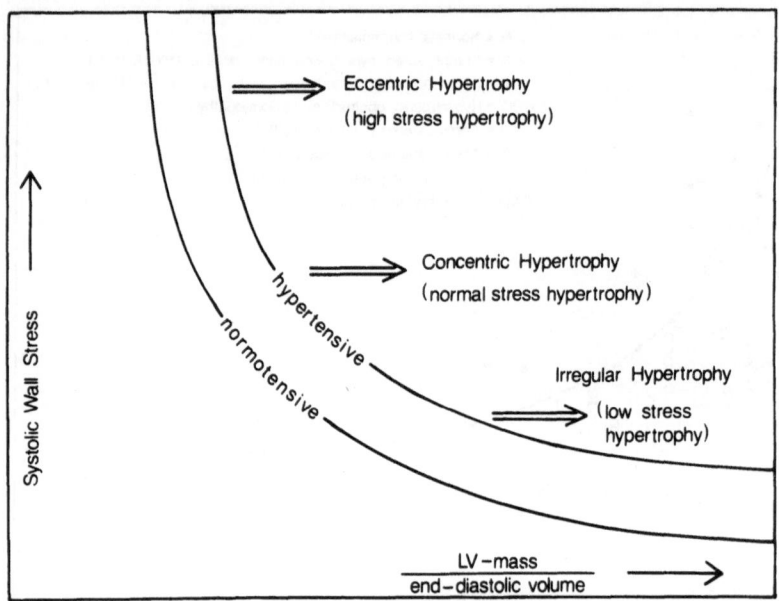

Fig. 8. Diagrammatic representation of the appropriateness of LV hypertrophy in chronic hypertrophic heart disease in man

From the metabolic point of view, high-stress hypertrophy has increased oxygen consumption per mass unit, with an impairment of LV function. In contrast, low-stress hypertrophy may have normal or even decreased oxygen consumption per LV mass unit at normal LV function. This may help to explain, for example, the existence of normal, decreased, or increased oxygen consumption per LV mass unit in chronic pressure or volume overload: despite large pressure load, the oxygen consumption may be normal or even decreased in aortic stenosis as long as heart size and systolic wall stress are normal or decreased respectively. On the other hand, the same pressure load may have high oxygen consumption, when LV dilatation occurs and when systolic wall stress increases [22–24].

Cardiac Consequences of Hypertensive Emergencies

An increase (hypertensive crisis) or decrease (antihypertensive treatment) in systolic pressure is associated with alterations in systolic wall stress, and hence in $M\dot{V}O_2$. However, pressure-induced stress alterations depend on the individual isobaric conditions, as well as on the initial mass to volume ratio (Fig. 9). An equal rise in pressure (for example, from 120 to 200 mmHg) (A' → B', Fig. 9) at a mass to volume ratio of 4 g/ml leads to a stress increase of only 80×10^3 dyn/cm^2, whereas the same rise in pressure (A → B) at a mass to volume ratio of 1.2 g/ml is followed by a considerable increase in stress of 180×10^3 dyn/cm^2. The same calculations and consequences as to systolic stress, and hence $M\dot{V}O_2$, are valid for therapeutically induced pressure reductions. This means that, from a diagnostic and prognostic point of view, a rise in systolic pressure in a dilated hypertensive heart causes a greater increase in peak systolic wall stress and in $M\dot{V}O_2$ than the same pressure increase in a non-dilated hypertensive heart. Because both stress and metabolic reserve are limited in man, the left ventricu-

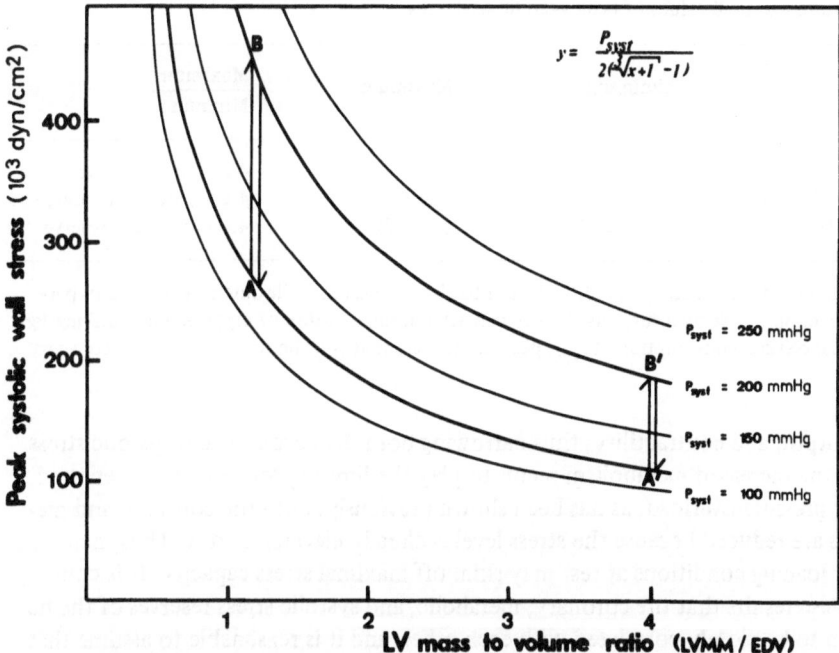

$$y = \frac{P_{syst}}{2(\sqrt[n]{x+1}-1)}$$

$P_{syst} = 250$ mmHg

$P_{syst} = 200$ mmHg

$P_{syst} = 150$ mmHg

$P_{syst} = 100$ mmHg

Fig. 9. Relation between left ventricular mass to volume ratio and systolic wall stress at different isobaric conditions; for further explanation with regard to hypertensive crisis see text

lar stress capacity is increasingly reduced with: (a) an increase in initial systolic stress, (b) a decrease in mass to volume ratio, and (c) an increase in systolic pressure. However, a therapeutic reduction in systolic pressure will lead to greater reduction in both stress and oxygen consumption in patients with left ventricular dilatation than in patients with concentric hypertrophy (Fig. 9). Thus the relation between mass to volume ratio and peak systolic wall stress elucidates the importance of pressure-dependent changes in systolic stress, and hence in myocardial stress and metabolic reserve [22–24].

Cardiac Reserve Capacities

A close relationship seems to exist between the coronary, metabolic, and systolic stress reserves of the left ventricle (Table 3) [23]. This obviously helps to explain the limited left ventricular function, or reserve capacity, or both in disorders associated with coronary (for example, in coronary artery disease), metabolic (for example, in hyperthyroidism), and systolic wall stress abnormalities (for example, in decompensated left ventricular pressure overload). Because the human heart works almost exclusively aerobically, an increase in left ventricular function may be accomplished, preferably by an increase in myocardial oxygen supply. In coronary artery disease, the coronary reserve is limited because of coronary stenosis. Accordingly, the coronary factor is the limiting link that diminishes the oxygen availability to the myocardium, thereby restricting both the metabolic and systolic stress reserves. In hyperthyroid heart disease an increased $M\dot{V}O_2$ occurs, due to excess increase in heart

Table 3. Minimal and maximal values of peak systolic wall stress

	Minimum	Maximum	Maximum / Minimum
T_{syst} (10^3 dyn/cm^2)[a]	100 ± 12	450 ± 46	4.5 = stress reserve
MVO_2 (ml/min × 100 g)[b]	5.2 ± 0.3	24 ± 2.9	4.6 = metabolic reserve
V_{cor} (ml/min × 100 g)[c]	79 ± 12	392 ± 26	4.9 = coronary reserve

All values (maximal versus minimal) $p < 0.001$. [a] Essential hypertension. [b] Chronic valvular and hypertensive pressure overload. [c] Normal subjects (before and after administration of dipyridamole, 0.5 mg/kg). MVO_2, myocardial oxygen consumption; T_{syst}, peak circumferential systolic wall stress; V_{cor}, coronary blood flow

rate, cardiac output, and contractility, thus narrowing both the coronary and systolic stress reserves. Here, the increased metabolism seems to play the limiting role. In decompensated left ventricular pressure overload, as has been shown previously, both the coronary and metabolic reserves are reduced because the stress level is already elevated at rest. Thus increased left ventricular loading conditions at rest may skim off maximal stress capacity. It is concluded from these results that the coronary, metabolic, and systolic stress reserves of the human heart seem to be closely correlated with each other, and it is reasonable to assume that determination of coronary reserve gives important insight into the left ventricular metabolic and working capacity reserves [23].

Coronary Haemodynamics in Hypertrophic Heart Disease

In the course of diagnostic coronary blood flow measurements, (a) coronary flow, (b) coronary resistance, and (c) coronary reserve (= ratio of coronary resistance at control conditions and under maximum coronary vasodilatation, as achieved by dipyridamole 0.5 mg/kg i.v.) [1, 27] were analysed in a total of 351 patients. Coronary reserve averaged 4.9 in the normals and was significantly reduced in patients with essential hypertension (Table 4). In the hypertensives with concomitant coronary artery disease, the coronary reserve was quantitatively similar to the coronary reserve of patients with normotensive coronary artery disease [20, 22]. However, even in young hypertrophied hypertensives without coronary atery disease, significant reduction in the coronary reserve was found, some 34% less than that in normal controls. This may be interpreted as implying an increased coronary and ischaemic

Table 4. Coronary hemodynamics: P_{cor}: coronary perfusion pressure; $avDO_2$: arteriocoronary venous oxygen difference; V_{cor}: coronary blood flow of the left ventricle; R_{cor}: coronary resistance; EH: essential hypertension; CAD: coronary artery disease

	P_{cor} (mmHg)	$avDO_2$ (vol%)	V_{cor} (ml/min · 100 g)	R_{cor} (mmHg · min · 100 g · ml^{-1})	Coronary reserve
Normal subjects (no. = 12)	82 ± 2	12.2 ± 0.1	71 ± 3	1.15 ± 0.04	4.9 ± 0.25
EH (no. = 63)	129 ± 8[†]	12.9 ± 0.2	83 ± 2[‡]	1.57 ± 0.06[†]	3.25 ± 0.3
CAD (no. = 38)	87 ± 5	12.8 ± 0.6	64 ± 3[§]	1.36 ± 0.09	1.78 ± 0.08

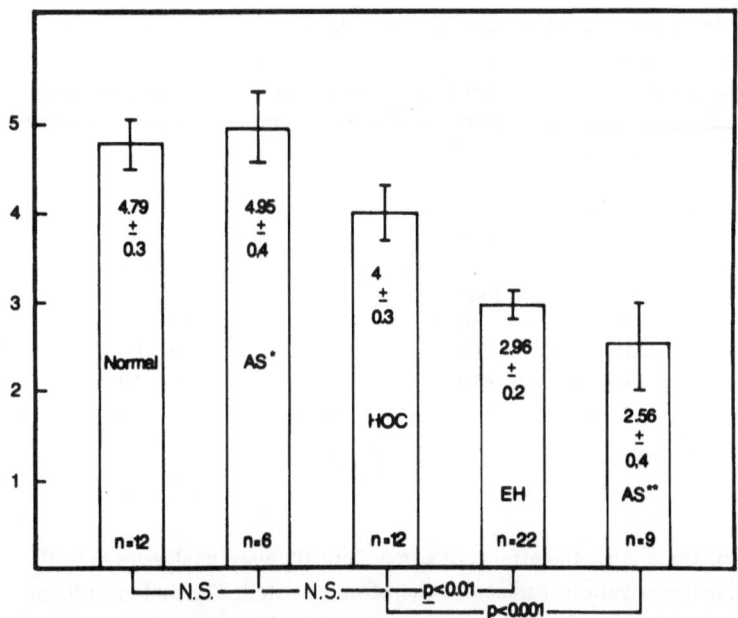

Fig. 10. Coronary reserves in normals (n = 12), in clinically compensated aortic stenosis (AS^X), in hypertrophic obstructive cardiomyopathy (HOC), in hypertensive hypertrophy at normal coronary arteriogram (EH) and in decompensated aortic stenosis (AS^{XX}). Note the significant reduction in coronary reserve in hypertensive hypertrophy (at normal myocardial oxygen consumption) when compared with non-hypertensive hypertrophy (AOC, AS^X). In decompensated aortic stenosis (AS^{XX}) with considerably increased oxygen consumption the coronary reserve is metabolically reduced

risk in patients with hypertensive LV hypertrophy, even without coronary artery stenosis. Thus one of the first vascular changes in essential hypertension seems to influence the coronary circulation.

This hypertensive-related reduction in coronary reserve seems not to be hypertrophy-dependent, but to be specific for hypertensive hypertrophy, since, except for decompensating aortic stenosis, normal coronary reserve is found in significant myocardial hypertrophy due to clinically compensated aortic stenosis and to hypertrophic obstructive or non-obstructive cardiomyopathy (Fig. 10) [10, 11]. Thus the vascular lesions as induced by high blood-pressure disease in the coronary vascular bed may considerably reduce coronary reserve on the arteriolar and capillary level, whereas hypertrophy itself may be without limiting significance with regard to oxygen supply to the myocardium.

Pharmacotherapeutic Interventions

Analgesics

Analgesics are often and necessarily used in intensive care medicine, for example in the postoperative period, in acute myocardial infarction, and in pericarditis, myocarditis, and other diseases. The therapeutic aim is the amelioration of pain without myocardial depression in these cardiac patients. Clinical observations have shown that decrease in left ventricular function may sometimes be present following the administration of different analgesics [13].

Table 5. Equianalgesic potency related to 50% depression of contractility[a]

	Equianalgesic doses		Bath concentrations that produced 50% depression of contractility [μg/ml]	Relative contractile depressant potency
	mg	potency		
Morphine	10	1	2000	1
Fentanyl	0.1– 0.2	50 –100	50–100	2– 4
Piritramide	5 –10	1 – 2	1000	1– 2
Pentazocine	30	0.3	50	60
Meperidine	70	0.1– 0.2	100	100–200
Tilidine	100	0.1– 0.4	400	10– 50

[a] Related to 50% reduction of dl/dt_{max}

A systematic survey of the contractile effects of some clinically used analgesics in both experimental and clinical catheterization studies was therefore initiated. The main results of these experimental studies show that there is, in clinically comparable dose-ranges, no difference in contractile depressant potency of morphine, fentanyl, and piritramide, whereas significant contractile depression is present for meperidine, that is for pethidine (or dolantin) (Table 5) [15, 17]. Thus myocardial and contractile depression would not be expected following the administration of large doses of morphine, fentanyl, or piritramide. In contrast, meperidine should be regarded with caution for use in cardiac patients because of its strong contractile depressant effects [15, 17].

Similar results were found for clinical studies with meperidine in chronic valvular and coronary disease, where marked depression of cardiac output, stroke volume, and of the maximum rate of left ventricular pressure development occurred (Fig. 11) [16]. In contrast to meperidine or pethidine, however, tilidine (Fig. 12), morphine, and fentanyl exhibited no contractile depressant effects using therapeutic and equi-analgesic doses in man. Thus differentiated therapy with equi-analgesic doses of cardioneutral analgesics in possible, and may be important for analgesic treatment of the altered myocardial function in the cardiac patient.

Digitalis Glycosides

Digitalis glycosides are, except for anti-arrhythmic management of atrial flutter, clinically used in order to support or improve the impaired function of the failing heart. This seems to be an empirically valid indication. However, digitalis glycosides are also often given, without a real, rational indication, as prophylactic treatment in patients without cardiac failure, e.g. in patients with arterial hypertension and coronary artery disease. To examine this problem the effects of intravenous digoxin (0.01 mg/kg body wt) were studied in clinically compensated, *concentrically hypertrophied* hypertensives with normal coronary arteriogram with regard to ventricular function and coronary haemodynamics.

Before digoxin, ventricular function, as evidenced by contraction velocity, pressure-related, and ejection phase indexes, was quite normal (Table 6) [22]. Fifty minutes following digoxin a marked increase in the maximum rate of pressure development (by 19.4%) occur-

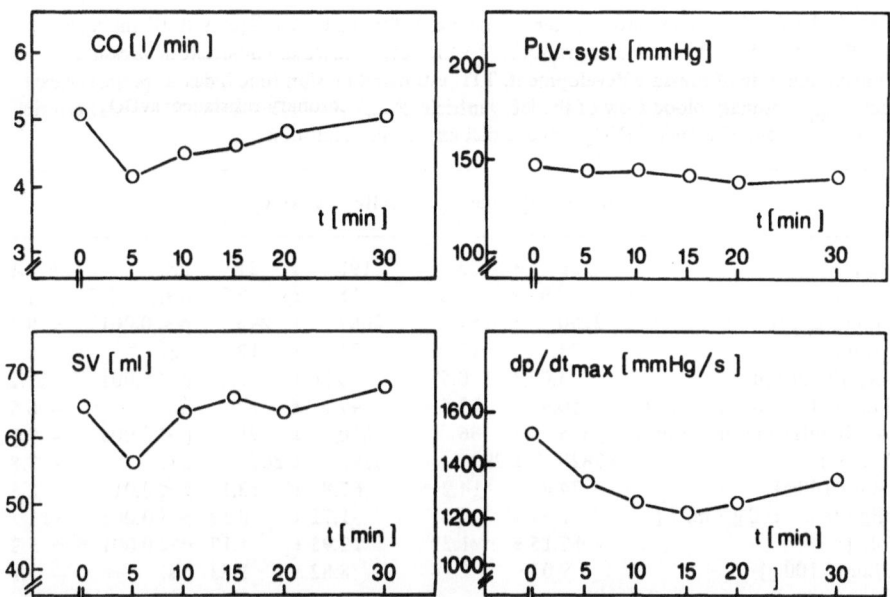

Fig. 11. Effects of meperidine (pethidine) (1 mg/kg i.v. 5 min) in man (n = 7). Points represent mean values of all measurements. Note the considerable (and statistically significant) myocardial depression following meperidine. *CO*, cardiac output; P_{LV}, systolic pressure in the left ventricle; *SV*, stroke volume; dp/dt_{max}, maximum rate of pressure generation in the left ventricle

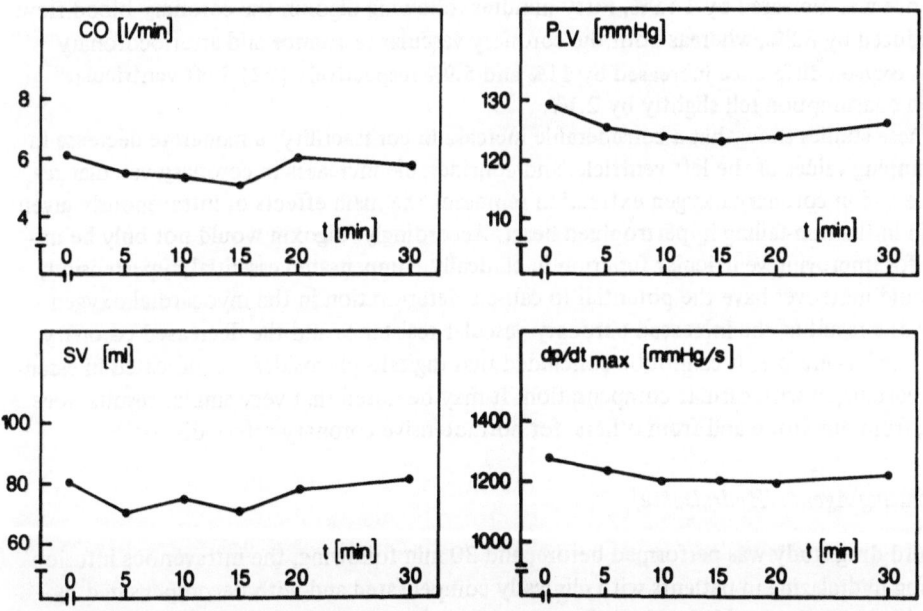

Fig. 12. Effects of tilidine (1.5 mg/kg i.v. 5 min) on ventricular function in man (n = 10). Note that at equi-analgesic doses there are no contractile depressant effects in comparison with meperidine. *CO*, cardiac output, P_{LV}, systolic pressure in the left ventricle; *SV*, stroke volume; dp/dt_{max}, maximum rate of pressure generation in the left ventricle

Table 6. Ventricular dynamics and coronary hemodynamics before and after digoxin (0.01 mg/kg body weight, i.v.). PLV: systolic left ventricular pressure; PLVED: left ventricular end-diastolic pressure; dp/dt_{max}: maximum rate of pressure development. TTI: estimated tension time index as pressure-heart rate product; V_{cor}: coronary blood flow of the left ventricle; R_{cor}: coronary resistance; $avDO_2$: arterio-coronary venous oxygen difference; MVO_2: myocardial oxygen consumption

	Before digoxine		After digoxine		P	%
P_{LV} [mmHg]	196	± 23	198	± 21	n.s.	+ 1.1
P_{LVED} [mmHg]	15.9	± 3.8	15.7	± 3.1	n.s.	− 1.2
dp/dt_{max} [mmHg/sec]	2250	± 287	2687	± 243	p < 0.001	+19.4
Heart rate [l/min]	74	± 13	71	± 12	n.s.	− 5.2
Cardiac index [l/min · m²]	3.67	± 0.57	3.26	± 0.58	p < 0.001	−11.2
Stroke volume index [ml/beat · m²]	50.9	± 12.5	47.6	± 12	n.s.	− 6.5
Cardiac work [mmHg · ml/min · m²]	675	± 86	610	± 91	p < 0.005	− 9.7
~TTI (~P_{syst} · n)	13828	± 2927	13296	± 2652	n.s.	− 3.8
V_{cor} [ml/min · 100 g]	74.4	± 14.2	67.8	± 13.1	p < 0.01	− 8.8
R_{cor} [mmHg · min · 100 g · ml⁻¹]	1.54	± 0.21	1.71	± 0.19	p < 0.001	+11
$avDO_2$ [Vol%]	12.15	± 1.29	12.95	± 1.17	p < 0.001	+ 5.9
MVO_2 [ml/min · 100 g]	9.03	± 2.14	8.82	± 1.83	n.s.	− 2.1

red. However, the cardiac index fell by 11.2%, and — resulting from the changes in the mean systolic pressure and cardiac index — the external cardiac work decreased by 9.7%. Heart rate and stroke index were reduced by 5.2% and 6.5% respectively (Table 6). Corresponding to the arterial pressure elevation and the reduction in the cardiac index, the total peripheral resistance was increased by 14.9%. Fifty minutes following digoxin the coronary blood flow was reduced by 8.8%, whereas both the coronary vascular resistance and arteriocoronary venous oxygen difference increased by 11% and 5.9% respectively [22]. Left ventricular oxygen consumption fell slightly by 2.1%.

These studies show that a considerable increase in contractility, a moderate decrease in the pumping values of the left ventricle, and considerable increases in coronary vascular resistance and in coronary oxygen extraction represent the main effects of intravenously given digoxin in the non-failing hypertrophied heart. Accordingly, digoxin would not only be unsuited for improving ventricular function in clinically compensated essential hypertension, but would moreover have the potential to cause a deterioration in the myocardial oxygen supply as a result of the increased coronary vascular resistance and the decreased coronary blood flow. Therefore, it cannot be concluded that digitalis glycosides are indicated in essential hypertension with cardiac compensation. It may be noted that very similar results were found, from our group and from others, for normotensive coronary artery disease.

Vasodilating Agents (Hydralazine)

The third drug study was performed before, and 30 min following, the intravenous infusion of 20 mg hydralazine in patients with clinically compensated and with decompensated hypertensive heart disease. Under the influence of hydralazine, the left ventricular systolic pressure decreased by 16%, and left ventricular end-diastolic pressure decreased by 21% (Table 7) [22]. There were no significant changes in heart rate, nor in the maximum left ventricular pressure development. Cardiac index and stroke volume index were enhanced by

Table 7. Left ventricular dynamics and coronary hemodynamics before and after hydralazine (20 mg i.v.). Abbreviations see Table 6

	Before hydralazine	After hydralazine	P	%
P_{LV} [mmHg]	167.2 ± 8.43	140.24 ± 16.40	<0.001	−16.12
P_{LVED} [mmHg]	15.42 ± 3.45	1.25 ± 4.12	<0.01	−27.04
dp/dt_{max} [mmHg/sec]	1836.33 ± 513.51	1988.66 ± 823.42	n.s.	+ 8.30
Heart rate [l/min]	75.0 ± 16.0	80.0 ± 16.0	n.s.	+ 6.8
Cardiac index [l/min · m²]	2.61 ± 0.38	3.25 ± 0.43	<0.001	+24.24
Stroke volume index [ml/beat · m²]	37.02 ± 9.76	43.83 ± 10.24	<0.005	+18.40
Cardiac work [mmHg · ml/min · m²]	447.55 ± 58.73	480.64 ± 70.51	n.s.	+ 7.39
~TTI (P_{syst} · HR)	1088.18 ± 243.68	920.18 ± 138.64	<0.01	−15.44
V_{cor} [ml/min · 100 g]	59.42 ± 12.84	83.86 ± 33.09	<0.02	+41.13
R_{cor} [mmHg · min · 100 g · ml⁻¹]	1.71 ± 0.57	1.09 ± 0.40	<0.01	−36.14
avDO₂ [Vol%]	13.47 ± 1.80	10.97 ± 1.63	<0.001	−18.58
MVO_2 [ml/min · 100 g]	8.47 ± 2.34	9.10 ± 3.12	n.s.	+ 7.51

x ± SD, n = 10

24% and 18% respectively, whereas external cardiac work remained nearly unaltered as a consequence of reduction of systolic blood-pressure and increase in cardiac output. The product of mean systolic pressure and heart rate significantly decreased by 15%.

Coronary blood flow was considerably enhanced by 41% (from 59 to 83 ml/min × 100 g) (Table 7) [22]. The coronary vascular resistance decreased by 36% (from 1.71 to 1.09 units), and the arteriocoronary venous oxygen difference was markedly reduced. Myocardial oxygen consumption of the left ventricle was almost unchanged. All these haemodynamic changes were still more pronounced in the failing heart.

The results demonstrate that hydralazine leads to: (a) effective ventricular unloading, as evidenced by reduction in both end-diastolic and systolic left ventricular pressure; (b) considerable augmentation of left ventricular ejection pump function; and (c) marked increase in coronary blood flow without significantly changing myocardial oxygen consumption. With regard to these results, vasodilating drugs of the hydralazine type can be considered of high therapeutic value in heart failure, if preservation and/or improvement of ventricular function without alterations in myocardial energy demand are desired.

Summary

Some recent advances in cardiovascular pathophysiology are described on the basis of cardiac catheterization studies in more than 900 patients with hypertensive, coronary congestive, valvular, and myocardial disease.

1. Chronic pressure overload has smaller (mean) ventricular size than chronic volume overload. Left ventricular function is inversely related to both left ventricular volume (size) and systolic wall stress.

2. Systolic wall stress represents the main determinant of the ventricular after-load. Systolic wall stress is directly correlated with myocardial oxygen consumption.

3. Systolic wall stress is an important result of the appropriateness and degree of cardiac hy-

pertrophy. In the course of chronic heart disease, at least two types of inappropriate hypertrophy may occur (low-stress hypertrophy and high-stress hypertrophy).
4. Morphine, fentanyl, and piritramide have no direct myocardial depressant potency. In
contrast, meperidine (pethidine) has strong negatively inotropic effects and should be can-
tiously used in patients with heart disease.
5. In the non-failing heart, intravenous digoxin may depress both cardiac ejection function
and coronary blood flow (reduced oxygen availability?). The use of digoxin should be recommended with reservation in these patients.
6. Hydralazine produces marked improvement of ventricular function and of oxygen availability to the myocardium of the failing and of the non-failing heart. The only minor increase
in myocardial energy demand may be due to the effective systolic unloading (wall stress reduction, decrease in outflow impedance) which counterbalances the energy costs associated
with increased cardiac function.

The results are discussed with special reference to clinical considerations relevant to the
cardiac patient in anaesthesia.

References

1. Braunwald E, Ross J, Sonnenblick EH (1968) Mechanisms of contraction of the normal and failing
   heart. Little, Brown & Co, Boston
2. Braunwald E (1971) Control of myocardial oxygen consumption. Physiological and clinical considerations. Am J Cardiol 27:416–432
3. Bretschneider HJ (1967) Aktuelle Probleme der Koronardurchblutung und des Myokardstoffwech-
   sels, vol 15. Stuttgart, Regensburg Ärztl Fortbild, pp 1–27
4. Bürger SB, Strauer BE (1977) Dynamics of left ventricular hypertrophy and contraction in spontaneously hypertensive rats (Abstr). Circulation [Suppl III] 56:III–234
5. Bürger SB, Strauer BE (1978) Left ventricular geometry and wall stress in various stages of hypertrophy due to spontaneous essential hypertension (Abstr). Circulation [Suppl II] 57, 58:II–158
6. Gaasch WH, Battle WE, Oboler HH, Banas JS, Levine HJ (1972) Left ventricular stress and compliance in man. Circulation 45:746–762
7. Greene DG, Carlisle R, Grant C, Bunnell I (1967) Estimation of left ventricular volume by one-
   plane cineangiography. Circulation 35:61–69
8. Hood WP (1971) Dynamics of hypertrophy in left ventricular wall of man. In: Alpert NR (ed)
   Cardiac hypertrophy. Academic Press, New York, pp 445–452
9. Hugenholtz PG, Kaplan E, Hull E (1969) Determination of left ventricular wall thickness by an-
   giocardiography. Am Heart J 78:513–522
10. Kochsiek K, Heiss HW, Tauchert M, Strauer BE (1971) Koronarreserve und Sauerstoffverbrauch
    bei hypertrophischer obstruktiver Cardiomyopathie. Verh Dtsch Ges Inn Med 27:880–883
11. Kochsiek K, Tauchert M, Cott L, Neubaur J (1970) Die Koronarreserve bei Patienten mit Aorten-
    vitien. Verh Dtsch Ges Inn Med 76:214–218
12. Linzbach HJ (1960) The heart failure from the point of view of quantitative anatomy. Am J Cardiol
    5:370
13. Lowenstein E, Hallowell P, Levine FH, et al. (1969) Cardiovascular response to large doses of intra-
    venous morphine in man. New Engl J Med 281:1389
14. Sandler E, Dodge HT (1963) Left ventricular tension and stress in man. Circ Res 13:91–104
15. Strauer BE (1972) Contractile responses to morphine, piritramide, pethidine and fentanyl: A com-
    parative study on the isolated ventricular myocardium. Anesthesiology 37:304
16. Strauer BE (1973) Die Wirkung von Pethidin auf Herzmechanik und Kontraktilität des menschli-
    chen Herzens. Klin Wochenschr 51:1105
17. Strauer BE (1975) Dynamik, Koronardurchblutung und Sauerstoffverbrauch des normalen und
    kranken Herzens. Karger, Basel

18. Strauer BE, Scherpe A (1975) Myocardial mechanics and oxygen consumption in experimental hyperthyroidism. In: Roy PE, Harris P (eds) The cardiac sarcoplasm. University Park Press, Baltimore, pp 495–502

19. Strauer BE, Scherpe A (1975) Experimental hyperthyroidism IV. Myocardial muscle mechanics and oxygen consumption in eu- and hyperthyroidism. Basic Res Cardiol 70:246–255

20. Strauer BE (1977) Die quantitative Bestimmung der Koronarreserve in der Diagnostik koronarer Durchblutungsstörungen. Internist (Berlin) 18:579

21. Strauer BE, Beer K, Heitlinger K, Höfling B (1977) Left ventricular systolic wall stress as a primary determinant of myocardial oxygen consumption: comparative studies in patients with normal left ventricular function, with pressure and volume overload and with coronary heart disease. Basic Res Cardiol 72:306–313

22. Strauer BE (1980) Hypertensive heart disease. Springer, Berlin Heidelberg New York

23. Strauer BE (1979) Myocardial oxygen consumption in chronic heart disease: Role of wall stress, hypertrophy and coronary reserve. Am J Cardiol 44:731

24. Strauer BE (1979) Ventricular function and coronary hemodynamics in hypertensive heart disease. Am J Cardiol 44:999

25. Strauer BE (1976) Änderungen der Kontraktilität bei Druck- und Volumenbelastungen des Herzens. Vortr Dtsch Ges Kreislaufforsch

26. Strauer BE (ed) (1981) The heart in hypertension. International Boehringer Mannheim Symposium Springer, Berlin Heidelberg New York

27. Tauchert M (1973) Koronarreserve und maximaler Sauerstoffverbrauch des menschlichen Herzens. Basic Res Cardiol 68:1–83

Anaesthesia in Coronary Heart Disease

G. Smith

Ischaemic heart disease is a major cause of morbidity and mortality in the population of western Europe and North America. Its prevalence is illustrated by the fact that over 40% of adult males in the age-range 45—55 die as a consequence of the disease. Furthermore, the problem of dealing with this condition is rendered more difficult by the fact that only one in ten patients with ischaemic heart disease may exhibit symptoms. As surgery is being performed on an increasingly ageing population, and the incidence of the disease is high among the elderly, anaesthetists are encountering the condition with increasing frequency.

Several retrospective epidemiological studies from the United States have confirmed that patients with ischaemic heart disease present an increased risk of developing peri-operative myocardial infarction. In summary, in the population over the age of 30 years, the overall peri-operative myocardial infarction rate is of the order of 0.13%, increasing in males over the age of 50 years to 0.6%. Where there has been one previous myocardial infarction prior to surgery, the risk of developing a subsequent peri-operative myocardial infarction increases to 6% of the overall population [1—4]. In addition, there is good evidence that the more recent the first myocardial infarction in respect of time of operation, the higher is the rate of further reinfarction after surgery. The risk of further reinfarction is greatest within a 6-month interval.

In a study by Goldman and his colleagues in 1978 [5], on patients over 40 years of age, the incidence of post-operative infarction was found to be 3% where there was no infarction prior to surgery. Where one infarction had occurred 2—5 years prior to surgery, the reinfarction rate increased to 4%. An infarction occurring 6 months to 2 years prior to surgery was associated with a peri-operative reinfarction rate of 8%, and where the infarction had occurred within 6 months of surgery, there was a dramatic increase in the reinfarction rate. In agreement with other studies, it was found that the overall mortality rate for the first infarction after surgery is approximately 19%, but this increased to over 50% for a reinfarction occurring after surgery.

By discriminant function analysis, various factors were determined which correlated with the development of post-operative cardiac complications. Each was assigned a score describing its relative importance, and the factors with the highest scores included:
1. Triple heart sounds or elevation of the jugular venous pressure
2. A myocardial infarction occurring within the previous 6 months
3. Abnormal rhythm
4. In excess of five ventricular extrasystoles occurring prior to surgery.

Factors to which a low score was ascribed included:
1. Age in excess of 70 years
2. Emergency surgery
3. Poor general medical condition
4. Intrathoracic or intra-abdominal procedures.

None of these clinical studies has selected any individual anaesthetic agent or technique as being particularly hazardous, and the overall conclusions that are to be drawn from all the epidemiological studies are that for elective surgery it is essential to treat cardiac failure and arrhythmias medically and postpone surgery for at least 6 months after a myocardial infarction.

Although it is conceivable that events occurring in the post-operative period, where there is less control than in the operative period, are more likely to be responsible for the development of post-operative myocardial infarction, it is important to consider what are the most appropriate anaesthetic techniques for the large population at risk with frank or silent ischaemic heart disease.

Events occurring during anaesthesia may induce ischaemia by upsetting the balance between oxygen supply and oxygen demand in the myocardium (Table 1). Oxygen supply to the myocardium is determined by coronary perfusion pressure and coronary vascular resistance, which is autoregulated by the level of myocardial metabolic activity. Oxygen content is determined by haemoglobin concentration, arterial PO_2, and haemoglobin saturation, and it is obviously essential to obtain an optimum haemoglobin and avoid hypoxaemia in patients with ischaemic heart disease.

The major determinants of oxygen demand are myocardial contractility and left ventricular wall tension [6]. Heart rate is probably the next most important factor, and external cardiac work the least important. Standard clinical teaching in managing patients with ischaemic heart disease maintains the necessity of avoiding increases in oxygen demand by preventing excessive sympatho-adrenal activity (by sedating a patient well pre-operatively), avoiding tachycardia and hypertension induced by light anaesthesia and pain, and avoiding cardiac overfilling as might occur with over-enthusiastic intravenous infusions or in patients with cardiac failure.

Coronary perfusion is determined by the coronary perfusion pressure and coronary vascular resistance. Coronary vascular resistance is dependent not only on the intrinsic tone of the small coronary vessels, but also upon the extent of compression produced by contraction of the ventricular muscle during systole. The extent of this compression is determined by left ventricular wall tension, left ventricular end-diastolic pressure, and heart rate. Thus the subendocardial circulation is at greater risk of developing ischaemia than is the epicardial circulation, and during the development of cardiac failure, endocardial ischaemia precedes de-

Table 1. Determinants of myocardial oxygen supply and demand

Oxygen supply	Oxygen demand
Coronary perfusion pressure	Myocardial contractility
Coronary vascular resistance	Left ventricular wall tension
Oxygen content: haemoglobin	Heart rate
PaO_2	External cardiac work (cardiac output × mean arterial
S_aO_2	pressure)

velopment of transmural ischaemia. Recently, the use of the radioisotope-labelled micro-sphere technique has enabled investigators to determine the distribution of blood flow be-tween the subendocardial and subepicardial circulations. Both thoracic epidural anaesthesia [7] and halothane anaesthesia [8] have been shown to improve the endocardial/epicardial distribution ratio.

In the last 10 years there have been a large number of investigations into the effects of anaesthetic drugs and techniques on coronary perfusion and myocardial oxygen consump-tion in experimental animals. Halothane has been subjected to the greatest number of inves-tigations in a variety of different experimental models, and it has been shown that although this drug produces profound reductions in coronary and myocardial blood flow, changes in oxygen extraction are minimal [9, 10, 11]. Studies of myocardial oxygen consumption of lactate have also indicated that halothane is not associated with any impairment of myocard-ial oxygenation in the normal myocardium [11, 12]. Recently it has been confirmed that halothane in end-tidal concentrations of 0.7% and 1.5% produced considerable reduction in myocardial oxygen consumption and myocardial blood flow in the human. However, oxygen extraction decreased significantly with the higher concentration of halothane, despite a re-duction in mean arterial pressure to a maximum of 60 mmHg [13].

Studies on other anaesthetic drugs, including enflurane [14], Althesin [15], thiopentone [16] and ketamine [17, 18], in experimental animals or the human, have shown also that although these drugs may produce profound changes in coronary blood flow and myocardial oxygen consumption, the oxygen supply/demand relationship is maintained. Thus the changes are produced secondarily to alteration in metabolic demand, and changes in oxygen extraction do not occur or are minimal. The exception to this statement appears to be the anaesthetic induction agent propanidid, which was found to produce a marked but ephem-eral coronary vasodilatation resulting in an appreciable transient reduction in coronary vascular resistance [35].

More recently, attention has turned to the effect of anaesthetic agents and techniques on the myocardial oxygen supply/demand relationship in animals with experimentally in-duced myocardial ischaemia. The author has been involved in several studies using the canine model described by Marshall and Parratt [19]. In this model, blood flow is measured in the left main coronary artery using an electromagnetic flowmeter, and oxygen consumption in normal myocardial tissue calculated from the product of this flow and (arterial minus coro-nary sinus) oxygen content. Changes in this normal area are compared with blood flow and oxygen consumption changes occurring in an ischaemic area of myocardium produced by one-stage ligation of the anterior descending branch of the left main coronary artery. In this area, blood flow is measured using a radioisotope clearance technique, and oxygen consump-tion calculated using blood samples drawn from a collateral vein.

With this model it has been demonstrated (unpublished studies) in a group of six dogs, that elevation of arterial PCO_2 from 37.6 to 68.4 mmHg was associated with an increase in mean arterial pressure from 88 to 104 mmHg, together with a significant increase in blood flow to normal myocardium and an increase in total cardiac output. However, blood flow in the ischaemic area decreased despite an increase in ischaemic oxygen consumption ("coro-nary steal"), and these changes were accompanied by a deterioration in the extent of ST de-pression on the ECG. Restoration of normocapnia was accompanied by improvement in blood flow to the ischaemic area and improvement in the ECG.

Similarly, the author has also demonstrated (unpublished studies) in a group of seven greyhounds that sodium nitroprusside also produced coronary steal from an ischaemic area.

The drug was infused as an 0.01% solution in a dose sufficient to cause a reduction in mean arterial pressure from 96 to 53 mmHg and a small, non-significant increase in heart rate from 139 to 148 beats/min. There was no change in cardiac output, mean coronary blood flow to the normal area of myocardium was unchanged, and the availability/consumption ratio in normal myocardium improved slightly but not to a significant extent. In the ischaemic area of myocardium, myocardial blood flow diminished from 44 to 23 ml/100 g/min, but oxygen consumption diminished by a corresponding amount and there was no significant change in the availability/consumption ratio. When, however, sodium nitroprusside was infused in a larger dose to cause a reduction in mean arterial pressure from 87 to 39 mmHg, although there was an increase in the availability/consumption ratio in the normal area of myocardium, there was a decrease in the ratio in the ischaemic area of myocardium. The change in the ratio between the two areas was significantly different, indicating a worsening of oxygenation in the ischaemic area in comparison with the normal area of myocardium.

These unpublished observations confirm previous studies by Chiarello and his colleagues [20], who noted that whilst nitroglycerin improved the extent of ST elevation in ten patients with an acute transmural anterior myocardial infarction, nitroprusside infused to produce similar haemodynamic changes as those following nitroglycerin caused an increase in the extent of ST segment elevation. These observations led to a formal study on 14 open-chested dogs, in which coronary artery occlusion was carried out and regional myocardial blood flow measured using a microsphere technique. Nitroprusside was found to increase the extent of ST elevation and reduce myocardial blood flow in the ischaemic area, whereas nitroglycerin reduced ST segment elevation and increased regional myocardial blood flow in the ischaemic area, and also increased the endocardial/epicardial ratio in the ischaemic area. These observations suggest that nitroglycerin may be preferable to sodium nitroprusside when reductions of pre-load and after-load are required during anaesthesia in patients with coronary artery disease.

Using the Marshall and Parratt model, Smith and colleagues have shown that halothane appears to have a beneficial effect on oxygen supply/demand relationships in acute experimental myocardial ischaemia [21]. Despite producing a 42% reduction in mean arterial pressure in a group of eight greyhound dogs, halothane 1% inspired produced a significant improvement in the ratio oxygen availability/oxygen consumption in the ischaemic in comparison with the normal area, and this was accompanied by a significant improvement in venous drainage PO_2 from the ischaemic collateral vein in comparison with coronary sinus blood. Although the mechanism of this effect was not open to investigation, suspicion rested heavily upon the 15% reduction in heart rate which occurred.

Two other recently published studies also suggest that halothane has a beneficial effect on oxygen supply/demand relationships in acute myocardial ischaemia in the dog. Bland and Lowenstein [22], by summating ST segment elevation, demonstrated that halothane 0.75% decreased the severity of myocardial ischaemia induced by constricting the left anterior descending coronary artery of the dog. More recently, Verrier and his colleagues [8] have shown that in the dog in which a coronary artery is gradually constricted, there is greater coronary vascular reserve under halothane than under nitrous oxide anaesthesia. Coronary vascular reserve is defined as the difference in blood flow between that in a stated situation and that which can be achieved by maximum vasodilatation using an infusion of carbochromen. It should be noted in particular that Verrier indicated in his recent article that if the heart was paced to produce an increase in heart rate in the halothane group to match that occurring in the nitrous oxide group, the advantage of halothane disappeared and coronary vascular reserve became identical for both halothane and nitrous oxide anaesthesia.

During maximum vasodilatation induced by carbochromen, there is a linear relationship between pressure and flow. Extrapolation of this line back to zero flow produces a pressure at which flow ceases. This zero flow pressure intercept (waterfall pressure) has been found to be considerably higher than right atrial pressure, left atrial pressure, or coronary sinus pressure [8, 23]. This waterfall pressure is highest in the subendocardium and least in the subpericardium, and is a reflection of the tissue pressure. Waterfall pressure was found to be lower during halothane than nitrous oxide anaesthesia [8]. The use of waterfall pressure rather than left or right atrial pressure in the calculation of vascular resistance may reconcile previous conflicting data in which halothane has been found to produce either small increases [9, 24] or decreases [25, 26] in coronary vascular resistance.

The beneficial effects produced by halothane anaesthesia may be accounted for by reductions in: (a) tension in the wall of the ventricle; (b) total amount of ventricular wall tension by diminution in heart rate; and (c) myocardial oxygen consumption by reduction in heart rate, myocardial contractility, and ventricular wall tension. It should be noted that an increase in left ventricular end-diastolic pressure or intraluminal pressure would diminish blood flow in the subendocardial plexus. In all three experimental studies already quoted [8, 21, 22], halothane did not produce an increase in left ventricular end-diastolic pressure, although during controlled human studies of the effect of halothane on coronary blood flow, 1.5% end-tidal halothane concentration was associated with a significant increase in left ventricular end-diastolic pressure [13].

Thus, there appears to be common agreement that in experimental myocardial ischaemia, halothane has a beneficial effect. The mechanism of this effect is probably dependent mainly on the reduction in heart rate, and there is no suggestion that halothane has any specific effects in improving myocardial ischaemia. Recently, in a prospective study of patients undergoing coronary artery bypass surgery, there was less intra-operative ischaemia in patients receiving halothane anaesthesia than in a group receiving morphine anaesthesia, as assessed by ECG monitoring [27]. This is consistent with the view that provided undue hypotension is avoided, halothane is an appropriate agent for patients with myocardial ischaemia.

Unfortunately, although these animal studies may enable us to understand the principles on which the haemodynamic state of patients should be maintained, they do not provide any additional guidance on the limits of change in systemic arterial pressure, heart rate, left ventricular end-diastolic pressure, or any other haemodynamic factor which can be tolerated by patients with ischaemic heart disease. For this one has to turn to clinical studies, but at the present time there is little useful information.

It is known that induction of anaesthesia may be beneficial in reducing the extent of ischaemia in patients with impending myocardial infarction [28]. It is also known that ischaemia develops commonly in patients with ischaemic heart disease undergoing anaesthesia, and that it occurs most frequently at endotracheal intubation with concomitant systemic arterial hypertension [29].

Because animal studies are unhelpful in attempting to define the levels of haemodynamic variables which should be maintained during anaesthesia, considerable attention has focused recently on attempting to define clinical predictors of myocardial ischaemia. Because the heart rate/systolic arterial pressure product (RPP) correlates during exercise with myocardial oxygen consumption in the conscious patient with angina [30], it has been recommended that the RPP should not be allowed to exceed 12 000 during anaesthesia [31]. Recently, however, it has been shown that during anaesthesia, the RPP is a poor correlate both of myocardial oxygen consumption in man [13] and of the development of myocardial ischaemia in clinical anaesthesia [32]. Among other studies which have demonstrated this is a recent one utilizing discriminant function analysis. In patients undergoing coronary artery bypass surgery under halothane anaesthesia, it was shown that pulmonary artery wedge pressure, central venous pressure (CVP), RPP, and arterial pressure singly were poor predictors of ischaemia. However, a combination of hypotension with raised central venous pressure (as may occur in cardiac failure), or a combination of hypotension with tachycardia, were good predictors of the development of ischaemia [32]. Similarly, Thomson and his colleagues demonstrated [33] in a similar group of patients that whilst RPP did not correlate with peri-operative ischaemia, there was a good correlation between diastolic pressure time index/ systolic pressure time index (DPTI/SPTI) and intra-operative ischaemia. In addition, lower values of this index pre-operatively correlated with those patients who demonstrated ischaemic changes peri-operatively. Unfortunately, because of the heterogeneity of ischaemic heart disease, it may be impossible to predict in advance the optimum values of haemodynamic variables for any individual patient. Assessment of the balance between myocardial oxygen supply and demand is the aim of the anaesthetist [34]. At the present time the only useful means of detecting an imbalance is by the use of the ECG, particularly the V5 configuration.

It is concluded that currently the best advice in managing patients with coronary artery disease is to:

(1) Maintain systemic arterial pressure at pre-operative angina-free levels

(2) Maintain the lowest heart rate compatible with maintenance of cardiac output

(3) Suppress any sympatho-adrenal activity which may be induced by pre-operative apprehension, pain, or unduly light levels of anaesthesia

(4) Maintain cardiac filling pressures in the same range as the pre-operative angina-free levels by careful monitoring of central venous pressures and, if available or indicated, pulmonary capillary wedge pressure.

References

1. Knapp RB, Topkins MJ, Artusio JF (1962) The cerebrovascular accident and coronary occlusion in anesthesia. JAMA 182:332
2. Topkins MJ, Artusio JF (1964) Myocardial infarction and surgery, a five year study. Anesth Analg (Cleve) 23:716
3. Steen PA, Tinker JH, Tarhan S (1978) Myocardial reinfarction after anesthesia and surgery. JAMA 239:2655
4. Tarhan S, Moffitt EA, Taylor WE et al. (1972) Myocardial infarction after general anesthesia. JAMA 220:1451
5. Goldman L, Caldera DL, Southwick FS, et al. (1978) Cardiac risk factors and complications in non-cardiac surgery. Medicine 57:357
6. Braunwald E (1971) Control of myocardial oxygen consumption: physiologic and clinical considerations. Am J Cardiol 27:416
7. Klassen GA, Bramwell RS, Bromage PR, et al. (1980): Effect of acute sympathectomy by epidural anesthesia on the canine coronary circulation. Anesthesiology 52:8
8. Verrier ED, Edelist G, Consigny PM, et al. (1980) Greater coronary vascular reserve in dogs anesthetized with halothane. Anesthesiology 53:445

9. Smith G, Vance JP, Brown DM, et al. (1974) Changes in canine myocardial blood flow and oxygen consumption in response to halothane. Br J Anaesth 46:821

10. Merin RG, Kumazawa T, Luka NL (1976) Myocardial function and metabolism in the conscious dog and during halothane anesthesia. Anesthesiology 44:402

11. Merin RG, Verdouw PD, de Jong JW (1977) Dose-dependent depression of cardiac function and metabolism by halothane in swine (*Sus scrofa*). Anesthesiology 46:417

12. Merin RG (1969) Myocardial metabolism in the halothane-depressed canine heart. Anesthesiology 31:20

13. Sonntag H, Merin RG, Donath U, et al. (1979) Myocardial metabolism and oxygenation in man awake and during halothane anesthesia. Anesthesiology 51:204

14. Merin RG, Kumazawa T, Luka NL (1976) Enflurane depresses myocardial function, perfusion and metabolism in the dog. Anesthesiology 45:501

15. Sonntag H, Schenk HD, Regensburger D, et al. (1973) Effects of Althesin (Glaxo CT1341) on coronary blood flow and myocardial metabolism in man. Acta Anaesthesiol Scand 17:218

16. Sonntag H, Hellberg K, Schenk HD, et al. (1975) Effects of thiopental (Trapanal) on coronary blood flow and myocardial metabolism in man. Acta Anaesthesiol Scand 19:69

17. Folts JD, Alfonso S, Rowe GG (1975) Systemic and coronary haemodynamic effects of ketamine in intact anaesthetized and unanaesthetized dogs. Br J Anaesth 47:686

18. Smith G, Thorburn J, Vance JP, et al. (1979) The effects of ketamine on the canine coronary circulation. Anaesthesia 34:555

19. Marshall RJ, Parratt JR (1973) The effects of dipyridamole on blood flow and oxygen handling in the acutely ischaemic and normal canine myocardium. Br J Pharmacol 49:391

20. Chiariello M, Gold HK, Leinbach RC, et al. (1976) Comparison between the effects of nitroprusside and nitroglycerin on ischemic injury during acute myocardial infarction. Circulation 54:766

21. Smith G, Rogers K, Thorburn J (1980) Halothane improves the balance of oxygen supply to demand in acute experimental myocardial ischaemia. Br J Anaesth 52:577

22. Bland JHL, Lowenstein E (1976) Halothane-induced decrease in experimental myocardial ischaemia in the non-failing canine heart. Anesthesiology 45:287

23. Klocke FJ, Ellis AK, Orlick AE (1980) Sympathetic influences on coronary perfusion and evolving concepts of driving pressure, resistance and transmural flow regulation. Anesthesiology 52:1

24. Vance JP, Brown DM, Smith G, et al. (1979) Coronary blood flow responses to hypoxia in the presence and absence of halothane. Br J Anaesth 51:193

25. Vatner SF, Smith NT (1974) Effects of halothane on left ventricular function and distribution of regional blood flow in dogs and primates. Circ Res 34:155

26. Domenech RJ, Macho P, Valdes J, et al. (1977) Coronary vascular resistance during halothane anesthesia. Anesthesiology 46:236

27. Kistner JR, Miller ED, Lake CL, et al. (1979) Indices of myocardial oxygenation during coronary-artery revascularisation in man with morphine versus halothane anesthesia. Anesthesiology 50:324

28. Estafanous FG, Viljoen JF (1974) Effect of induction of anaesthesia and ventilation on e.c.g. signs of ischaemia in patients with acute coronary artery insufficiency. Anesth Analg (Cleve) 53:610

29. Roy WL, Edelist G, Gilbert B (1979) Myocardial ischaemia during non-cardiac surgical procedures in patients with coronary artery disease. Anesthesiology 51:393

30. Robinson BF (1967) Relation of heart rate and systolic blood pressure to the onset of pain and angina pectoris. Circulation 35:1073

31. Gaines GY, Giesecke AH (1980) Hypotension during noncardiac anesthesia in the cardiac patient. In: Brown BR Jr (ed) Anesthesia and the patient with heart disease. FA Davis Company, Philadelphia, p 101

32. Lieberman RW, Orkin FK, Schwartz AJ, et al. (1980) Predictors of ischaemia during CABG with halothane. Anesthesiology 53:S96

33. Thomson IR, Lappas DG, Emerson CW, et al. (1980) Pre-op DPTI/SPTI: Predictor of intra-op ischaemia? Anesthesiology 53:S107

34. Smith G (1976) The coronary circulation and anaesthesia (Editorial). Br J Anaesth 48:933

35. Smith G, Vance JP, Brown DM (1973) The effect of propanidid on myocardial blood flow and oxygen consumption in the dog. Br J Anaesth 45:691

The Anaesthetic Management of Coronary and Cardiac Surgery

D.G. Lappas

Introduction

So much has been written about techniques for the anaesthetic management of patients undergoing open-heart surgery, that the principles of proper anaesthetic use are often forgotten. In the anaesthetic management of the cardiac surgical patient it is extremely important to know the pathophysiology of the cardiovascular lesion and the functional condition of the myocardium [17]. The broad range of anaesthetic drugs tolerated by the diseased heart makes the choice of anaesthetic far less important to the patient than the care with which it is administered.

Numerous studies have been published which describe and evaluate the cardiovascular effects of anaesthetic drugs [2, 5, 6, 14, 16, 22, 24, 28]. The data are conflicting, and there is often confusion among anaesthesiologists. Interpretation of the cardiovascular effects of various anaesthetics requires consideration of the following points. First, it must be remembered that many of the data accumulated in the literature have been the result of studies in a normal, healthy population. The patient with significant cardiac disease will often not respond to anaesthetics in the same way as the normal person. Secondly, the therapeutic regimen used prior to the induction of anaesthesia may significantly attenuate or enhance the circulatory effects of the anaesthetic drugs chosen. Thirdly, in the intra-operative management of the patient it is extremely important to know the functional starting point. Finally, it has been found that when two anaesthetics are used together, the resultant cardiovascular effect may not be the simple sum of the effects of each drug [14, 25, 27, 28].

We have little evidence that particular anaesthetic drugs or techniques offer special advantages to the patient at risk with a cardiovascular disorder [1]. In fact, better understanding of fundamental haemodynamic peculiarities characteristic of the primary cardiac lesion is likely to prove overwhelmingly more important for an ultimate improvement in survival rates [3, 4].

Bearing these points in mind, we will discuss briefly the pathophysiology associated with the various valvular lesions and with ischaemic heart disease. Obviously, an in-depth and detailed discussion of all the cardiovascular effects of the various anaesthetics is an immense subject well beyond the scope of this article. The major points, however, will be included in the coverage of the anaesthetic considerations relevant to cardiac surgical patients. In the approach to patients with valvular heart disease, the anaesthetist should bear in mind those circulatory variables that he is able to influence [26]. For instance, he cannot change the condition of the valvular lesion, but he can affect heart rate, intravascular volume [23], ventricular filling pressures, and vascular resistance.

Aortic Stenosis

Aortic valvular stenosis is the classic example of chronic pressure overload due to obstruction of left ventricular ejection. Progressively, the heart responds to the increased pressure load by undergoing concentric hypertrophy of the ventricular wall, while the ventricular chamber size does not change.

Ventricular compliance is reduced and small changes in volume are associated with disproportionate alterations in ventricular filling pressure. Atrial contraction and sinus rhythm are important, accounting for up to 40% of ventricular filling via the atrial booster pump effect. At the early stage of the disease, stroke volume and cardiac output remain in the normal range. Progressively, however, left ventricular failure develops and the stroke volume and cardiac output are greatly reduced.

In the absence of symptoms, anaesthesia is usually well tolerated, whereas patients with established symptomatology are at high risk [18, 27]. Since the main lesion is obstruction to left ventricular ejection, preservation of myocardial contractility is of paramount importance. Therefore, inhalation anaesthetics and barbiturates should be used with extreme caution, if at all. The maintenance of good perfusion pressure is important, so that perfusion of the hypertrophic myocardium can be accomplished. Adequate intravascular volume and preservation of normal sinus rhythm and rate are essential in preserving stroke volume and arterial pressure.

Aortic Insufficiency

The speed of development and progression of aortic regurgitation is related to its cause. Thus patients with aortic regurgitation resulting from rheumatic fever have an asymptomatic latent period of up to 20 years, while patients with regurgitation following infective endocarditis have early symptoms. Acute heart failure often occurs following valvular infection, aortic dissection, or aortic trauma.

Aortic insufficiency imposes a volume overload on the left ventricle as the regurgitant stream from the aorta is added to normal ventricular filling from the left atrium. The ventricle adapts to this increased load by undergoing eccentric hypertrophy, that is, increasing both chamber size and ventricular wall thickness. The ventricle becomes more compliant and large increases in volume do not affect the pressure significantly. Left ventricular filling pressure remains normal, while the total stroke volume is increased. The total stroke volume (the amount ejected by the left ventricle) includes the forward stroke volume, that portion that goes to the periphery, as well as the regurgitant volume. The enormous volume load, however, is not detrimental to the myocardium in terms of oxygen requirement, since the velocity of contraction is increased with a rapid decline in wall tension. Progressively, as contractility becomes impaired, stroke volume falls, as does ejection fraction, while left ventricular filling pressure increases. Therefore, the increase in peripheral vascular resistance will affect forward ejection, i.e. stroke volume.

In acute aortic insufficiency there is a sudden increase in left ventricular end-diastolic pressure because the normal ventricle, both in size and compliance, is suddenly exposed to a large regurgitant flow of blood. As a result, acute heart failure develops. In the absence of severe aortic regurgitation and congestive heart failure, anaesthesia and operation are tolerated well. In these patients, however, the arterial pressure is very labile, and drugs used in

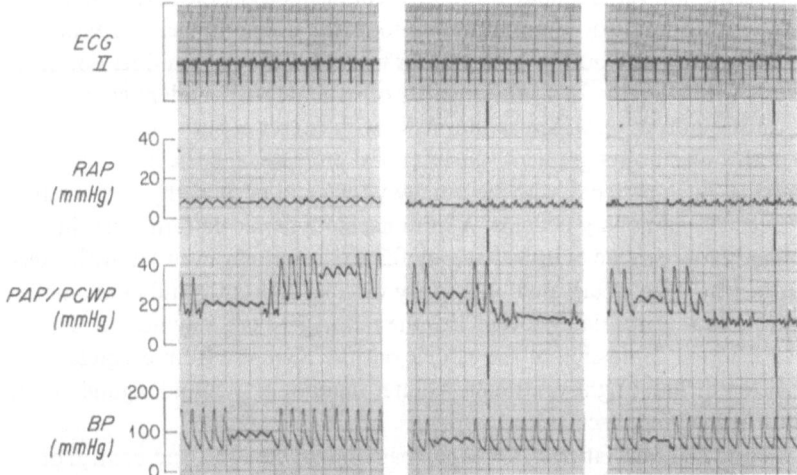

Fig. 1. Haemodynamic improvement with sodium nitroprusside (*second and third columns from the left*) in a 62-year-old patient with severe mitral and aortic regurgitation during open-heart surgery. Infusion of nitroprusside produced a progressive decrease in right atrial (*RAP*), pulmonary artery (*PAP*), and pulmonary capillary wedge (*PCWP*) pressures. Mean PAP decreased from 36 to 22 mmHg and mean PCWP from 20 to 10 mmHg, while the amplitude of the regurgitant waves in PCWP tracing fell. Systolic arterial blood-pressure (*BP*) decreased from 155 to 125 mmHg, while mean arterial pressure decreased from 90 to 75 mmHg. The haemodynamic improvement with nitroprusside can be attributed to a decrease in regurgitant volume, secondary to a fall in peripheral vascular resistance, since cardiac output increased (from 4.2 to 5.1 l/min). Heart rate showed a small decrease

anaesthesia which have known hypotensive properties should be given very slowly or in low concentrations. Heart rate should be slightly elevated, since bradycardia predisposes to ventricular distention and subsequent pulmonary congestion. Vasodilator drugs [11] (i.e. nitroprusside, nitroglycerin, hydralazine), by decreasing impedance to left ventricular ejection, increase forward flow and decrease regurgitant volume (Fig. 1). Conversely, vasoconstrictors decrease effective cardiac output and should be avoided whenever possible.

Mitral Stenosis

Mitral stenosis, except for the rare congenital form, is almost always a sequel of rheumatic disease and symptoms develop gradually over the years. The principal defect is an obstruction to left atrial emptying. This alters haemodynamics in three major respects: filling of the left ventricle, left atrial dynamics, and pulmonary function and circulation. Across the mitral valve an abnormal diastolic gradient develops. Thus left ventricular diastolic pressure is normal or low, while left atrial pressure is elevated. As a result of elevated atrial pressure, pulmonary venous and pulmonary capillary pressures increase. The rise in pulmonary artery pressure is often passive, but in addition, arteriolar constriction (reactive pulmonary hypertension) appears in some patients, and may lead to severe pulmonary hypertension far above that responding to the elevated left atrial pressure.

The haemodynamic pattern of mitral stenosis varies from a combination of normal cardiac output with a large mitral gradient, to a low fixed output with a relatively small gradient. The clinical presentation varies among these different haemodynamic patterns. In the majority of patients with moderate or severe mitral stenosis, the pulmonary capillary wedge pressure is elevated and the cardiac output is normal, or nearly so, at rest, but does not increase proportionately with exercise. In a small number of patients with moderately severe mitral stenosis the cardiac output may increase normally with exercise, but there is a consequent marked rise in the mitral valve gradient, the left atrial pressure, and the pulmonary capillary wedge pressure. Such patients, who are usually young and in sinus rhythm, are at risk of developing an acute pulmonary oedema. A third haemodynamic pattern exists in patients with a distinctly low cardiac output that may fail to rise or may even fall with exertion. In these patients, who have an elevated pulmonary vascular resistance and pulmonary hypertension, mitral stenosis is invariably severe, but the mitral gradient may not be as high as expected because of severe depression of the cardiac output. Sequelae from progressive pulmonary hypertension include: right ventricular failure, functional tricuspid regurgitation, and permanent lesion in the lung vasculature.

Tachycardia and/or atrial fibrillation often accompany mitral stenosis, and control of heart rate is very important. Since the filling of the ventricle is difficult due to the stenosis of the valve, shortening of the diastolic period with tachycardia will greatly affect ventricular volume. Anaesthetic and other drugs that cause tachycardia should therefore be avoided. Inhalation anaesthetics in low concentration may be given cautiously. With pre-existing pulmonary hypertension, possible deleterious effects of anaesthetics on the pulmonary circulation must be remembered. Nitrous oxide should be avoided in the presence of pulmonary hypertension because it can cause pulmonary vasoconstriction leading to a further increase in pulmonary artery pressure. Thus the drug may cause right ventricular decompensation. Large doses of narcotics (fentanyl, morphine) given at a slow infusion rate are tolerated well. In patients with low cardiac output and severe mitral stenosis, inhalation anaesthetics should be avoided.

Mitral Insufficiency

Pure mitral regurgitation commonly results from one of several other disorders, including mitral valve prolapse, ruptured chordae, papillary muscle dysfunction, calcified mitral annulus, and bacterial endocarditis. The most frequent cause of clinically significant mitral regurgitation is nonetheless rheumatic valve disease.

In mitral regurgitation, a portion of the left ventricular blood is ejected into the low-pressure left atrium. Compensation occurs initially through more complete left ventricular emptying, and later through left ventricular dilation. In long-standing mitral regurgitation, the left ventricular compliance is commonly increased so that left ventricular volume may be increased with little or no elevation of left ventricular end-diastolic pressure. Cardiac output may thus be maintained for years, despite severe mitral regurgitation. Pulmonary capillary wedge and pulmonary artery pressures may remain normal or slightly elevated in the patient with a large compliant left atrium. Severe pulmonary hypertension is much less commonly encountered with mitral regurgitation than with mitral stenosis.

Acute mitral insufficiency from ruptured chordae tendinae or an infarcted papillary muscle is not well tolerated, and frequently leads to severe cardiac failure and pulmonary oedema. Vasodilation therapy and inotropic support are often required during anaesthesia. Again, depression of myocardial contractility, increase in systemic and pulmonary vascular resistance, and tachyarrhythmias are not tolerated well. If pulmonary hypertension exists, similar considerations apply as described for mitral stenosis.

Ischaemic Heart Disease

Patients with a history of coronary artery disease are particularly susceptible to peri-operative myocardial ischaemia, which can produce infarction, life-threatening arrhythmias, or congestive heart failure. Myocardial oxygenation is a function of the relationship of myocardial oxygen demand to myocardial oxygen supply [3, 9]. The major determinants of myocardial oxygen demand are heart rate, ventricular wall tension, and contractility. Myocardial oxygen supply is a function of coronary blood flow, blood oxygen availability, abnormal regional perfusion, and heart rate [10].

The clinical and haemodynamic picture in patients with coronary artery disease can vary significantly [12]. For example, a large percent age of these patients have normal haemodynamics and cardiac function until an ischaemic episode occurs. These patients tolerate anaesthetics well. On the contrary, if there is congestive heart failure, several anaesthetic drugs may affect cardiac performance significantly. It is therefore important to distinguish these patients, since they are at high risk.

Patients with a history of ischaemic heart disease may develop haemodynamic changes during a general anaesthetic, prone to upset the delicate balance between myocardial metabolic requirements and available blood flow [21]. An anaesthetic-induced reduction in arterial blood-pressure due to a direct or neurohumorally-mediated influence on heart rate, myocardial contractile performance, arteriolar resistance vessel tone, or venous compliance, may affect myocardial perfusion. A massive sympathetic discharge elicited upon stimulation by laryngoscopy, endotracheal intubation, or surgical incision may increase significantly the work of the myocardium, and thus myocardial oxygen requirements (Fig. 2). This re-

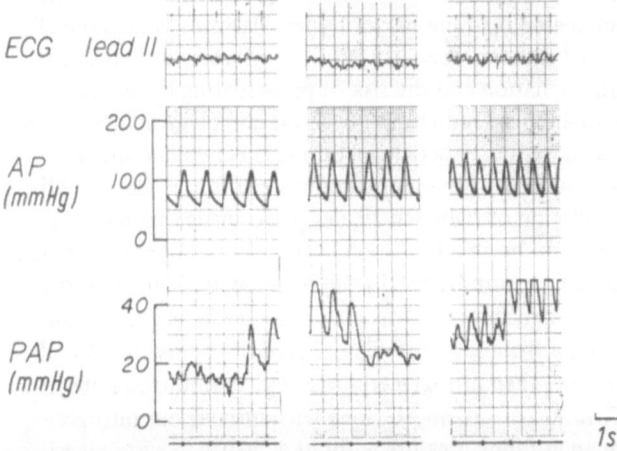

Fig. 2. The effect of an acute increase in arterial blood-pressure (*AP*) and heart rate on pulmonary artery (PAP) and pulmonary capillary wedge pressure during operation for myocardial revascularization but before extracorporeal bypass. The patient exhibited a progressive rise in pulmonary arterial and wedge pressure. Note the appearance of pulsus alternans on the AP tracing on the *far right column*. These changes are indicative of left ventricular dysfunction

sponse is mediated via one or more of the mechanisms described. In both instances, corona-ry blood flow to muscle supplied by a narrowed vessel may be affected sufficiently to initi-ate ischaemia de novo, and, if sustained, myocardial infarction. Optimal therapy during anaesthesia includes control of heart rate, as well as systemic arterial and pulmonary capilla-ry wedge pressures.

There is little evidence that particular anaesthetic drugs or techniques offer special ad-vantages to the patient at risk from an ischaemic myocardium [15]. Arguments generated in favour of a specific anaesthetic technique are derived from data accrued from observations made on patients or drawn from animal models, neither source being beyond criticism or continued controversy. One rule does seem to apply with remarkable consistency: patients with coronary artery disease tolerate poorly a cavalier approach to pronounced fluctuations in systemic blood-pressure. The risk of intra-operative ischaemic injury of the myocardium can be reduced by preventing or promptly treating any haemodynamic change caused by anaesthesia or surgical stimulation which may alter the balance between myocardial metabo-lic requirements and available blood flow [7, 13, 19].

Most volatile anaesthetics and drugs administered intravenously to induce sleep reduce myocardial contractile performance [25, 27]. Some compounds also exercise a direct effect on resistance and venous capacitance vessels, or alter their response to sympathetic stimuli. None of the responses are clinically significant unless the result is a reduction in the quality of myocardial perfusion, either through a diminution in the pressure gradient for perfusion (i.e. the difference between aortic and left ventricular diastolic pressures) or the duration of diastole.

The use of large quantities of fentanyl has been suggested as an alternative to volatile anaesthetics, and reported to achieve a level of anaesthesia adequate to protect against the consequences of sympathetic stimulation. The disadvantage associated with all potent syn-thetic narcotics is their prolonged duration of action, with a requirement for extended post-operative mechanical ventilation, an argument not necessarily valid if the patient is haemo-dynamically unstable. All narcotics increase venous compliance by peripheral block of sympathetic stimuli; this response is directly related to the dose used. Requirements for in-travascular component therapy are increased, and the risk of hypervolaemia arises as the ef-fect of the narcotic on venomotor tone begins to wane [23]. Coronary artery disease limits the adjustments possible through autoregulation and the risk of perpetuating ischaemia is created following an acute sympathetic-induced reduction in venous compliance, increase in arteriolar tone, or abbreviation of diastole often experienced during general anaesthesia.

Reduction in peripheral venous compliance (venoconstriction) results in a central redi-stribution of blood volume, with stimulation of right ventricular performance such that a potentially ischaemic left ventricle may not be able to respond. Thus, both pulmonary blood volume and left ventricular end-diastolic pressure (LVEDP) will increase, with an accentua-tion of ischaemia and ventricular failure. An acute and sustained increase in left ventricular filling pressure must be brought under control using vasodilators [13]. If the rise in LVEDP is secondary to increased venomotor tone, then nitroglycerin therapy, as an intravenous in-fusion, appears preferable [8, 20]. Titration of venomotor tone with intravenous nitrogly-cerin allows for an appropriate decrease in filling pressure without a change in systemic ar-tery pressure (Fig. 3).

An acute increase in arteriolar tone leading to systemic arterial hypertension is usually accompanied by an increase in LVEDP, whether induced pharmacologically or by a sympa-thetic stimulus (Fig. 2). A rise in arterial pressure at low LVEDP is not likely to result in myo-

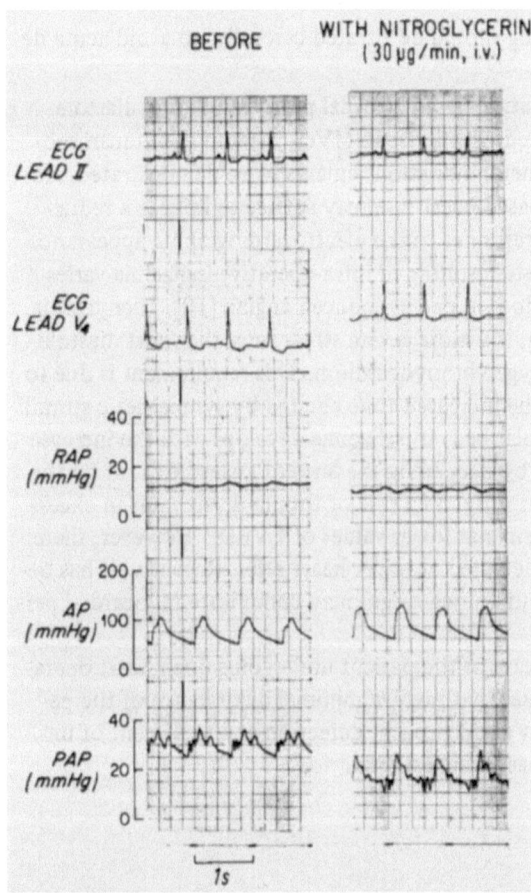

Fig. 3. The effect of nitroglycerin infusion on haemodynamics and the electrocardiogram in a patient during operation for myocardial revascularization. Nitroglycerin caused a significant reduction in right atrial (RAP) and pulmonary arterial (PAP) pressures, while arterial blood-pressure (AP) increased. The decrease in systolic and diastolic PAP in the presence of an increased AP can be attributed to improved left ventricular ejection due to relief of myocardial ischaemia with nitroglycerin. In addition, nitroglycerin increased venous capacitance as indicated by the decrease in RAP

cardial ischaemia. On the contrary, an acute elevation in LVEDP during a hypertensive response runs the risk of perpetuating ischaemia. Wall stress generated during isovolumic contraction and ejection sets the limits for O_2 requirements, while quality of myocardial perfusion or O_2 supply is adjusted according to the gradient between aortic diastolic and LV diastolic pressures and duration of diastole. A high LVEDP implies a high wall stress and lesser endocardial perfusion, perhaps at constant O_2 demand; a high aortic diastolic pressure may increase isovolumic wall stress, but it will also improve the myocardial perfusion gradient. There is amazingly little evidence to suggest that acute arterial hypertension is detrimental as long as filling pressure is not allowed to increase. In fact, an elevated aortic pressure is of lesser consequence than an increase in heart rate in patients with fixed coronary obstruction, probably because the added O_2 demand for the ejection phase is less of a burden than a reduction in the duration of diastolic coronary blood flow. If systemic hypertension must be treated, vasodilators such as nitroprusside are extremely useful. Since nitroprusside is a potent vasodilator, the infusion rate of the drug should be titrated carefully, to avoid acute decrease of the arterial pressure.

An increase in heart rate limits the duration of myocardial perfusion during diastole. Whether the increased frequency is associated with a rise in MVO_2/beat in the human subjected to the sympathetic stimuli of anaesthetic induction remains to be demonstrated. Abbreviation of diastole secondary to an increased heart rate may suffice to initiate a reduction in LV end-diastolic compliance as a forerunner to the electrocardiographic appearance of ST segment changes. The critical heart rate resulting in intra-operative ischaemia varies substantially from patient to patient, as it does in pacing-induced angina [10]. Tachycardia, owing to peri-operative sympathetic stimuli, is a more severe stress since the short diastole is accompanied by a greater demand for oxygen in myocardium. This requirement is due to the additional cardiac burden imposed by the increased tone elicited by sympathetic stimuli in both the resistance and capacitance vascular bed. If ischaemia develops with the increase of heart rate, it should be controlled either by deepening the level of anaesthesia, or by the intravenous administration of a beta-blocker drug. As a rule of thumb, heart rates in excess of 90 beats/min are likely to result in ischaemia at lower values of LVEDP. However, there are instances where ECG ischaemia can be detected at lower heart rates. Recently, it has become apparent that coronary vasospasm of unknown origin may complicate myocardial perfusion.

In conclusion, optimal intra-operative care of the patient undergoing open-heart operation is best attained by anaesthetic techniques that involve minimal disturbance of the patient's resting haemodynamic state, and that allow prompt detection and treatment of unexpected variations from the normal response to anaesthesia.

References

1. Bassell GM, Lin YT, Oka Y, Becker RM, Frater RWM (1978) Circulatory response to tracheal intubation in patients with coronary artery disease and valvular disease. Bull NY Acad Med 54:842–848
2. Bland JHL, Lowenstein E (1976) Effect of halothane on myocardial ischaemia. Anesthesiology 45: 287–293
3. Braunwald E (1971) Control of myocardial oxygen consumption. Physiologic and clinical consideration. Am J Cardiol 27:416–432
4. Cohn JM (1973) Blood pressure and cardiac performance. Am J Med 55:351–361
5. Dowdy EG, Kaya KL (1968) Studies of the mechanism of cardiovascular responses to ketamine. Anesthesiology 29:931–943
6. Eger EI, Smith NT, Stoelting RK, Cullen DJ, Kadis LB, Whitcher CE (1970) Cardiovascular effects of halothane in man. Anesthesiology 32:396–409
7. Ellrodt G, Chew CYC, Singh BN (1980) Therapeutic implications of slow-channel blockade in cardiovascular disorders. Circulation 62:669–679
8. Epstein SE, Kent KM, Goldstein RE, Borer JS, Redwood DR (1975) Reduction of ischaemic injury by nitroglycerin during acute myocardial infarction. New Engl J Med 292:29–35
9. Hoffman JIE (1978) Determinants and prediction of transmural myocardial perfusion. Circulation 58:381–391
10. Gobel FL, Norstrom LA, Nelson RR (1978) The rate-pressure product as an index of myocardial oxygen consumption during exercise in patients with angina pectoris. Circulation 57:549–555
11. Greenberg BH, DeMots H, Murphy E, Rahimtoola SH (1981) Mechanism of improved cardiac performance with arteriolar dilators in aortic insufficiency. Circulation 63:263–268

12. Johnson RA, Zir LM, Harper RW, Leinbach RC, Hutter AM Jr, Pohost GM, Block PC, Gold HK (1979) Patterns of haemodynamic alteration during left ventricular ischaemia in man. Relation to angiographic extent of coronary artery disease. Br Heart J 41:441–451
13. Kotter V, von Leitner ER, Wunderlich J, Schroder R (1977) Comparison of haemodynamic effects of phentolamine, sodium nitroprusside, and glyceryl trinitrate in acute myocardial infarction. Br Heart J 39:1196–1204
14. Lappas DG, Buckley MJ, Laver MB, Daggett WM, Lowenstein E (1975) Left ventricular performance and pulmonary circulation following addition of nitrous oxide to morphine during coronary artery surgery. Anesthesiology 43:61–69
15. Lappas DG, Geha D, Fischer JE, Laver MB, Lowenstein E (1975) Effect of large doses of intravenous morphine upon filling pressures of the heart and pulmonary circulation of patients with coronary artery disease. Anesthesiology 42:153–159
16. Lappas DG, Lowenstein E, Waller J, Fahmy NR, Daggett WM (1976) Haemodynamic effects of nitroprusside infusion during coronary artery operation in man. Circulation [Suppl III] 54:III–4
17. Lappas DG, Powell JW, Daggett W H (1977) Cardiac dysfunction. Anesthesiology 47:117–135
18. Lowenstein E, Hallowell P, Levine FH, Daggett WM, Austen WG, Laver MB (1969) Cardiovascular response to large doses of intravenous morphine in man. N Engl J Med 281:1389–1393
19. Nies AS, Shand DG (1975) Clinical pharmacology of propranolol. Circulation 52:6–12
20. Ogilvie RI (1978) Effect of nitroglycerin on peripheral blood flow distribution and venous return. J Pharmacol Exp Ther 207:372–380
21. Robinson BF (1967) Relation of heart rate and systolic blood pressure to the onset of angina pectoris. Circulation 35:1073–1083
22. Smith NT, Eger EI, Stoelting RK, Whayne TF, Cullen D, Kadis LB (1970) The cardiovascular and sympathomimetic responses to the addition of nitrous oxide to halothane in man. Anesthesiology 32:410–421
23. Stanley TH, Stanford W, Armstrong R, Cline R (1973) The effects of high dose morphine are fluid and blood requirements in open-heart operations. Anesthesiology 38:536–541
24. Stanley TH, Stanford W, Armstrong R, Cline R (1974) The effect of morphine anesthesia in blood requirements during and after valve replacement and coronary artery bypass grafting. Ann Thorac Surg 17:368–376
25. Stoelting RK (1972) Haemodynamic effect of gallamine during halothane nitrous oxide anesthesia. Anesthesiology 36:612–615
26. Stoelting RK, Gibbs PS (1973) Haemodynamic effects of morphine and morphine nitrous oxide in valvular heart disease and coronary artery disease. Anesthesiology 38:45–52
27. Stoelting RK, Reiss RR, Longnecker DE (1972) Haemodynamic response to nitrous oxide-halothane and halothane in patients with valvular heart disease. Anesthesiology 37:430–435
28. Wong KC, Martin WE, Hornbein TF, Freund FG, Everett J (1973) The cardiovascular effects of morphine sulfate with oxygen and nitrous oxide in man. Anesthesiology 38:542–549

Influence of Inhalation Anaesthetics on the Autonomic Nervous System

M. Göthert

Introduction

Inhalation anaesthesia and various stressful events associated with surgery may severely alter the function of the autonomic nervous system. Almost all investigations of the influence of inhalation anaesthetics on autonomic nervous activity deal with the effects of these drugs on the sympatho-adrenal system, and on the baroreceptors which are the sensory organs for the afferent limb of baroreceptor reflexes. This predominant interest in the sympathetic division of the autonomic nervous system is due to the attempts to relate the main side-effects of these drugs on the cardiovascular system to changes in autonomic nervous activity. Thus hypo- or hypertensive reactions may occur during inhalation anaesthesia; in this connection it is of interest that changes in blood-pressure due to alterations of arteriolar resistance can be related to an increase or decrease in sympatho-adrenal activity; by contrast, cholinergic impulses are virtually devoid of physiological significance in this respect. Furthermore, inhalation anaesthetics are known to cause a negative inotropic effect; again, the force of contraction of the cardiac ventricles is effectively controlled by the sympathetic but not by the parasympathetic nervous system. The present report will therefore concentrate on the effects of inhalation anaesthetics on the sympatho-adrenal system and on the baroreceptor reflexes. However, it should be pointed out that a reduction of the sympathetic tone causes a predominance of parasympathetic nervous activity. In this situation the administration of atropine is absolutely necessary to avoid serious dysfunction of various organ systems.

Controversial results concerning the influence of inhalation anaesthesia on plasma adrenaline (A) and noradrenaline (NA) have been reported, although the specificity and sensitivity of the methods used for determination of plasma catecholamines (CA) were considerably improved by introduction of radioenzymatic techniques. For instance, Roizen et al. [31] found a decrease in plasma NA in rats anaesthetized with halothane, whereas Da Prada et al. [8] observed an increase; Stokke et al. [37] reported no change and Balogh et al. [3] a slight increase in plasma CA during halothane-nitrous oxide anaesthesia in man. In all of these investigations radioenzymatic methods were used for determination of plasma CA.

In the present report the possible reasons for these and similar discrepancies found with other inhalation anaesthetics will be discussed. For this purpose some of the pharmacodynamic effects of these compounds on the baroreceptors and on discrete functional levels of the sympatho-adrenal system will be reviewed. It is not the intention to consider each compound as a pharmacological entity, but to analyse the principles and common features of their actions. Mainly data obtained with halothane, enflurane, and methoxyflurane will be reported, and a major part of this presentation will be devoted to personal experimental investigations in this field. Moreover, additional influences on the sympatho-adrenal system which occur during inhalation anaesthesia but which are not caused by these compounds themselves will be considered. Finally, by integration of all synergistic and antagonistic influences, conclusions will be drawn concerning the overall effects of inhalation anaesthetics on sympatho-adrenal activity, which are reflected by changes in plasma catecholamines.

Effects on Baroreceptors

A decrease in blood-pressure causes decreased stimulation of baroreceptors in the aorta and carotid sinus, resulting in a decreased impulse flow via afferent nerve fibres to the vasomotor centres in the brain-stem, and finally in an increased sympatho-adrenal output to the effector sites. Halothane and enflurane have been shown to cause a sensitization of the baroreceptors [4, 22]. Thus, at a given level of blood-pressure, the anaesthetics increase discharge via afferent fibres, and a higher level of blood-pressure than the real one is signalled to the central nervous system. On the other hand, since the main site of action of halogenated inhalation anaesthetics underlying the decrease in blood-pressure appears to be the cardiovascular system itself, an inhibition of impulse flow from the baroreceptors resulting in reflex activation of the sympatho-adrenal system only occurs if the hypotensive effect overcomes the sensitization of the baroreceptors.

Effects on the Central Nervous System

In cats halothane decreased the preganglionic sympathetic activity, but the anaesthetic had little effect on the response of preganglionic sympathetic neurones to baroreceptor stimulation [36]. These results indicate that the anaesthetic causes a depression of the central sympathetic tone, but that this effect is rather weak. Moreover, the authors postulate that the compound acts predominantly on the pressor elements of the medullary vasomotor centre. The results obtained with enflurane were very similar to those reported for halothane [24, 35], whereas the effects of methoxyflurane were less pronounced; with this anaesthetic a slight reduction in preganglionic sympathetic activity could only be observed in baroreceptor-denervated cats [34]. Interestingly, in cats anaesthetized with enflurane or methoxyflurane, addition of nitrous oxide caused an increase in pre-ganglionic sympathetic discharge [24].

Effects on Sympathetic Ganglia and the Adrenal Medulla

There is no doubt that halothane is capable of blocking transmission in sympathetic ganglia. This has already been established by early work of Biscoe and Millar [5] in cats and rabbits, and of Price and Price [29] in dogs (in this connection see also the reviews by Alper and Flacke [1] and Gardier [10]). Interestingly, halothane markedly inhibited the response to dimethylphenylpiperazinium (DMPP), a nicotinic receptor agonist, leaving unchanged the response to McN-A-343, a muscarinic receptor agonist; these findings indicate that halothane specifically inhibits the responses mediated by post-synaptic nicotinic ganglionic receptors [2]. Although there exist only few reports on the effect of methoxyflurane on sympathetic

Table 1. Inhibitory effects produced by inhalation of 1.7–1.9 MAC of various anaesthetics on catecholamine secretion from the cat adrenal medulla. Values are mean percentages of pre-anaesthetic levels

	Basal (nonstimulated) secretion		Secretion evoked by splanchnic nerve stimulation	
	Adrenaline	Noradrenaline	Adrenaline	Noradrenaline
Halothane, 1.5%[a]	26	12	15	7
Enflurane, 2.2%[b]	19	25	30	18
Methoxyflurane, 0.4%[c]	17	6	30	14

[a] [15]; [b] [17]; [c] [9]

ganglionic transmission, the latter appears also to be blocked by this anaesthetic, as demonstrated by Ovadia et al. [28] in dogs. By contrast, 80% nitrous oxide did not produce a ganglionic blockade in this species of animal [11]. In order to examine the influence of inhalation anaesthetics on the catecholamine release from the adrenal medulla, we carried out experiments in cat adrenals in situ and in isolated bovine adrenals.

In cats which had received pentobarbital as a basal anaesthetic, inhalation of halothane 0.7%–1.5% caused a concentration-dependent inhibition of basal A and NA release (measured by determination of the CA in blood samples drawn from the adrenolumbar vein; Table 1). The A and NA secretion evoked by splanchnic nerve stimulation was also strongly decreased by halothane 1% and 1.5%, indicating that the compound acts directly on the synapse between spanchnic nerve fibres and chromaffin cells (Table 1). The decrease in nonstimulated release is therefore due not only to the central nervous inhibition of the sympathoadrenal system just described, but also to this peripheral site of action. In agreement with the inhibitory effect of halothane on stimulation-evoked CA release, the anaesthetic also decreased the pressor effect of splanchnic nerve stimulation, whereas the pressor effect of exogenous NA remained unaffected. In a similar way to halothane, enflurane also caused a decrease both in basal and in stimulation-evoked secretion of catecholamines from the cat adrenal medulla in situ (Fig. 1; Table 1). The same holds true for methoxyflurane (Table 1; an inhibition of non-stimulated CA release from the adrenal medulla was also found by Li et al. [23]).

The rather improbable possibility that an inhibition of CA synthesis by clinically relevant concentrations of halothane and methoxyflurane substantially contributes to the decrease in release was ruled out by in vitro experiments with tyrosine hydroxylase and dopamine-ß-hydroxylase, prepared from bovine adrenals [33]. However, experiments in perfused bovine adrenals proved to be suitable for further elucidation of the site and mechanism of action underlying the inhibition of adrenal medullary CA secretion. Since halothane in a concentration-range corresponding to that used in surgical anaesthesia inhibited the acetylcholine (ACh)-induced CA release (Fig. 2; [12]), it may be concluded that the anaesthetic acts directly on the chromaffin cell and that the release mediated by acetylcholine receptors is impaired. In order to find out whether nicotinic and/or muscarinic receptors are involved, the effects of halothane on the release induced by the nicotinic receptor agonist DMPP and by the muscarinic receptor agonist pilocarpine were studied [20]. There is no doubt that un-

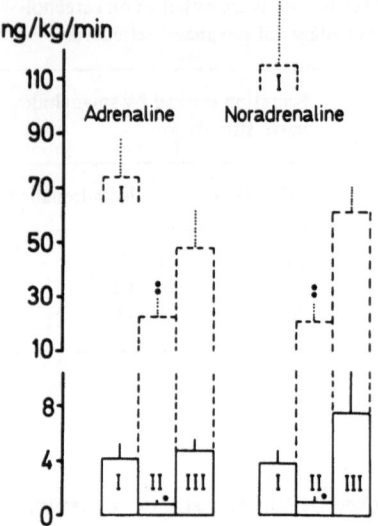

Fig. 1. Basal and stimulation-evoked release of adrenaline and noradrenaline from the cat adrenal medulla in situ before (*I*), during (*II*), and after (*III*) anaesthesia with 2.2% enflurane. For details of the experimental conditions, see [17]. Basal catecholamine release is represented by the *columns* marked by the *solid lines*. Both for adrenaline and noradrenaline, only the *top of the column* representing the pre-anaesthetic release evoked by splanchnic nerve stimulation is shown, whereas values of stimulation-evoked secretion during and after enflurane anaesthesia are represented by the *full areas of the columns* marked by the *broken lines*. Both basal and stimulation-evoked secretion were significantly decreased (*p < 0.05; **p < 0.001) compared to the corresponding original levels before anaesthesia. Means (+ SEM) of six to eight experiments are given

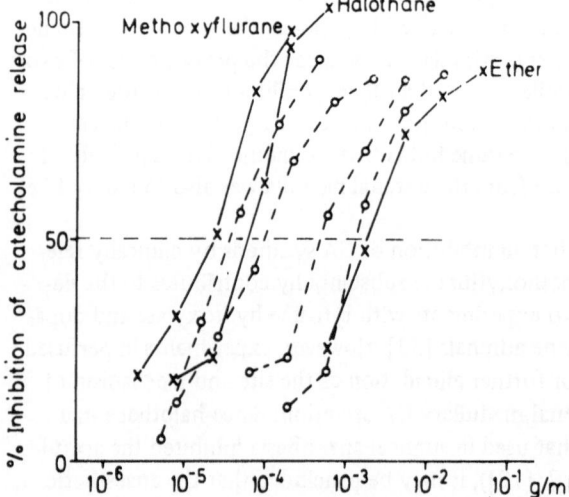

Fig. 2. Inhibitory effects of inhalation anaesthetics (*solid lines*) and aliphatic alcohols on the acetylcholine (10 μg/ml)-induced catecholamine secretion from perfused bovine adrenals. The results obtained with alcohols are represented by the *broken lines* (from left to right: hexanol, pentanol, butanol, and propanol). Means of at least three experiments are given

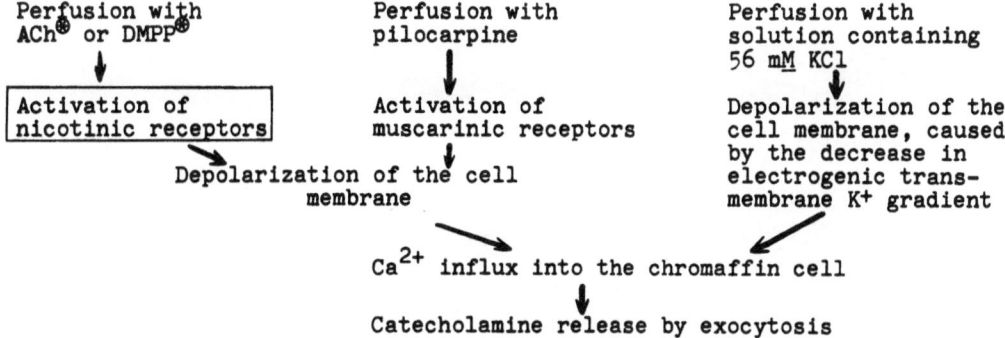

Fig. 3. Stimulus-release coupling: events on the cell membrane of chromaffin cells. *ACh*, acetylcholine; *DMPP*, dimethylphenylpiperazinium

der physiological conditions, activation of the nicotinic receptor represents the main pathway for stimulation of catecholamine release. Halothane strongly inhibited the DMPP-evoked release, leaving that evoked by pilocarpine unaffected. The anaesthetic also did not alter the release evoked by 56 mM KCl. Similar results were obtained in corresponding experiments with enflurane [18]. From these findings conclusions can be drawn as to the precise site of action of the anaesthetics in the cell membrane of the chromaffin cells. Figure 3 shows a schematic representation of stimulus-release coupling in the chromaffin cells. Since Ca^{2+} influx is a common pathway with all methods of stimulation used, it can be assumed that Ca^{2+} influx via a common channel or any subsequent step is not impaired by the drugs. Depolarization of the cell membrane occurs after activation of both nicotinic and muscarinic receptors, thus excluding the possibility that the selective inhibition of release evoked by nicotinic receptor activation is due to an interaction with depolarization, at least if one assumes that the latter is caused by a common mechanism. By exclusion of other possibilities, therefore, it appears that the inhibition is due to an interaction of the anaesthetics with the nicotinic receptor itself or with an ionic channel specifically associated with the receptor protein. As expected, halothane caused not a competitive but a non-competitive inhibition of the release evoked by acetylcholine [20]. Further experiments revealed that not only inhalation anaesthetics but also other hydrophobic drugs cause an inhibition of the ACh-evoked release (Fig. 2). The inhibitory potencies of these compounds expressed in terms of their IC_{50} values (i.e. those concentrations producing 50% inhibition of ACh-evoked release) was proportional to their membrane/buffer partition coefficients (i.e. their hydrophobic properties [19]). Taken together, it may be concluded that the inhibition by anaesthetics of the ACh-evoked CA release may be due to hydrophobic interaction of the drugs, either with the receptor protein itself or with an ionic channel closely associated with the receptor. In the first case a conformational change would be induced, which in turn would impair receptor-agonist interaction, whereas in the latter a decreased influx of ions (probably Na^+ and/or Ca^{2+}) would occur.

Effects on the Terminal Sympathetic Nerve Fibres

The effects of inhalation anaesthetics on NA release from terminal sympathetic nerve fibres was investigated in isolated, perfused rabbit hearts with an intact post-ganglionic sympathe-

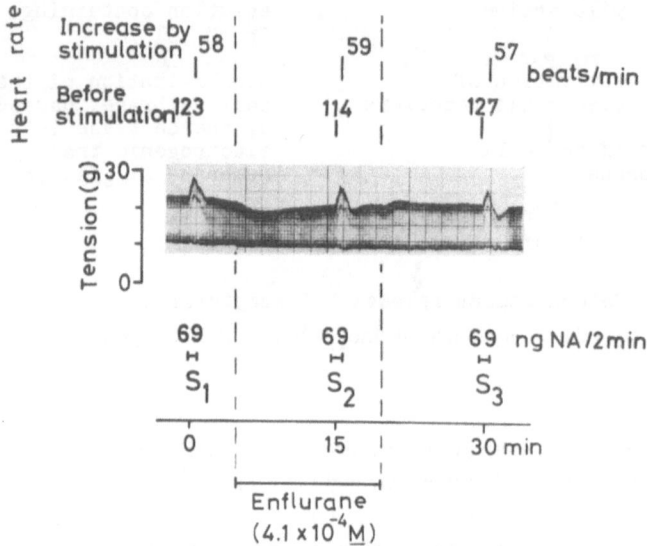

Fig. 4. Effects of enflurane on the stimulation-evoked noradrenaline output from a perfused rabbit heart with an intact sympathetic nerve supply. $S_1 - S_3$ indicate the 1-min periods of electrical nerve stimulation. Enflurane was present in the perfusion fluid during the time indicated by the *vertical broken lines*. It is evident that both the impulse-evoked noradrenaline release and the resulting increase in heart rate and tension development are not altered by the anaesthetic

tic nerve supply. Figure 4 shows that enflurane did not alter the NA output in response to electrical stimulation of the nerve fibres and the stimulation-evoked increase in both heart rate and tension. This result was reproducible at concentrations up to 1.24 mM [16]. In the same preparation halothane also failed to produce a significant change of stimulated NA output [13]. Similar results were also obtained with halothane in the dog heart in vivo by Price et al. [30]. Indirect determination of the NA release from isolated sympathetically innervated cat atria also revealed that halothane had no effect on the release induced by nerve impulses: the anaesthetic did not alter the positive chronotropic response to either exogenous NA or stimulation of the sympathetic nerves [26].

In contrast, another indirect study in which the isolated saphenous vein of dogs was used indicated that halothane inhibited the evoked release of NA [25]; the compound considerably depressed the increase in tension of the venous strips induced by electrical field stimulation, but did not alter that in response to NA. Direct evidence for a decrease in NA release evoked by nerve impulses was obtained in an investigation by Roizen et al. [32], who used the isolated guinea-pig vas deferens-hypogastric nerve preparation; halothane inhibited the release of NA evoked by electrical nerve stimulation, but it did not decrease the stimulation-induced release of dopamine-ß-hydroxylase. This dissociation between CA and enzyme release has been suggested to be due to the possibility that halothane may enhance binding of NA to the vesicular membrane.

It is difficult to explain the discrepancies concerning the effect of halothane on electrically evoked release of NA. One possible explanation could be that the discrepancies are due to tissue differences. For a more comprehensive review of the effects of inhalation anaesthetics on NA release from noradrenergic nerve fibres, see Göthert [14].

Table 2. Influence of inhalation anaesthetics on the neuronal uptake of noradrenaline (NA)

	Removal of NA[a] (% of the amount infused)
Controls (n = 10)	41 ± 3.5
Halothane 1.13 μM (n = 10)	33.3 ± 3.2 (N.S.)[b]
Enflurane 1.24 μM (n = 6)	46 ± 4 (N.S.)[c]
Methoxyflurane 0.047 μM (n = 6)	36.8 ± 7.4 (N.S.)[c]

[a] Removal of exogenous NA (10 ng/ml) by isolated rabbit hearts was measured. NA was present in the perfusion fluid for 10 min. The anaesthetics were added to this fluid 10 min before and during perfusion with NA.
[b] Göthert [13]; [c] Göthert et al. [21]

Four processes are competing for the NA, released from the sympathetic nerve fibres: (a) binding to adrenoceptors, (b) neuronal reuptake, (c) extraneuronal uptake, and (d) diffusion from the synaptic cleft into the bloodstream. Inhalation anaesthetics do not alter the interaction between NA and adrenoceptors (see reviews by Alper and Flacke [1] and Gardier [10]). Furthermore, as shown in Table 2, halothane, enflurane, and methoxyflurane do not significantly alter the neuronal uptake of NA. Similar results were obtained by Naito and Gillis [26] and Brown et al. [6] in cat ventricle slices and guinea-pig atria respectively; these authors reported that halothane, enflurane, and methoxyflurane did not substantially affect the accumulation of labelled NA by the isolated tissues. Since, in addition, no data are available which indicate that inhalation anaesthetics may affect extraneuronal uptake, the amount of NA diffusing into the bloodstream probably reflects very well the amount of NA released. Therefore, in the absence of an influence of inhalation anaesthetics on inactivation of catecholamines, determination of plasma CA appears to be suitable for the evaluation of the activity of the sympatho-adrenal system.

Synopsis of Factors Possibly Influencing the Sympatho-adrenal System During Inhalation Anaesthesia

Before the results of the pharmacological experiments on discrete functional levels of the sympatho-adrenal system are compared with those of determination of plasma catecholamines, it is worthwhile giving a synopsis of the main factors which may influence the sympatho-adrenal system during inhalation anaesthesia (Fig. 5). As outlined in the previous sections, there is strong evidence that the inhalation anaesthetics halothane, enflurane, and methoxyflurane inhibit sympatho-adrenal function at the level of the central nervous system and at the level of sympathetic ganglia and adrenal medulla. It is still doubtful whether these compounds also cause a direct inhibitory action on the terminal sympathetic nerve fibres; if present at all, this effect would be rather weak. Reflex activation of the sympatho-adrenal system due to the anaesthetic-induced decrease in blood-pressure is also rather weak, or it may not even occur at all, because the anaesthetics sensitize the baroreceptors, as has been described.

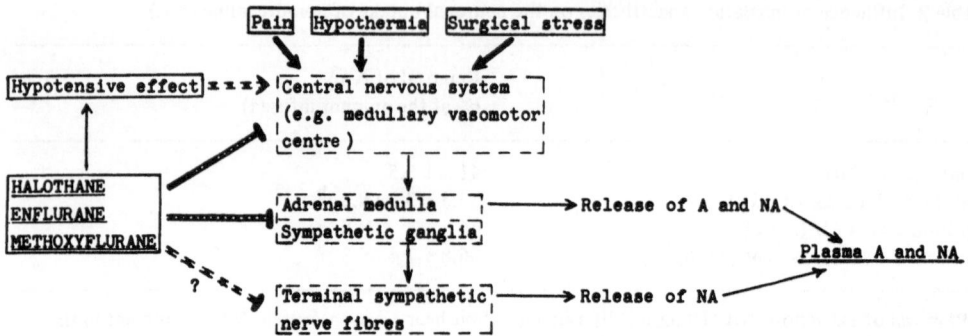

Fig. 5. Stimulatory (→) and inhibitory (■□■□■□■□■□■□■) effects which may influence the sympatho-adrenal system during anaesthesia with halothane, enflurane, or methoxyflurane. A, adrenaline; NA, nor-adrenaline

On the other hand, strong excitatory effects on the sympatho-adrenal function via its central nervous division can be brought about by influences which are not directly caused by the anaesthetics themselves, but which also occur during anaesthesia. Some of these influences can be summarized by the term "surgical stress". Furthermore, induction of hypothermia also causes a pronounced activation of the sympatho-adrenal system. The same holds true for pain, which may stimulate the sympatho-adrenal function, particularly during low stages of anaesthesia. In conclusion, at any moment during inhalation anaesthesia, the overall activity of the sympatho-adrenal system is dependent on the prevalance of either the inhibitory or the excitatory influences or on the balance between them. This overall sympatho-adrenal activity is evaluated by determination of plasma catecholamines.

Changes in Plasma Catecholamines Due to Pharmacodynamic Effects of Inhalation Anaesthetics and Stressful Events During Anaesthesia

The influence of an inhalation anaesthetic, namely methoxyflurane, on plasma catecholamines during activation of the sympatho-adrenal system by hypothermia (30 °C) has been studied by Ottermann et al. [27] in patients undergoing cardiovascular surgery. During anaesthesia with methoxyflurane, hypothermia increased plasma A by about 160% and plasma NA by about 40%, when compared to the corresponding values measured under methoxyflurane anaesthesia at a normal body temperature (controls). After withdrawal of the anaesthetic, the differences between the two groups were even more pronounced: In the post-operative phase of rewarming (at 34 °C), the concentrations of A and NA were increased by as much as 450% and 90% respectively, as compared to the controls. When the course of changes within both groups is considered, there is a slight tendency towards an increase in plasma CA compared to the pre-anaesthetic levels in the controls, and a very pronounced, progressive increase compared to the pre-anaesthetic, pre-hypothermia level in the hypothermia group. The authors conclude that hypothermia produces a strong activation of the whole sympatho-adrenal system, which is not prevented by methoxyflurane anaesthesia; however, they admit that the even more pronounced increase in plasma CA during withdrawal of methoxyflurane may be due to the disinhibition of the sympatho-adrenal activity, which in turn may be caused by the elimination of the anaesthetic. Indeed, this point deserves more attention, since according to the results presented in the previous sections it is likely that the hypothermia-induced increase in plasma CA would be much more pronounced in the absence of the anaesthetic; however, this suggestion cannot be confirmed experimentally in man.

Nevertheless, indirect evidence for this proposal can be provided by reanalysing our data obtained in the cat adrenal medulla. Figure 1 shows the influence of enflurane on the basal CA release and on the secretion evoked by splanchnic nerve stimulation; in this connection it is of interest that according to preliminary results of Ottermann et al. [27] enflurane caused very similar effects on plasma CA when the same condition were applied as in the study carried out with methoxyflurane. In Fig. 1 only the top of the columns representing stimulation-evoked CA release before anaesthesia (I) is shown, whereas the stimulation-evoked release during (II) and after enflurane anaesthesia (III) is represented by the full areas of the columns marked by the broken lines. Thus it is evident at first sight that in spite of the pronounced inhibitory effect of enflurane on the synapse between splanchnic nerve and chromaffin cell, the stimulated release during enflurane anaesthesia is much higher than the basal release before anaesthesia. Furthermore, it can be concluded from the data presented here that the stimulation-evoked CA release would actually have been much higher in the absence of the anaesthetic (the difference in scale between the upper and lower part of Fig. 1 should be noted). Taken together, the pattern shown in Fig. 1 is indeed very similar to that obtained by Ottermann et al. [27] in their investigation of the influence of methoxyflurane on the hypothermia-induced increase in plasma CA.

With these findings in mind, it is no longer surprising that the results obtained during anaesthesia with halothane quoted in the introduction are controversial. It has been shown by Bühler et al. [7] that A and NA in plasma of handled and restrained rats are much higher than the concentrations found in the plasma of undisturbed, freely moving animals. In their study of the influence of halothane on plasma CA, Roizen et al. [31] determined their control values in handled, restrained rats. The blood samples were drawn 4–6 h after halothane anaesthesia from the carotid arteries cannulated during anaesthesia. Further control values were determined 3 weeks later in blood obtained by decapitation of the animals. It is easy to understand that, compared to these control values obtained under both stressful conditions, plasma NA was found to be decreased by halothane. By contrast, Da Prada et al. [8] obtained their blood samples from freely moving rats in which the jugular vein was chronically catheterized. In these animals, plasma NA was very low under control conditions, and the effect of halothane was an increase. Stressful events before or during anaesthesia, independent of the pharmacodynamic effects of the anaesthetic, probably also explain the differences between the results of clinical studies in man.

Finally, it may be concluded from all the data presented here and from the schematic representation shown in Fig. 5 that the inhibitory effect of the halogenated inhalation anaesthetics may under certain conditions protect the organism from excessive sympatho-adrenal activation caused by stressful events which may occur during anaesthesia.

Summary

In spite of considerable improvement in specificity and sensitivity of the methods used for determination of plasma catecholamines (CA) by introduction of radioenzymatic techniques, controversial results as to the influence of inhalation anaesthesia on plasma adrenaline (A) and noradrenaline (NA) have been reported; e.g. in some investigations of the effects of halothane anaesthesia, decreased levels were found, whereas most authors reported unchanged or even increased concentrations of A and NA. Discrepancies also exist between most of these results and those obtained in experiments on various species of animals in which the influence of inhalation anaesthetics on discrete functional levels of the central and peripheral sympatho-adrenal system was examined. It has been reported that halothane, enflurane, and methoxyflurane produce a decrease in pre-ganglionic sympathetic activity, a ganglionic blockade, and an inhibition of both basal and stimulation-evoked release of adrenal medullary catecholamines, indicating that the direct effects of these drugs on the sympatho-adrenal system are inhibitory.

However, the overall effect of inhalation anaesthesia on CA release from the terminal sympathetic nerve fibres and the adrenal medulla is not only due to these direct inhibitory effects, but is also strongly influenced by, for example, surgical stress and anaesthetic induced changes of cardiovascular function. As a result of these antagonistic influences, unchanged, decreased, or increased plasma CA may be found, depending on the prevalance of either the inhibitory or the excitatory influences, or on the balance between them.

References

1. Alper MH, Flacke W (1969) The peripheral effects of anesthetics. Ann Rev Pharmacol 9:273–296
2. Alper MH, Fleisch JH, Flacke W (1969) The effects of halothane on the responses of cardiac sympathetic ganglia to various stimulants. Anesthesiology 31:429–436
3. Balogh D, Hammerle AF, Hörtnagel H, Brücke T, Stadler-Wolffersgrün R (1979) Plasma-Katecholamine bei Halothan-N$_2$O-Anaesthesie und Neuroleptanalgesie. Intra- und postoperative Vergleichsstudie. Anaesthesist 28:517–522
4. Biscoe TJ, Millar RA (1964) The effect of halothane on carotid sinus baroreceptor activity. J Physiol (Lond) 173:24–37
5. Biscoe TJ, Millar RA (1966) The effect of cyclopropane, halothane and ether on sympathetic ganglionic transmission. Br J Anaesth 38:3–12
6. Brown BR, Tatum EN, Crout JR (1972) The effects of inhalation anesthetics on the uptake and metabolism of 1-^{3}H-norepinephrine in guinea-pig atria. Anesthesiology 36:263–267
7. Bühler HU, Da Prada M, Haefely WE, Picotti GB (1978) Plasma adrenaline, noradrenaline and dopamine in man and different animal species. J Physiol (Lond) 276:311–320
8. Da Prada M, Picotti GB, Carruba MO, Haefely WE (1979) Plasma catecholamine, normetanephrine and p-octopamine levels: Stress- and drug-induced changes in rat. In: Usdin E, Kopin IJ, Barchas J (eds) Catecholamines: basic and clinical frontiers, vol I. Pergamon, Oxford New York, pp 915–917
9. Dreyer C, Bischoff D, Göthert M (1974) Effects of methoxyflurane anesthesia on adrenal medullary catecholamine secretion: inhibition of spontaneous secretion and secretion evoked by splanchnic-nerve stimulation. Anesthesiology 41:18–26
10. Gardier RW (1972) Autonomic nervous system. In: Chenoweth MB (ed) Modern inhalation anaesthetics. Handbook of experimental pharmacology, vol XXX. Springer, Berlin Heidelberg New York, pp 123–148
11. Garfield JM, Alper MH, Gillis RA, Flacke W (1968) A pharmacological analysis of ganglionic actions of some general anesthetics. Anesthesiology 29:79–92

12. Göthert M (1972) Die Sekretionsleistung des Nebennierenmarks unter dem Einfluß von Narkotika und Muskelrelaxantien. Anaesthesiol Resusc 70:

13. Göthert M (1974) Effects of halothane on the sympathetic nerve terminals of the rabbit heart. Differences in membrane actions of halothane and tetracaine. Naunyn Schmiedebergs Arch Pharmacol 286:125–143

14. Göthert M (1979) Modification of catecholamine release by anaesthetics and alcohols. In: Paton DM (ed) The release of catecholamines from adrenergic neurons. Pergamon, Oxford New York, pp 241: 261

15. Göthert M, Dreyer C (1973) Inhibitory effect of halothane anaesthesia on catecholamine release from the adrenal medulla. Naunyn Schmiedebergs Arch Pharmacol 277:253–266

16. Göthert M, Kennerknecht E (1976) Effects of general anaesthetics on the cell membrane of sympathetic nerve terminals: an investigation of the mechanism of action of anaesthetics. Excerpta Medica International Congress Series No. 387. 6th world congress of anaesthesiology, Mexico-City, April 24–30, 1976. Abstract No. 145 (F5–1/2). Excerpta Medica Amsterdam

17. Göthert M, Wendt J (1977) Inhibition of adrenal medullary catecholamine secretion by enflurane. 1. Investigations in vivo. Anesthesiology 46:400–403

18. Göthert M, Wendt J (1977) Inhibition of adrenal medullary catecholamine secretion by enflurane. 2. Investigations on isolated bovine adrenals: site and mechanism of action. Anesthesiology 46: 404–410

19. Göthert M, Schmoldt A, Thielecke G (1974) Zum Wirkungsmechanismus von Inhalationsnarkotica auf die Katecholaminfreisetzung aus dem Nebennierenmark. Anaesthesist 23:137–141

20. Göthert M, Dorn W, Loewenstein I (1976) Inhibition of catecholamine release from the adrenal medulla by halothane. Site and mechanism of action. Naunyn Schmiedebergs Arch Pharmacol 294: 239–249

21. Göthert M, Kennerknecht E, Thielecke G (1976) Inhibition of receptor-mediated noradrenaline release from the sympathetic nerves of the isolated rabbit heart by anaesthetics and alcohols in proportion to their hydrophobic property. Naunyn Schmiedebergs Arch Pharmacol 292:145–152

22. Hagenau W, Pietsch D, Arndt JO (1976) Der Effekt von Halothan und Enflurane sowie von Propanidid und Ketamin auf die Aktivität der Barorezeptoren des Aortenbogens decerebrierter Katzen. Anaesthesist 25:331–341

23. Li TH, Shaul MS, Etsten BE (1968) Decreased adrenal venous catecholamine concentrations during methoxyflurane anesthesia. Anesthesiology 29:1145–1152

24. Millar RA, Warden JC, Cooperman LH, Price HL (1970) Further studies of sympathetic actions of anaesthetics in intact and spinal animals. Br J Anaesth 42:366–378

25. Muldoon SM, Vanhoutte PM, Lorenz RR, Van Dyke RA (1975) Venomotor changes caused by halothane acting on the sympathetic nerves. Anesthesiology 43:41–48

26. Naito H, Gillis CN (1968) Anesthetics and response of atria to sympathetic nerve stimulation. Anesthesiology 29:259–266

27. Ottermann U, Dudziak R, Appel E, Palm D (1979) Die Wirkung von Hypothermie und Methoxyflurane-Narkose auf die sympathonervale und sympathoadrenale Aktivität bei Herzoperationen. Anaesthesist 28:551–556

28. Ovadia LO, Li TH, Etsten BE (1969) Mechanisms of ganglionic transmission during methoxyflurane and halothane anesthesia. Anesthesiology 30:349

29. Price HL, Price ML (1967) Relative ganglion-blocking potencies of cyclopropane, halothane and nitrous oxide and the interaction of nitrous oxide with halothane. Anesthesiology 28:349–353

30. Price HL, Warden JC, Cooperman LH, Price ML (1968) Enhancement by cyclopropane and halothane of heart rate responses to sympathetic stimulation. Anesthesiology 29:478–483

31. Roizen MF, Moss J, Henry DP, Kopin IJ (1974) Effects of halothane on plasma catecholamines. Anesthesiology 41:432–439

32. Roizen MF, Thoa NB, Moss J, Kopin IJ (1975) Inhibition by halothane of release of norepinephrine, but not of dopamine-ß-hydroxylase, from guinea pig vas deferens. Eur J Pharmacol 31:313–318

33. Schmoldt A, Göthert M (1974) Einfluß von Narkotika auf die Katecholaminsynthese im Nebennierenmark. Anaesthesist 23:10–13

34. Skovsted P, Price HL (1969) The effects of methoxyflurane on arterial pressure, preganglionic sympathetic activity and barostatic reflexes. Anesthesiology 31:515–521

35. Skovsted P, Price HL (1972) The effect of ethrane on arterial pressure, preganglionic sympathetic activity and barostatic reflexes. Anesthesiology 36:257–262
36. Skovsted P, Price ML, Price HL (1969) The effects of halothane on arterial pressure, preganglionic sympathetic activity, and barostatic reflexes. Anesthesiology 31:507–514
37. Stokke DB, Christensen NJ, Hole P, Andersen PK, Juhl B (1978) Plasma catecholamines during equipotent anaesthesia with cyclopropane and halothane-N_2O in man. Anaesthesist 27:469–474

Interactions of Cardiovascular Drugs with Inhalational Anaesthetics

P. Foëx, G.R. Cutfield and C.M. Francis

Introduction

The incidence of arterial hypertension and of coronary heart disease is very high. Many patients presenting for elective or emergency surgery and requiring anaesthesia are therefore treated with antihypertensive or anti-anginal medication. The possibility of interactions between cardiovascular drugs and inhalational anaesthetics must, therefore, be envisaged. Three main categories of drugs will be discussed in this review. Firstly, the antihypertensive agents; secondly, the adrenergic beta-receptor antagonists; and, thirdly, the more recently introduced calcium influx blockers. Interactions with other cardiovascular drugs, such as digitalis and anti-arrhythmic agents, will not be discussed.

Antihypertensive Medication

Arterial hypertension is most commonly associated with a normal cardiac output, and the high blood-pressure thus reflects increased systemic vascular resistance. The increase in systemic vascular resistance may be attributed to several factors. Reduction of arterial distensibility secondary to thickening of the arterial wall is an important determinant of high resistance to blood flow that is caused directly by reduction of intraluminal diameter [1, 2]. The loss of arterial distensibility decreases the capability of the arterial bed to behave as an elastic reservoir and to convert the highly pulsatile flow generated by the cardiac pump into a more continuous flow. This basic function of the larger arteries is lost in hypertensive disease [3]. Arteriolar constriction is another cause of high vascular resistance. It may occur in response to increased sympathetic nervous discharge or increased circulating vasoconstrictors (e.g. noradrenaline, renin, mineralocorticoids). The lack of circulating vasodilators (e.g. prostaglandins) may also be incriminated.

   With the exception of the adrenergic beta-receptor antagonists, most of the drugs used in the treatment of arterial hypertension act by dilating the arterioles. This effect may be caused either by their action on the sympathetic nervous system or by their direct action on the arteriolar smooth muscle. Reserpine, methyldopa, and clonidine appear to act essentially centrally. The mechanism involved includes depletion of catecholamine stores in the central nervous system and in effectors such as heart, adrenals, and arterial smooth muscle. Stimulation of alpha-2-adrenergic receptors in the brain-stem and medulla may also play a role. Stimulation of these receptors causes inhibition of central sympathetic outflow. Bethanidine, debrisoquin, and guanethidine are alpha-adrenergic neuron blockers. They impair transmission in post-ganglionic sympathetic fibres or block transmission at sympathetic nerve endings. Vasodilatation is most pronounced when the patient is in the upright position and during exercise. Postural hypotension and exercise-induced hypotension suggest profound blockade of circulatory reflexes [4].

Alpha-adrenergic receptor antagonists block the action of noradrenaline and adrenaline at the vascular receptor sites. They are used essentially in the treatment of hypertensive crises, in the preparation for surgery of phaeochromocytoma, and in the treatment of peripheral vasospasm. Phentolamine is a short-acting competetive antagonist, while thymoxamine, an agent used in the treatment of vasospasm, is a competitive antagonist with more prolonged action. Phenoxybenzamine is a non-competitive, long-acting alpha-adrenergic receptor antagonist. Labetalol combines alpha- and beta-adrenergic antagonist properties and is used in the treatment of arterial hypertension.

Relaxation of vascular smooth muscle may be achieved by administration of agents such as hydralazine and prazosin (long-term treatment) or diazoxide and sodium nitroprusside (hypertensive emergencies). Minoxidil, another peripheral vasodilator, is used in the treatment of severe hypertension but causes fluid retention.

Recently, another approach to reducing arterial tone has been suggested. Inhibition of an angiotensin-converting enzyme reduces conversion of angiotensin I into angiotensin II, and thus causes reduction of blood-pressure. Captopril is an orally active angiotensin-converting enzyme inhibitor currently being investigated for the treatment of arterial hypertension [5].

Diuretics are extensively used in the management of arterial hypertension. Their exact mode of action is not entirely clear. Reduction of plasma volume occurs in the early stage of their administration, but not during prolonged treatment. Vasodilatation due to reduction of sensitivity of the arterioles to noradrenaline may explain their efficacy in hypertension. Their effect on total body potassium stores must be borne in mind, since further losses of potassium are likely to occur during the post-operative period.

Anaesthesia

For many years considerable concern has been expressed by anaesthetists that increasingly potent antihypertensive drugs may profoundly disturb circulatory homeostasis during anaesthesia. After reports of circulatory collapse during induction of anaesthesia in reserpinized patients [6], and of bradycardia and hypotension during anaesthesia [7, 8], many authors have advocated that all antihypertensive drugs should be withdrawn before surgery [9, 10, 11]. As it became apparent that the problems of anaesthesia for the hypertensive patients are primarily those related to the association of ischaemic heart disease and cerebrovascular disease, and not those of pharmacological interactions between anaesthetic agents and antihypertensive medications, the validity of this practice has been questioned [12, 13, 14, 15].

Detailed studies of the cardiovascular and respiratory responses to anaesthesia have been carried out in treated and in untreated hypertensive patients [14, 16, 17, 18]. The antihypertensive medication consisted mostly of the association of reserpine, methyldopa, or bethanidine with a thiazide diuretic. Comparisons of the haemodynamic values in the two groups of patients showed that the reduction of arterial pressure and systemic vascular resistance caused by halothane supplementing nitrous oxide in oxygen were smaller in treated than in untreated patients (Fig. 1). Concern has often been expressed that because the anti-

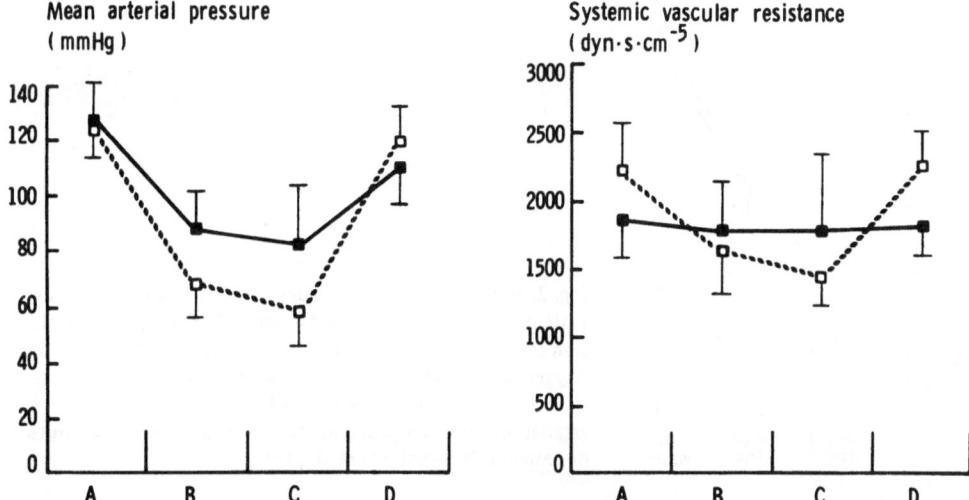

Fig. 1. In treated (■——■) and untreated (□••••□) hypertensive patients, haemodynamic values (expressed as mean and SEM) have been recorded in the awake state (*A*), under anaesthesia (nitrous oxide/oxygen supplemented by halothane) before (*B*) and after surgery (*C*), and finally in the awake state after surgery (*D*). Mean arterial pressure fell to a lesser extent in the treated than in the untreated patients. Systemic vascular resistance remained essentially unchanged in the treated patients. After Prys-Roberts et al. [14]

hypertensive drugs interfere with sympathetic reflexes, their maintenance could cause profound reductions of cardiac output during anaesthesia. Comparisons of treated and untreated hypertension showed cardiac output to be reduced to the same extent in the two groups of patients (Fig. 2). In the same studies the incidence of dysrhythmias and of electrocardio-

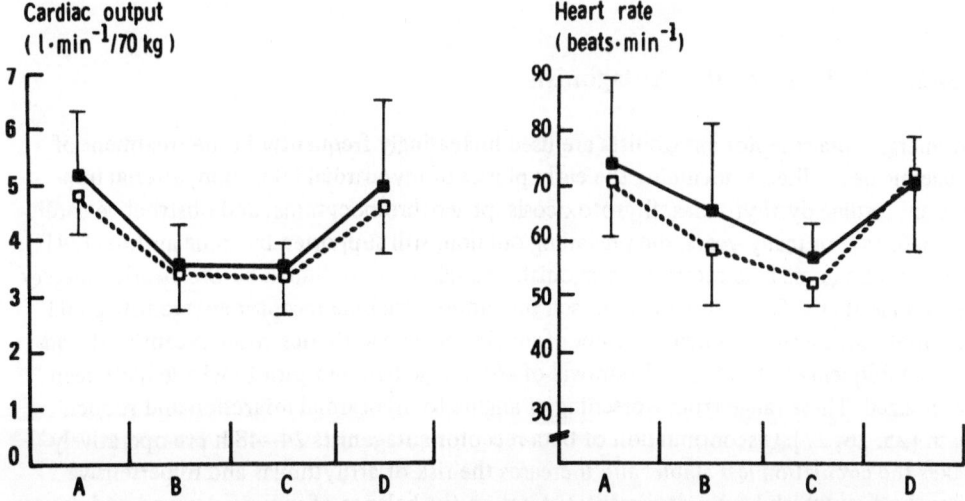

Fig. 2. In treated (■——■) and untreated (□••••□) hypertensive patients, values for cardiac output were almost identical in the awake state and under anaesthesia. Heart rate was slower under anaesthesia than in the awake state. At each stage the values were slightly higher in treated than in untreated patients. The haemodynamic values are given as on Fig. 1. After Prys-Roberts et al. [14]

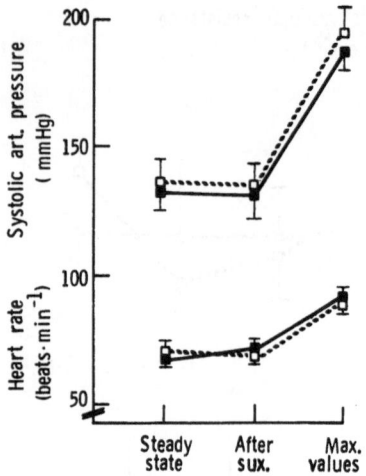

Fig. 3. In treated (■——■) and untreated (□···□) hypertensive patients, the effects of laryngoscopy and endotracheal intubation carried out under steady-state anaesthesia (nitrous oxide/oxygen supplemented by halothane) and facilitated by suxamethonium (*sux*) have been recorded. The increases in systolic arterial pressure and heart rate were similar in the two groups of patients. Prys-Roberts et al. [16]

graphic signs of myocardial ischaemia was found to be lower in the treated hypertensive patients. The hypertensive responses to laryngoscopy and endotracheal intubation were, however, hardly reduced in the treated hypertensive patients (Fig. 3). Following these studies demonstrating not only the absence of adverse interactions between halothane and antihypertensive drugs, but also the greater stability of the cardiovascular system of treated hypertensive patients, we have systematically advocated maintenance of antihypertension up until and including the morning of surgery, [14, 19, 20, 21]. This attitude is now widely accepted and most authors [22, 23] recommend maintenance of antihypertensive treatment. So far there has been no documented evidence of adverse interactions between the modern inhalational agents and antihypertensive medication. It should be stressed, however, that hypertensive patients, even if they are treated, may have an unstable cardiovascular system. Adequate monitoring is an essential part of their management.

Adrenergic Beta-receptor Antagonists

Adrenergic beta-receptor antagonists are used increasingly frequently in the treatment of ischaemic heart disease, including the early phases of myocardial infarction, arterial hypertension, cardiac dysrhythmias, thyrotoxicosis, phaeochromocytoma, and obstructive cardiomyopathies. For many years, the prevailing opinion, still supported by some authors [24] was that adrenergic beta-receptor antagonists should be discontinued before elective surgery under anaesthesia. Concern was expressed that adrenergic beta-receptor antagonists could potentiate the negative inotropic effect of inhalational anaesthetics. More recently, the adverse consequences of sudden withdrawal of adrenergic beta-receptor blockade have been emphasized. These range from worsening of angina to myocardial infarction and sudden death [25, 26, 27]. Discontinuation of beta-receptor antagonists 24—48 h pre-operatively makes the circulation less stable, and increases the risk of arrhythmias and hypertensive crises, both of which have a detrimental effect on the balance of oxygen demand and oxygen supply [28]. Conversely, maintenance of adrenergic beta-receptor blockade throughout the peri-operative period benefits the patients submitting for cardiac or non-cardiac surgery [29, 30, 31, 32].

Adrenergic beta-receptor antagonists also have a place in the anaesthetic management of many groups of patients, and are used to prevent and treat some of the manifestations of sympathetic over-activity that may develop during anaesthesia and surgery. They are used for the prevention and treatment of dysrhythmias associated with: laryngoscopy, endotracheal intubation, and bronchoscopy [29, 33]; catecholamines [34, 35]; or developing during dental surgery [36, 37], neurosurgery of the posterior fossa [38], cardiac and vascular surgery [39], or surgery of the thyroid gland [40] and of phaeochromocytoma [41]. They also minimize tachycardia caused by deliberately induced hypotension [42] and hypothermia [43]. Beta-adrenoceptor antagonists are effective in the prevention and treatment of hypertensive crises caused by anaesthetic or surgical manoeuvres [29, 31, 32, 44].

By providing more stable cardiovascular conditions and by protecting the myocardium against excessive increases in oxygen demand, beta-adrenoceptor antagonists contribute particularly to the safe anaesthetic management of patients with cardiovascular diseases. However, these powerful therapeutic agents may modify the cardiovascular responses of the surgical patient both under anaesthesia and during the post-operative period. Detailed knowledge of drug interactions is of considerable importance for the choice of the anaesthetic agents that are most suitable in the case of patients on adrenergic beta-receptor blockers, and also for the choice of the adrenergic beta-receptor blockers to be used during the peri-operative period.

Inhalational Anaesthetics

All inhalational anaesthetic agents exert a negative inotropic effect on the isolated heart muscle [45]. At concentrations corresponding to 1 MAC, depression of active force ranges between 12% for cyclopropane to about 40% for halothane, enflurane, methoxyflurane, and isoflurane. During clinical anaesthesia, the negative inotropic effect of the inhalational agents may be masked by the positive inotropic effect of sympathetic activation. The latter may be caused by the agent itself, e.g. diethyl ether and cyclopropane, or by surgical manoeuvres. By themselves, the modern anaesthetic agents do not increase sympathetic activity [46, 47] unless hypercapnia, hypoxia, or hypovolaemia are allowed to develop.

Halothane

When intermittent positive pressure ventilation is used, halothane causes dose-dependent reductions of cardiac output and arterial pressure [48, 49] because of its negative inotropic effect. Unless other factors, (i.e. hypercapnia, hypoxia, haemorrhage, severe anaemia, deliberate haemodilution, or administration of catecholamines) are responsible for increased sympathetic activity, adrenergic beta-receptor antagonists do not modify the cardiovascular responses to halothane anaesthesia.

In hypertensive patients, no adverse interaction has been observed between halothane and either intravenous practolol or oral pre-treatment with practolol. Arterial pressure and cardiac output were well maintained by comparison with values recorded in hypertensive patients not given beta-adrenoceptor antagonists. Both oral and intravenous practolol were shown to prevent hypertensive responses to laryngoscopy and intubation, and to decrease the incidence of dysrhythmias [29]. Adrenergic beta-receptor blockade thus appeared to protect the heart against the effects of sympathetic over-activity. In patients with coronary heart disease, the responses to halothane anaesthesia of patients treated with propranolol

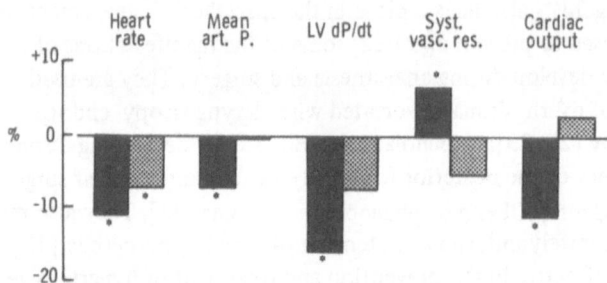

Fig. 4. In dogs, the effects of equipotent doses of metoprolol (1 mg • kg^{-1} i.v.) and practolol (2 mg • kg^{-1} i.v.) have been expressed as percent age change from control. Significant reductions of heart rate, arterial pressure, LV *dP/dt* and cardiac output, together with a significant increase of systemic vascular resistance, were observed after metoprolol (denoted by *solid black column*). After practolol (*shaded column*) only the reduction of heart rate reached statistical significance. After Burt and Foëx [52] and Prys-Roberts et al. [51]

have also been compared to those of untreated patients. No significant difference in arterial pressure or cardiac output was observed between the two groups thus confirming the lack of adverse interaction between adrenergic beta-receptor blockade and halothane anaesthesia [50].

Studies using the cardiovascular system of the dog as the experimental model have shown that under halothane anaesthesia practolol causes a significant but small reduction of heart rate (−14%), but no significant alterations of cardiac output, myocardial performance, and systemic vascular resistance [51]. Metoprolol, given in equipotent doses (Fig. 4), however, caused significant reductions of heart rate, cardiac output, and myocardial performance [52]. Both practolol and metoprolol are cardioselective beta-adrenoceptor antagonists. An important difference between the two agents is that metoprolol is a pure antagonist, while practolol is a partial agonist. Presence of partial agonist properties may minimize the effect of beta-1-adrenoceptor blockade on the circulation. In the case of non-selective beta-adreno-ceptor blockade the effects on the circulation of the partial agonist oxprenolol [53, 54] are of very small magnitude, at doses causing a ten-fold shift of the isoprenaline dose-response curve (Fig. 5).

Enflurane

Like halothane, enflurane causes dose-dependent reductions of arterial pressure and cardiac output due to myocardial depression when administered under normocapnic intermittent positive pressure ventilation [55, 56]. Similarly, enflurane causes dose-dependent reductions of pre-ganglionic sympathetic activity [46], and inhibits catecholamine secretion by the adrenal medulla [57]. Since there is no direct evidence of adrenergic stimulation caused by enflurane, adrenergic beta-receptor blockade should not modify the haemodynamic responses to enflurane anaesthesia. This is borne out by observations in patients treated with propranolol up to less than 12 h before operation. In these patients, enflurane anaesthesia was well tolerated [58]. However, in experimental studies, adrenergic beta-receptor blockade with propranolol has been shown to increase the negative inotropic effect of enflurane [55]. While at 1 MAC enflurane propranolol caused significant reductions of cardiac performance and arterial pressure, but not of cardiac output, at 1.5 MAC cardiac output was substantially reduced

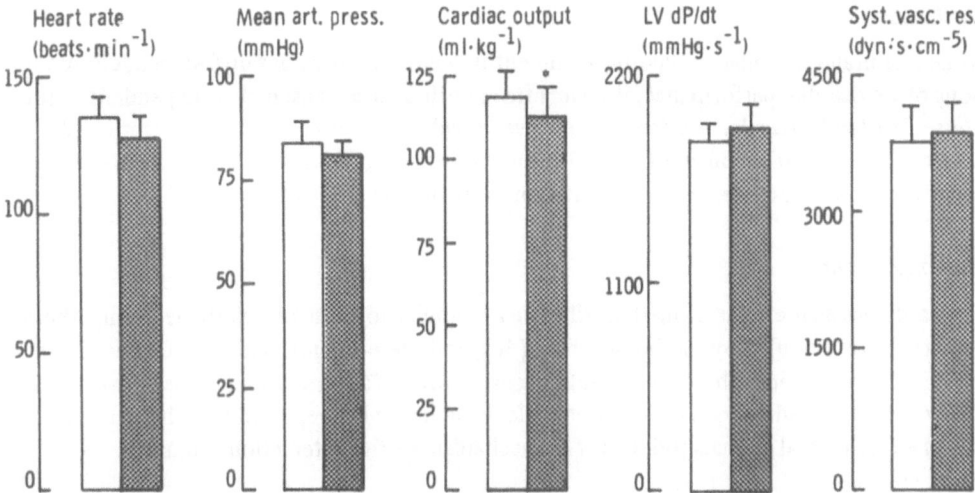

Fig. 5. In ten dogs anaesthetized with halothane, the intravenous administration of oxprenolol had little effect on the circulation. Though statistically significant, the reduction of cardiac output after oxprenolol was only by 4%. The *open columns* represent mean values (and SEM) before and the *shaded column* the mean values after oxprenolol. P. Foëx and W.A. Ryder, unpublished observations

and systemic vascular resistance was markedly elevated after beta-blockade. This adverse interaction between beta-blockade with propranolol and enflurane anaesthesia has not been confirmed by our recent study of the effect of oxprenolol (Fig. 6) under enflurane anaesthesia [59]. Doses of oxprenolol equipotent to those of propranolol previously reported were used. The dose-dependent depression of the circulation due to enflurane (from 0.5 to 1.5 MAC) was not modified by oxprenolol. Propranolol and oxprenolol are both non-selective adrenergic beta-receptor blockers. While propranolol is a pure antagonist, oxprenolol is a partial antagonist [54], and the lack of adverse interaction between oxprenolol and enflurane may be attributed to this characteristic of the agent.

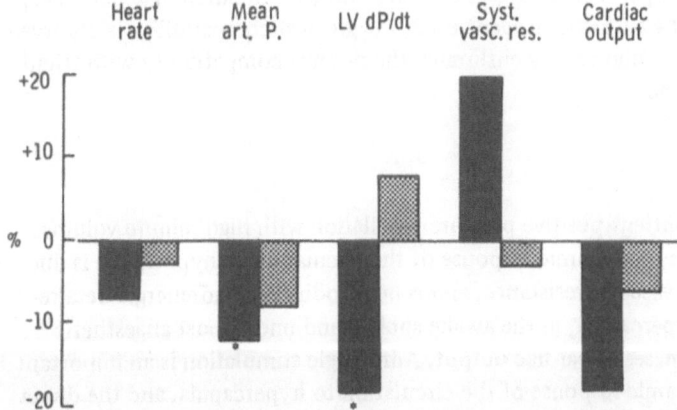

Fig. 6. In dogs anaesthetized with enflurane (1 MAC), the effects of equipotent doses of intravenous propranolol (0.3 mg · kg^{-1}, *solid black columns*) and oxprenolol (0.3 mg · kg^{-1}, *shaded columns*) have been represented as percentage change from control values. The effect of propranolol on the circulation was more pronounced than that of oxprenolol. After Horan et al. [55] and Cutfield et al. [59]

Isoflurane

While isoflurane is similar to halothane and enflurane in that it causes dose-dependent reductions of myocardial performance, it differs from both by also causing dose-dependent reductions of systemic vascular resistance. Thus over a wide range of concentrations isoflurane does not reduce cardiac output [60, 61]. Adrenergic beta-receptor blockade has only minimal effect on the responses of the circulation to isoflurane anaesthesia [61, 62].

Methoxyflurane

The cardiovascular effects of methoxyflurane are similar to those of halothane. Sympathetic activity is not modified by methoxyflurane [46], and therefore no adverse interaction with adrenergic beta-receptor blockade should occur. However, adverse interactions between methoxyflurane and adrenergic beta-receptor blockade have been reported both in man [63] and in experimental animals [64, 65]. The mechanism of this interaction is unclear.

Hypovolaemia

Hypovolaemia causes increases in sympathetic activity. Therefore, blockade of the adrenergic beta-receptors may be expected to modify the response of the circulation to acute hypovolaemia. Experimental studies of the effect of adrenergic beta-receptor blockade on the response of the circulation to standardized unreplaced blood loss have been carried out under various anaesthetic agents [51, 55, 61, 64]. While under anaesthesia with halothane supplementing nitrous oxide in oxygen neither practolol nor propranolol appeared to modify the responses of the circulation to haemorrhage, under enflurane anaesthesia beta-receptor blockade markedly increased the circulatory depression due to hypovolaemia. Under isoflurane anaesthesia, tolerance to blood loss was found to be unaffected by propranolol. Even in the presence of prolonged pre-treatment with very high doses of propranolol or oxprenolol, the responses of the circulation to blood loss were found to be no different from those observed in untreated animals [66, 67] when the challenge was applied under halothane anaesthesia. Under trichloroethylene anaesthesia, however, blood loss was more poorly tolerated in the beta-blocked animals. These experiments suggest that the influence of adrenergic beta-receptor blockade depends upon the anaesthetic agent used; the greatest compatibility is observed with halothane and isoflurane, followed by enflurane, the poorest compatibility with trichloroethylene and methoxyflurane.

Carbon Dioxide

Hypocapnia caused by intermittent positive pressure ventilation with high minute volumes reduces cardiac output. The hypodynamic response of the circulation to hypocapnia is due mostly to increased systemic vascular resistance, and is not modified by adrenergic beta-receptor blockade [53, 68]. Hypercapnia, in the awake subject and under most anaesthetic agents, causes significant increases of cardiac output. Adrenergic stimulation is an important determinant of the hyperdynamic response of the circulation to hypercapnia, and the direct myocardial depressant effect of CO_2 on the heart muscle is completely compensated for by the effect on the heart of beta-receptor stimulation. Blockade of the adrenergic beta-receptors suppress this support, and thus reduce cardiac output [67, 68] unless the agent is a partial agonist [53]. In the latter case the reduction of cardiac output is not significant.

Myocardial Ischaemia

Most of the experimental studies of the effects of volatile anaesthetic agents have been carried out on normal hearts and have examined global cardiac performance. A few studies have examined aspects of regional cardiac function in animals in which acute myocardial ischaemia had been induced by complete occlusion of one or several coronary arteries. Halothane has been shown to decrease the severity of ischaemia following repeated reversible occlusions of a branch of the left anterior descending coronary artery [69], and to decrease infarct size after coronary artery ligation [70]. However, studies of the effects of anaesthesia on myocardium supplied by a narrowed coronary artery may be more relevant to the problem of anaesthesia for patients with ischaemic heart disease than studies of the effects of anaesthesia after complete occlusion of a major coronary artery. Recently the effects of graded concentration of halothane [71, 72, 73] and of enflurane [74] on global and regional myocardial function have been studied in dogs, before and after critical constriction of the left anterior descending coronary artery (Fig. 7). Critical constriction was defined as the maximum degree of tightening of a micrometer-controlled snare that was compatible with a normal pattern of contraction and abolished 95% of the hyperaemic response to 10 s of complete occlusion of the constricted vessel. Regional wall function was evaluated by observing segment length throughout the cardiac cycle. This was measured with miniature ultrasonic length transducers implanted in subendocardial muscle. With this experimental model it has been possible to examine the responses to stepped increases of either halothane or enflurane concentration. Increasing the concentration of either of these agents caused dose-dependent reductions of global cardiac performance and of segment shortening. However, regional myo-

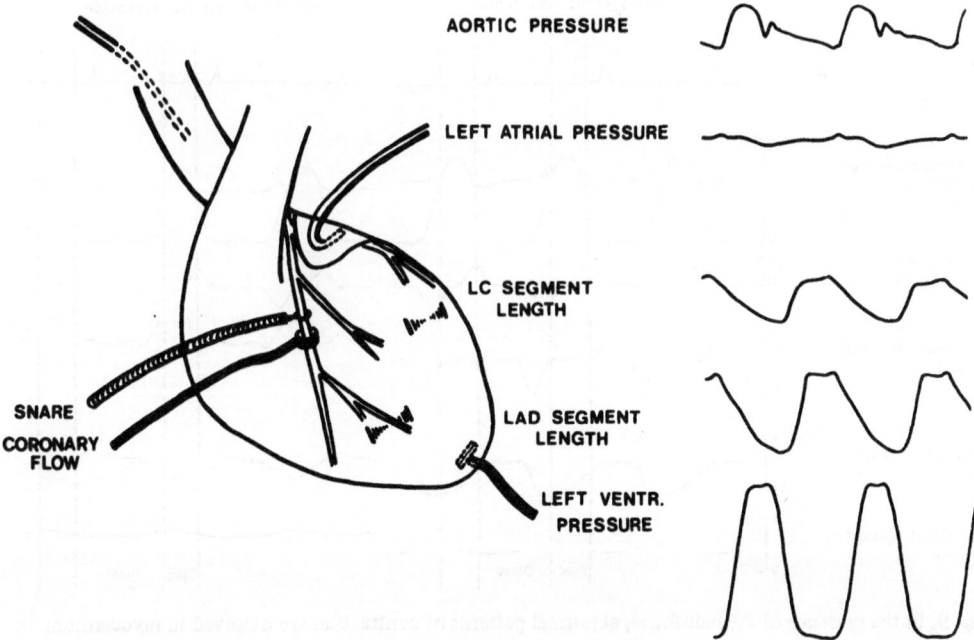

Fig. 7. Experimental model used for studies of the effects of volatile anaesthetic agents on myocardium supplied by critically narrowed coronary arteries. The snare placed around the left anterior descending coronary artery is controlled by a micrometer

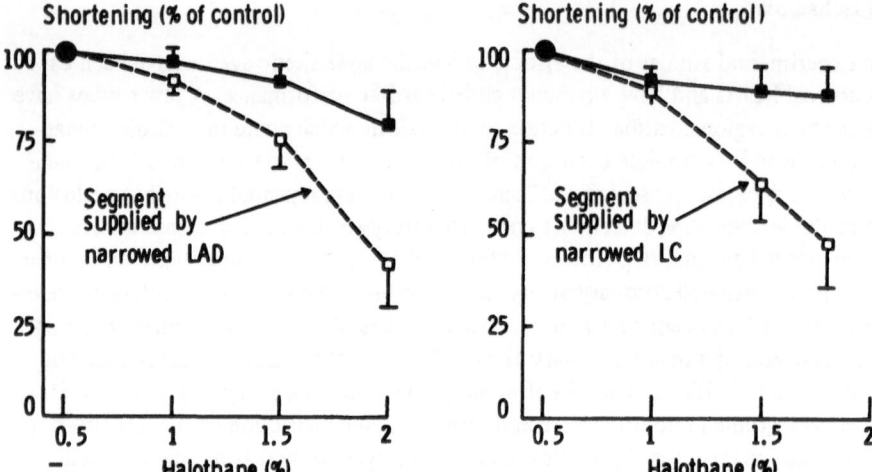

Fig. 8. The effects of stepped increases of halothane concentrations have been studied in dogs after critical constriction of either the left anterior descending coronary artery (*LAD*, left-hand panel) or the left circumflex coronary artery (*LC*, right-hand panel), and expressed as mean values (and SEM). The *solid symbols* relate to performance of control segments supplied by normal coronary vessels. Halothane causes substantially more depression of the myocardium supplied by narrowed vessels. After Lowenstein et al. [73] and Francis et al. [103]

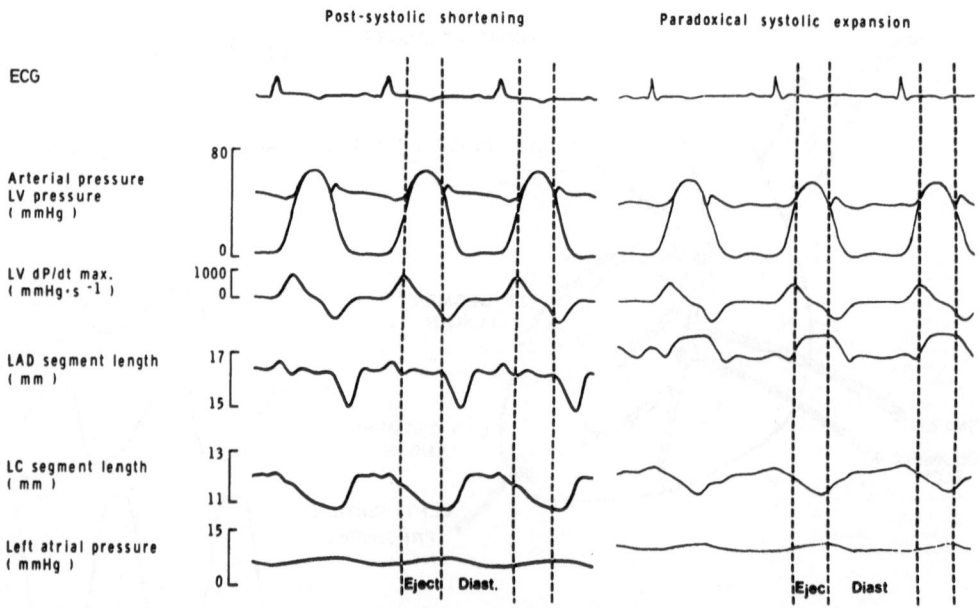

Fig. 9. In the presence of 2% halothane, abnormal patterns of contraction are observed in myocardium supplied by a critically narrowed left anterior descending coronary artery (*LAD*). Inspection of the length signals indicates the presence of post-systolic shortening (*left*) and paradoxical systolic lengthening (*right*) in the area supplied by the critically narrowed LAD. *LV dP/dt max*, maximum rate of pressure generation in the left ventricle; *LC*, left circumflex coronary artery

cardial depression was found to be considerably more severe in areas supplied by the narrowed coronary arteries than in areas supplied by normal coronary vessels (Fig. 8). Moreover, abnormal patterns of contractions were observed. Regional dysfunction, when present, was characterized by post-systolic shortening and by paradoxical expansion of the segment supplied by the narrowed vessel (Fig. 9). These features are similar to those observed in the case of myocardial ischaemia [75, 76]. That halothane and enflurane cause myocardial depression at both regional and global level is not surprising. However, the greater degree of depression of myocardium supplied by the narrowed but not occluded coronary artery needs to be explained; particularly important is the observation of alterations suggestive of myocardial ischaemia. Both halothane and enflurane cause dose-dependent reductions of diastolic arterial pressure accompanied by dose-dependent increases in left ventricular end-diastolic pressure. They thus cause substantial reductions of the coronary perfusion pressure gradient. In territories supplied by narrowed arteries, autoregulation of coronary blood flow has been suppressed and coronary blood flow is directly proportional to the coronary perfusion pressure gradient. If oxygen demand decreases less than oxygen supply, signs of myocardial ischaemia may develop. Indeed, in the case of both volatile agents, reductions of arterial pressure, as well as depression of contractility, contribute to the reduction of oxygen demand. However, the increase in end-diastolic tension is a factor that simultaneously contributes to a reduction in the coronary perfusion pressure and an increase in oxygen demand. Moreover, the subendocardium, the area where wall motion was determined, is the area most likely to have compromised blood flow when perfusion pressure decreases and end-diastolic wall tension increases. Stepped increases of concentration of volatile agents may thus cause imbalance between oxygen supply and oxygen demand, and this would explain the patterns of dysfunction that have been observed. If dysfunction is caused by an imbalance of oxygen demand and supply, then adrenergic beta-adrenoceptor blockade may be expected to exert a protective role. In the case of complete occlusion of coronary arteries, adrenergic beta-receptor blockade has been shown to improve regional myocardial function [75, 76]. Similarly, in the case of dysfunction caused by halothane [77] and by enflurane [78], improvement of shortening together with reduction of post-systolic shortening have been observed after administration of oxprenolol (Figs. 10 and 11). The fact that adrenergic beta-receptor blockade with oxprenolol appears to protect the myocardium against the effect of halothane and enflurane, and minimizes the risk of paradoxical wall motion, reinforces our view that adrenergic beta-receptor blockade is an important part of the anaesthetic management of patients with ischaemic and hypertensive heart disease.

Calcium Influx Blockers

In the cardiovascular system, calcium ions are of great importance. In myocardial cells and in specialized automatic and conducting cells, Ca^{2+} is involved in the genesis of cardiac action potentials, the excitation contraction coupling, and the control of energy storage and utilization. Movement of calcium ions across the membrane of smooth muscle alters smooth muscle tone, and thus the calibre (and resistance) of coronary and systemic arteries.

Over the last 20 years a number of agents that block the movement of calcium ions across cell membranes have been developed, and have been used in the treatment of cardiac arrhythmias, myocardial ischaemia (particularly when coronary artery spasm appears to play a role), hypertension, and hypertrophic cardiomyopathy. While the term "calcium antago-

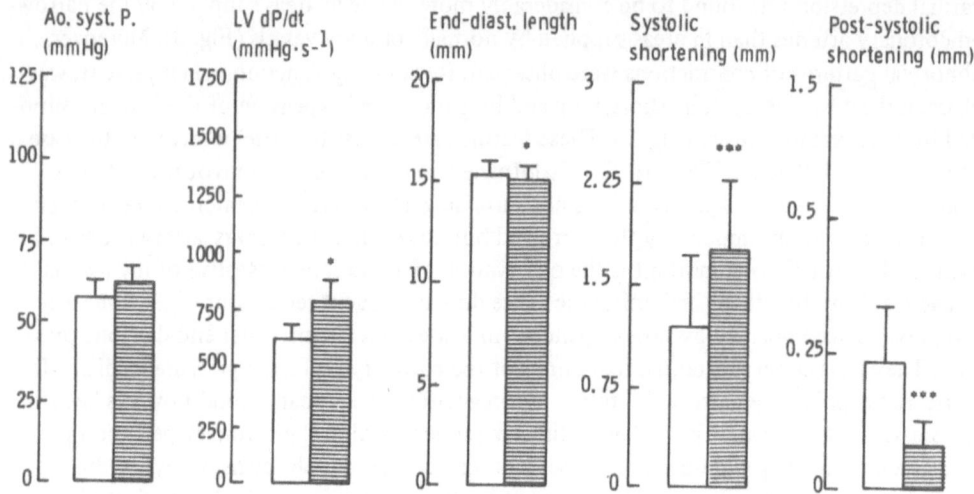

Fig. 10. In the presence of 2% halothane and of critical constriction of the left anterior descending coronary artery, oxprenolol improves global and regional myocardial function. After oxprenolol (0.3 mg · kg⁻¹ i.v.), systolic shortening is significantly increased while post-systolic shortening is significantly reduced. The *open columns* denote values before and the *shaded columns* after oxprenolol [77]. *Ao. syst. p,* aortic systolic pressure; *LV dP/dt,* left ventricular pressure generation rate

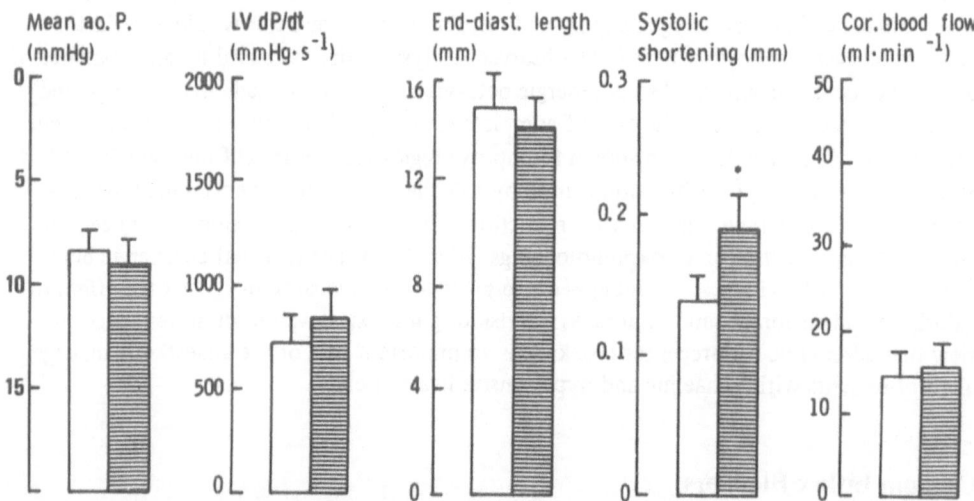

Fig. 11. In the presence of 3.3% enflurane, and of critical constriction of the left anterior descending coronary artery, oxprenolol improves regional function. After oxprenolol (0.3 mg · kg⁻¹ i.v.) systolic shortening is significantly increased in the area supplied by the critically narrowed coronary artery. The *open columns* denote values before and the *shaded columns* after oxprenolol [78]. *LV dP/dt,* left ventricular pressure generation rate; *Ao. P.,* aortic pressure

nists" has been widely used, this new class of drug should be referred to as "calcium influx blockers". These drugs lower intracellular calcium ion concentration by inhibiting the slow calcium influx that occurs during the plateau of the action potential. This inhibition, however, does not occur according to the traditional concepts of agonist-antagonist relationships. The calcium blockers have been subdivided into those altering the kinetics of calcium flux (verapamil) and those altering the total calcium conductance (nifidepine, diltiazem). This subdivision is based on differential effects on two gates in the calcium channel [79]. In the vascular smooth muscle, calcium blockers reduce intracellular calcium, but the mechanisms involved may be unrelated to the slow calcium current and thus differ from the effect on the myocardium [80].

Electrophysiology

Calcium channel blocking agents decrease the rate of sinus node discharge (negative chronotropic effect) and reduce conduction velocity through the atrioventricular node (negative dromotropic effect) [81]. Prolongation of atrioventricular nodal refractoriness and slowing of conduction explain the clinical effectiveness of verapamil in controlling supraventricular dysrhythmias dependent on re-entry involving the atrioventricular node. Experimental ventricular arrhythmias caused by coronary artery ligation are prevented by calcium blockers, but the role of these drugs in the management of ventricular arrhythmias complicating myocardial infarction is disputed. The place of calcium blockers in the treatment of dysrhythmias appears to be the control of supraventricular tachycardias, particularly re-entrant paroxysmal supraventricular tachycardias. Slowing of the ventricular rate in case of atrial fibrillation and atrial flutter is easily obtained, but the safety of using calcium blockers when these dysrhythmias are due to myocardial infarction needs further investigation. During halothane anaesthesia, intravenous verapamil has been shown to be effective in inhibiting ventricular and supraventricular dysrhythmias, but to be without effect on sinus tachycardia of adrenergic origin [82].

Myocardial Contractility

The net effect of the calcium blockers results from direct and reflex mediated actions. In denervated preparation, calcium blockers cause dose-dependent reductions of myocardial contractility that can be reversed by administration of calcium ions [83]. Myocardial oxygen consumption also decreases in a dose-dependent fashion. In the intact animal, however, reduction of peripheral vascular resistance may be substantial, and the resulting arterial hypotension may cause baroreceptor-mediated positive inotropic and chronotropic responses [84]. In this case the inotropic state of the myocardium may return to normal, tachycardia may be observed, and myocardial oxygen consumption is reduced because of the reduced afterload. The reflexly mediated responses to calcium blockers are suppressed by adrenergic beta-receptor antagonists. The negative inotropic effect of verapamil is potentiated by beta-adrenoceptor blockade [85], but not that of diltiazem [86]. The potential risk of a negative interaction between beta-blockers and calcium blockers has been emphasized [87], particularly in the case of their intravenous administration [88].

Coronary Circulation

Calcium blockers decrease smooth muscle tone in the coronary arteries, reduce coronary vascular resistance, and increase coronary blood flow [89]. This effect can be abolished only by increasing the extracellular calcium ion concentration and not by adrenergic beta-recep-

tor blockade. When administered soon after coronary artery ligation, calcium blockers augment coronary flow distal to the ligature. This enhanced collateral flow to the ischaemic area
may be caused by a reduction of coronary arteriolar resistance in vessels supplying the collat-
erals [90].

Ischaemic Myocardium

While agents that increase myocardial oxygen consumption have been found to increase infarct size, agents which reduce myocardial oxygen demand have a protective effect on the
acutely ischaemic myocardium [91]. Besides preventing ventricular fibrillation following coronary occlusion [92], verapamil significantly reduces epicardial ST segment elevations over
areas of ischaemic myocardium, and minimizes the haemodynamic deterioration caused by
ligation of the left anterior descending coronary artery [93, 94]. Increased collateral coronary blood flow is observed [94], but may not be the sole explanation of the improvement of
myocardial ischaemia after verapamil because administration of other coronary dilators,
such as dipyridamole, do not improve signs of ischaemia [95]. Peripheral vasodilatation and
hypotension are also unlikely to explain the beneficial effect of verapamil since, in the face
of ischaemia, hypotension aggravates ST segment alterations [91] and worsens function of
myocardium supplied by a narrowed coronary artery [72, 73]. The protective effect may be
due not only to effects on cardiac membranes but also to reduced intracellular uptake of calcium. Indeed, verapamil appears to protect the fine ultrastructure of heart muscle against
damage caused by hypoxia [96], and also to protect mitochondrial function [97]. However,
regional contractile function of myocardium made partially ischaemic is depressed by verapamil while function of normal myocardium is maintained [98]. In man, the effect of verapamil on myocardial performance in coronary disease has been found to be of negligible importance, possibly because cardiac depression is accompanied by vasodilatation and, therefore, reduction of left ventricular after-load [99].

Anaesthesia

With the growing interest in calcium blockers for the treatment not only of supraventricular
dysrhythmias but also of ischaemic heart disease and arterial hypertension, there may be a
substantial increase in the number of patients treated with calcium blockers presenting for
elective or emergency surgery and requiring anaesthesia. There have only been a few reports
of the interactions between calcium blockers and anaesthesia. Brichard and Zimmerman [82]
have used verapamil for the treatment of supraventricular and ventricular dysrhythmias observed under light halothane anaesthesia. They observed a reduction of both systolic and diastolic arterial pressures after verapamil 20 mg i.v. The reduction of blood-pressure lasted
5 min and was attributed to peripheral vasodilatation. In the absence of data concerning cardiac output and performance, hypotension could have been due to negative inotropy. Verapamil has also been used in a study of mechanisms of ketamine-induced hypertension [100].
Intravenous verapamil caused immediate falls in systolic pressure accompanied by moderate
reductions of the amplitude of finger and muscle plethysmograms, presumably reflecting
diminished contractility. In the experimental animal large doses of verapamil cause substantial reductions of arterial pressure that may be caused by the combination of vasodilation
and myocardial depression [101, 102].

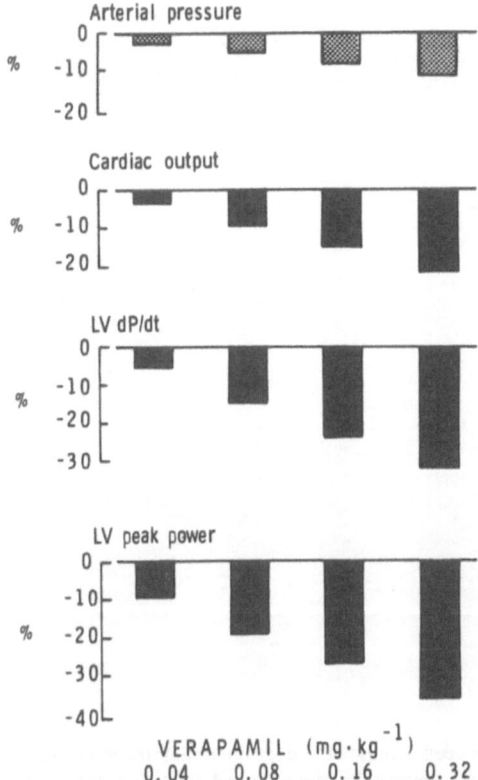

Fig. 12. The effects of verapamil on the circulation have been examined in dogs under halothane anaesthesia. Substantial dose-dependent reductions of cardiac output and of left ventricular performance have been noted. *LV dP/dt*, left ventricular pressure generation rate. P. Foëx, C.M. Francis, and G.R. Cutfield, unpublished observations

In a preliminary series of experiments we have examined the effects of verapamil on global and regional wall function, in dogs anaesthetized with halothane in oxygen, under normocapnic IPPV. While verapamil caused only modest changes of arterial pressure and did not modify heart rate, substantial dose-dependent reductions of global and regional performance, accompanied by reductions of cardiac output, were observed (Figs. 12 and 13). Myocardial depression was confirmed by the dose-dependent increases in left ventricular end-diastolic pressure and in end-diastolic segment length. Abnormal patterns of contraction were also observed following the higher doses of verapamil. The magnitude of the interaction between verapamil and halothane suggests that until further detailed studies are available, anaesthetists should be aware of the possibility of adverse interactions between calcium influx blockers and commonly used anaesthetic agents.

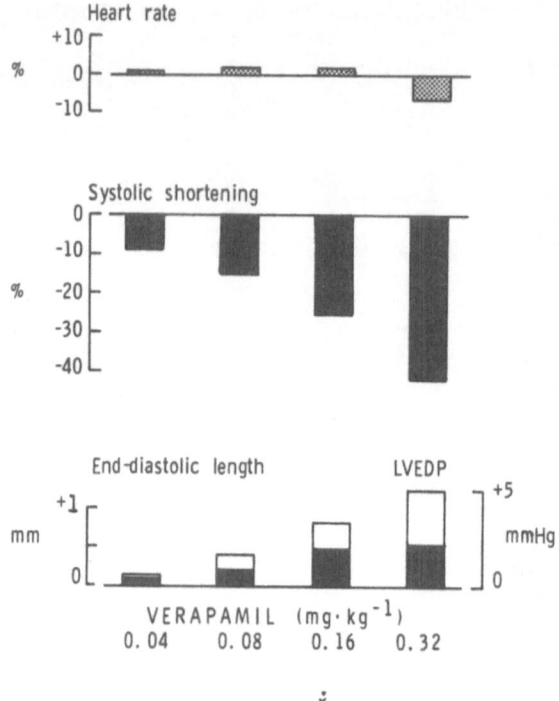

Fig. 13. The effects of verapamil on the circulation have been examined in dogs under halothane anaesthesia. Substantial reductions of systolic shortening have been observed, while both end-diastolic length and end-diastolic left ventricular pressure were recorded. On the lowest part of the diagram, the *solid columns* refer to end-diastolic length and the *open columns* to left ventricular end-diastolic pressure (*LVEDP*), P. Foex, C.M. Francis, and G.R. Cutfield, unpublished observations

References

1. Folkow B (1971) The haemodynamic consequences of adaptive structural changes of the resistance vessels in hypertension. Clin Sci 41:1
2. Folkow B (1978) Cardiovascular structural adaptation: its role in the initiation and maintenance of primary hypertension (The fourth Volhard Lecture). Clin Sci Mol Med [Suppl IV] 55:3
3. O'Rourke MF (1970) Arterial haemodynamics in hypertension. Circ Res [Suppl II] 26–27:123
4. Kirby B (1980) Drug therapy for hypertension and ischaemic heart disease. Int Anesthesiol Clin 18. 4:25
5. Ferguson RK, Vlasses PH, Koplin JR, Shirinian A, Burke JF, Alexander JC (1980) Captopril in severe treatment-resistant hypertension. Am Heart J 99:579
6. Smessaert AA, Hicks RG (1961) Problems caused by rauwolfia drugs during anesthesia and surgery. NY State J Med 61:2399
7. Coakley CS, Alpert S, Boling JS (1956) Circulatory responses during anesthesia of patients on rauwolfia therapy. JAMA 161:1143
8. Ziegler CH, Lovette JB (1961) Operative complications after therapy with reserpine compounds. JAMA 176:916
9. Leroy-Crandell D (1962) The anesthetic hazards in patients on antihypertensive therapy. JAMA 179:495

10. Rüdiger H, Linde I, Poppelbaum HF (1972) Antihypertensiva und Anaesthesie. Z Ärztl Fortbild 66:1187
11. Dundee JW (1958) Iatrogenic disease and anaesthesia. Br Med J 1:1433
12. Dingle HR (1966) Antihypertensive drugs and anaesthesia. Anaesthesia 21:151
13. Ominski AJ, Wollman H (1969) Hazards of general anesthesia in the reserpinized patient. Anesthesiology 30:443
14. Prys-Roberts C, Meloche R, Foëx P (1971) Studies of anaesthesia in relation to hypertension. I. Cardiovascular responses of treated and untreated patients. Br J Anaesth 43:122
15. Goldberg LI (1972) Anesthetic management of patients treated with antihypertensive agents or levodopa. Anesth Analg (Cleve) 51:625
16. Prys-Roberts C, Greene LT, Meloche R, Foëx P (1971) Studies of anaesthesia in relation to hypertension. II. Haemodynamic consequences of induction and endotracheal intubation. Br J Anaesth 43:531
17. Foëx P, Meloche R, Prys-Roberts C (1971) Studies of anaesthesia in relation to hypertension. III. Pulmonary gas exchange during spontaneous ventilation. Br J Anaesth 43:644
18. Prys-Roberts C, Foëx P, Greene LT, Waterhouse TD (1972) Studies of anaesthesia in relation to hypertension. IV. The effects of artificial ventilation on the circulation and pulmonary gas exchange. Br J Anaesth 44:335
19. Foëx P, Prys-Roberts C (1974) Anaesthesia and the hypertensive patient. Br J Anaesth 46:575
20. Prys-Roberts C (1976) Medical problems of surgical patients. Hypertension and ischaemic heart disease. Ann R Coll Surg Engl 58:465
21. Prys-Roberts C, Meloche R (1980) Management of anaesthesia in patients with hypertension or ischaemic heart disease. Int Anaesthesiol Clin 18. 4:181
22. Abrams LM, Chambers DA (1979) Pre-operative management. In: Kaplan JA (ed) Cardiac anesthesia. Grune & Stratton, New York, p 169
23. Brown BR (1980) Anesthetic considerations in essential hypertension. In: Brown BR (ed) Anesthesia and the patient with heart disease. F.A. Davis Company, Philadelphia, p 89
24. Hillis LD, Cohn PF (1978) Non-cardiac surgery in patients with coronary artery disease. Arch Intern Med 138:972
25. Slome R (1973) Withdrawal of propranolol and myocardial infarction. Lancet I:156
26. Miller RR, Olson HG, Amsterdam EA, Mason DT (1975) Propranolol withdrawal rebound phenomenon. N Engl J Med 293:416
27. Shand DG, Wood AJJ (1978) Propranolol withdrawal syndrome: why? Circulation 58:202
28. Slogoff S, Keats AS, Ott E (1978) Pre-operative propranolol therapy and aortocoronary bypass operation. JAMA 240:1487
29. Prys-Roberts C, Foëx P, Biro GP, Roberts JG (1973) Studies of anaesthesia in relation to hypertension. V. Adrenergic beta-receptor blockade. Br J Anaesth 45:671
30. Boudoulas H, Lewis RP, Snyder GL, Karayannacos P, Vasko JS (1979) Beneficial effect of continuation of propranolol through coronary bypass surgery. Clon Cardiol 2:87
31. Manners JM, Walters FJM (1979) Beta-adrenoceptor blockade and anaesthesia. Anaesthesia 34:3
32. Oka Y, Frishman W, Becker RM, Kadish A, Strom J, Matsumoto M, Orkin L, Frater R (1980) Clinical pharmacology of the new beta-adrenergic blocking drugs. Part 10. Beta-adrenoceptor blockade and coronary artery surgery. Am Heart J 99:255
33. Jenkins AV (1970) Adrenergic beta-blockade with ICI 50.172 (practolol) during bronchoscopy. Br J Anaesth 42:59
34. Katz RL (1965) Effects of alpha- and beta-adrenergic blocking agents on cyclopropane-catecholamine cardiac arrhythmias. Anesthesiology 26:289
35. Pöntinen PJ (1978) Cardiovascular effects of local adrenaline infiltration during halothane anaesthesia and adrenergic beta-receptor blockade in man. Acta Anaesthesiol Scand 22:130
36. Ryder W, Charlton JE, Gorman PBW (1971) Practolol and atropine medication in dental anaesthesia. Anaesthesia 26:508
37. Rollason WN, Russell JG (1980) Intravenous metoprolol and cardiac dysrhythmias. An evaluation in the management of dysrhythmias in outpatient dental anesthesia. Anesthesia 35:783
38. Whitby JD (1963) Electrocardiography during posterior fossa operation. Br J Anaesth 35:624
39. Moran JC, Caralps JM, Mulet J, Pifarre (1973) Propranolol and cardiac surgery. N Engl J Med 289:1254

40. Bird CC, Hayward I, Howells TH, Jones GD (1969) Cardiac arrhythmias during thyroid surgery. Anaesthesia 24:180

41. Bingham W, Elliot J, Lyons SM (1972) Management of anaesthesia for phaeochromocytoma. Anaesthesia 27:49

42. Hellewell J, Potts MW (1966) Propranolol during controlled hypotension. Br J Anaesth 38:794

43. Finlay WEI, Dykes WS (1968) Cardiac arrhythmias during hypothermia controlled by propranolol. Anaesthesia 23:631

44. Prys-Roberts C (1979) Hemodynamic effects of anaesthesia and surgery in renal hypertensive patients receiving large doses of beta-receptor antagonists. Anesthesiology 51:S122

45. Shimosato S, Etsten BE (1969) Effects of anesthetic drugs on the deart: a critical review of myocardial contractility and its relationship to haemodynamics. Clin Anesth 9. 3:17

46. Skovsted P, Price HL (1972) The effects of Ethrane on arterial pressure, preganglionic sympathetic activity and barostatic reflexes. Anesthesiology 36:257

47. Skovsted P, Sapthavichakul S (1977) The effect of isoflurane on arterial pressure, pulse rate, autonomic nervous activity and barostatic reflexes. Can Anaesth Soc J 24:304

48. Prys-Roberts C, Gersh BJ, Baker AB, Reuben SR (1972) The effects of halothane on the interactions between myocardial contractility, aortic impedance and left ventricular performance. I. Theoretical considerations and result. Br J Anaesth 44:634

49. Prys-Roberts C, Lloyd JW, Fisher A, Kerr JH, Patterson TJS (1974) Deliberate profound hypotension induced with halothane: studies of haemodynamics and pulmonary gas exchange. Br J Anaesth 46:105

50. Kopriva CJ, Brown ACD, Pappas G (1978) Haemodynamics during general anesthesia in patients receiving propranolol. Anesthesiology 48:28

51. Prys-Roberts C, Roberts JG, Foëx P, Clarke TNS, Bennett MJ, Ryder WA (1976) Interaction of anesthesia, beta-receptor blockade and blood loss in dogs with induced myocardial infarction. Anesthesiology 45:326

52. Burt G, Foëx P (1979) Effects of metoprolol on systemic haemodynamics, myocardial performance and the coronary circulation during halothane anaesthesia. Br J Anaesth 51:829

53. Foëx P, Ryder WA (1981) Interactions of adrenergic beta-receptor blockade (oxprenolol) and PCO_2 in the anesthetized dog. Influence of intrinsic sympathomimetic activity. Br J Anesth 53:19

54. Foëx P, Roberts JG, Saner CA, Bennett MJ (to be published) Oxprenolol and the circulation during anaesthesia in the dog: influence of intrinsic sympathomimetic activity. Br J Anaesth 53

55. Horan BF, Prys-Roberts C, Hamilton WK, Roberts JG (1977) Haemodynamic responses to enflurane anaesthesia and hypovolaemia in the dog and their modification by propranolol. Br J Anaesth 49:1189

56. Calverley RK, Smith NT, Prys-Roberts C, Eger EI, Jones CW (1978) Cardiovascular effects of enflurane anesthesia during controlled ventilation in man. Anesth Analg (Cleve) 57:619

57. Göthert M, Wendt J (1977) Inhibition of adrenal medullary catecholamine secretion by enflurane. Anesthesiology 46:400

58. Kaplan JA, Dunbar RW (1976) Propranolol and surgical anaesthesia. Anesth Analg (Cleve) 55:1

59. Cutfield GR, Francis CM, Foëx P, Ryder WA, Jones LA (to be published) The effects of oxprenolol on myocardial function during enflurane anaesthesia. Br J Anaesth 53

60. Stevens WC, Cromwell TH, Halsey MJ, Eger EI, Shakespeare TF, Bahlman SH (1971) The cardiovascular effects of a new inhalation anesthetic, forane, in human volunteers at constant arterial carbon dioxide tension. Anesthesiology 38:8

61. Horan BF, Prys-Roberts C, Roberts JG, Bennett MJ, Foëx P (1977) Haemodynamic responses to isoflurane anaesthesia and hypovolaemia in the dog, and their modification by propranolol. Br J Anaesth 49:1179

62. Philbin D, Lowenstein E (1976) Lack of beta-adrenergic activity of isoflurane in the dog: a comparison of circulatory effects of halothane and isoflurane after propranolol administration. Br J Anaesth 48:1165

63. Viljoen JF, Estafanous G, Kellner GA (1972) Propranolol and cardiac surgery. J Thorac Cardiovasc Surg 64:826

64. Saner CA, Foëx P, Roberts JG, Bennett MJ (1975) Methoxyflurane and practolol: a dangerous combination. Br J Anaesth 47:1025

65. Kaplan JA, Dunbar RW, Bland JW, Sumpter R, Jones EL (1975) Propranolol and cardiac surgery: a problem for the anesthesiologist. Anesth Analg (Cleve) 54:571

66. Roberts JG, Foëx P, Clarke TNS, Bennett MG, Saner CA (1976) Haemodynamic interactions of high-dose propranolol pretreatment and anaesthesia in the dog. III. The effects of haemorrhage during halothane and trichloroethylene anaesthesia. Br J Anaesth 48:411

67. Foëx P (1977) Beta-adrenergic blockade, arrhythmias and anaesthesia. Proc R Soc Med [Suppl II] 70:17

68. Foëx P, Prys-Roberts C (1974) Interactions of beta-receptor blockade and PCO_2 levels in the anaesthetized dog. Br J Anaesth 46:397

69. Bland JHK, Lowenstein E (1976) Halothane-induced decrease in experimental myocardial ischaemia in the nonfailing canine heart. Anesthesiology 45:287

70. Davis RF, DeBoer LWV, Rude RE, Lowenstein E, Maroko PR (1979) Beneficial effect of halothane on myocardial infarction size in dogs. Crit Care Med 7:134

71. Lowenstein E, Foëx P, Francis CM, Davies WL, Yusuf S, Ryder WA (1979) Narrowed coronary arteries, halothane, and paradox. Anesthesiology 51:S62

72. Francis CM, Lowenstein E, Davies WL, Foëx P, Ryder WA (1980) Effect of halothane on the performance of myocardium supplied by a narrowed artery. Br J Anaesth 52:236P

73. Lowenstein E, Foëx P, Francis CM, Davies WL, Yusuf S, Ryder W (to be published) Regional ischaemic ventricular dysfunction in myocardium supplied by a narrowed coronary artery with increasing halothane concentration in the dog. Anesthesiology

74. Cutfield GR, Francis CM, Foëx P, Lowenstein E, Davies WL, Ryder WA (1980) Myocardial function and critical constriction of the left anterior descending coronary artery: effects of enflurane. Br J Anaesth 52:953P

75. Theroux P, Ross J, Franklin D, Kemper WS, Sasayama S (1976) Regional myocardial function in the conscious dog during acute coronary occlusion and responses to morphine, propranolol, nitroglycerin and lidocaine. Circulation 53:429

76. Vatner SF, Baig H, Manders WT, Ochs S, Pagani M (1977) Effect of propranolol on regional myocardial function, electrograms, and blood gases in conscious dogs with myocardial ischaemia. J Clin Invest 60:353

77. Foëx P (1980) Beta-adrenergic blockade and anaesthesia. In: Burley DM, Birdwood GFB (eds) The clinical impact of beta-adrenoceptor blockade. Ciba Laboratories, Horsham, pp 75–96

78. Cutfield GR, Francis CM, Foëx P, Lowenstein E, Davies WL, Ryder WA (1981) Myocardial function and critical constriction of the left anterior descending coronary artery: protective effect of oxprenolol. Br J Anaesth 53:189P

79. Antman EM, Stone PH, Muller JE, Braunwald E (1980) Calcium channel blocking agents in the treatment of cardiovascular disorders. Part I: basic and clinical electrophysiologic effects. Ann Intern Med 93:875

80. Zelis R, Flaim SF (1981) "Calcium influx blockers" and vascular smooth muscle: do we really understand the mechanism. Ann Intern Med 94:124

81. Zipes DP, Fischer JC (1974) Effects of agents which inhibit the slow channel on sinus node automaticity and atrioventricular conduction in the dog. Circ Res 34:184

82. Brichard G, Zimmerman PE (1970) Verapamil in cardiac dysrhythmias during anaesthesia. Br J Anaesth 42:1005

83. Mangiardi LM, Hariman RJ, McAllister RG Jr, Bhargava V, Surawicz B, Shabetai R (1978) Electrophysiologic and haemodynamic effects of verapamil: correlation with plasma drug concentration. Circulation 57:366

84. Amlie JP, Landmark K (1978) The effect of nifedipine on the sinus and atrioventricular node of the dog heart after beta-adrenergic receptor blockade. Acta Pharmacol Toxicol (Copenh) 42:287

85. Walsh R, Badke F, O'Rourke R (1979) Differential effects of diltiazem and verapamil on left ventricular performance in conscious dogs. Circulation [Suppl II] 60:15

86. Newman RK, Bishop VS, Peterson DF, Leroux EJ, Horwitz LD (1977) Effect of verapamil on left ventricular performance in conscious dogs. J Pharmacol Exp Ther 201:723

87. Talano JV, Feerst D (1980) Verapamil. A new class of anti-arrhythmic agents with a variety of beneficial cardiovascular effects. Arch Intern Med 140:314

88. Opie LH (1980) Drugs and the heart. III. Calcium antagonists. Lancet I:806

89. Fleckenstein A (1977) Specific pharmacology of calcium in myocardium, cardiac pacemaker and vascular smooth muscle. Ann Rev Pharmacol Toxicol 17:149

90. Henry PD, Shuchleib R, Clark RE, Perez JE (1979) Effect of nifedipine on myocardial ischaemia: analysis of collateral flow, pulsatile heat and regional muscle shortening. Am J Cardiol 44:817

91. Maroko PR, Kjekshus JK, Sobel BE, Watanabe T, Covell JW, Ross J, Braunwald E (1971) Factors influencing infarct size following experimental coronary artery occlusions. Circulation 43:67

92. Kaumann AJ, Aramendia P (1968) Prevention of ventricular fibrillation induced by coronary ligation. J Pharmacol Exp Ther 164:326

93. Smith HJ, Singh BN, Nisbet HD, Norris RM (1975) Effects of verapamil on infarct size following experimental coronary occlusion. Cardiovasc Res 9:569

94. Luz PL da, Monteiro de Barros LF, Leite JJ, Pileggi F, Decourt LV (1980) Effect of verapamil on regional coronary and myocardial perfusion during acute coronary occlusion. Am J Cardiol 45:269

95. Bleifeld W, Wende W, Meyer J, Bussman WD (1975) Einfluß einer Vasodilatation durch Dipyridamol auf die Größe des akuten experimentellen Herzinfarktes. Z Kardiol 63:115

96. Nayler WG, Grau A, Slade A (1976) A protective effect of verapamil on hypoxic heart muscle. Cardiovasc Res 10:650

97. Nayler WG, Fassold E, Yepez C (1978) Pharmacological protection of mitrochondrial function in hypoxic heart muscle: effect of verapamil, propranolol and methylprednisolone. Cardiovasc Res 12:152

98. Smith HJ, Goldstein RA, Griffith JM, Kent KM, Epstein SE (1976) Regional contractility. Selectiv depression of ischemic myocardium by verapamil. Circulation 54:629

99. Ferlinz J, Easthope JL, Aronow WS (1979) Effects of verapamil on myocardial performance in coronary disease. Circulation 59:313

100. Johnstone M (1976) The cardiovascular effects of ketamine in man. Anesthesia 31:873

101. Oates HF (1979) Hypotensive action of nitroprusside and verapamil compared. Anesthesiology 51:363

102. Oates HF, Stocker LM, Stokes GS (1979) Verapamil as a hypotensive agent: a comparison in the anaesthetized rat, with hydralazine, diaozoxide and nitroprusside. Clin Exp Hypertens 1:473

103. Francis CM, Glazebrook C, Lowenstein E, Davies WL, Foëx P, Ryder WA (1980) Effect of halothane on the performance of the heart in the case of critical constriction of the left circumflex coronary artery. Br J Anaesth 52:631P

Microcirculatory Effects of Halothane and Enflurane

N. Franke, B. Endrich and K. Meßmer

Introduction

Halothane is widely used as a volatile anaesthetic since 1956 [3]. As an alternative, enflurane became available in 1963 [8]. Rapid, precise control of depth of anaesthesia, prompt recovery without sequelae, and a low incidence of side-effects are the main advantages of these drugs. While changes of central haemodynamics are well established, little information is available on how halothane and enflurane affect the microhaemodynamics, as well as the supply of oxygen and substrates to the tissue.

Microcirculatory effects of these drugs have only been established with regard to changes in vessel diameter [12], but not in terms of the density of erythrocyte-perfused capillaries. Furthermore, halothane and enflurane anaesthesia has always been performed in animals which had been anaesthetized already with at least one other drug. Therefore, the effects of both drugs on the microcirculation per se are hitherto unknown. As a consequence, a new experimental model was used for direct, quantitative studies of morphological and haemodynamic parameters of the microcirculation in the awake animal, during anaesthesia, and in the recovery period.

Material and Methods

A transparent skin flap chamber was implanted in 43 Syrian gold hamsters (body wt. 80–100 g). Permanent, indwelling catheters were introduced into carotid artery and jugular vein and advanced towards the right and left ventricle. The details of these methods are described elsewhere [4]. Seventy-two hours were allowed for recovery from anaesthesia and surgery. Prior to the experiment, the hamsters were immobilized in a transparent plastic tube, placed under the microscope and allowed to breathe spontaneously 30% O_2 in 70% N_2.

Control values from the awake animal were obtained 30 min after immobilization. All measurements were repeated 15 min, 30 min, and 60 min after induction of anaesthesia with 1 MAC halothane (1.1 vol.%) or enflurane (2 vol.%), and 10 min after the end of anaesthesia. At the beginning of anaesthesia, 15 hamsters received 0.5 ml oxypolygelatine (group I). In 16 hamsters of group II, oxypolygelatine was infused throughout anaesthesia in sufficient amounts to keep the central venous pressure at the control level. In 12 hamsters of group III, central venous pressure was kept constant by oxypolygelatine infusion throughout anaesthesia, and measurements of local pO_2 were taken in the awake animal and after 30 min of enflurane anaesthesia. Mean arterial pressure (MAP), central venous pressure (CVP), and heart rate (HR) were measured via the implanted catheters. For determinations of blood gases and acid-base status, blood (0.7 ml) was withdrawn from the arterial catheter and immediately replaced by the same amount of homologous blood.

Microscopic observation of the microcirculation was performed using intravital fluorescent microscopy after i.v. injection of 0.2 cc fluorescein-isothiocyanate (FITC) 5% bound to Dextran 150 000 to improve the poor contrast between blood-vessels and the surrounding subcutaneous tissue. The image received at the eyepiece was recorded by a video-camera and stored on video tape. Blood cell velocity measurements were carried out by a video photometric analyzer and on-line cross correlation [10]. Two photometric windows, which are sensitive to the scintillation of light, were positioned manually up-stream and down-stream in a given blood-vessel. These signals were processed on line with the delay to maximum cross correlation corresponding to the transit time of blood cells. Vessel diameters were measured by a video image shearing monitor [9], which was able to rotate the given television image and to shear the upper part of the picture against the lower part.

Functional capillary density, e.g. the density of erythrocyte-perfused capillaries, was analysed using stereological techniques [16]. For this purpose, pictures were taken directly from the TV-monitor and a mosaic was assembled from black and white prints. A precise drawing was made on a transparent sheet of paper. Counts were made of the total number of intersections between red cell perfused capillaries and grid lines within the given area of at least $1800 \times 800 \ \mu m$. From the number of intersections (N_c), total magnification (V), and the length of grid lines in both directions (L_G), the functional capillary density (L_A) was determined according to the following equation:

$$ L_A = \frac{\pi \cdot N_c \cdot V}{2 \, L_G} \qquad \frac{(\text{cm})}{(\text{cm}^2)} . $$

The local surface pO_2 was measured by means of a platinum multi-wire electrode [11, 13]. A histogram demonstrating the frequency distribution of at least 100 pO_2 values from different spots on the preparation was computed [11]. Since halothane is reduced on the platinum electrode and mimics oxygen [14], pO_2 measurements were performed during enflurane anaesthesia only. Student's t-test for paired data was used for statistical analysis.

Results

Anaesthesia with both Halothane and Enflurane (1 MAC) abolished spontanous arteriolar vasomotion. In group I (volume replacement with 0.5 ml oxypolygelatine), MAP, CVP, and HR (Fig. 1) decreased after the onset of anaesthesia and reached the control values again during recovery. No differences in the macrohaemodynamic response to halothane and enflurane could be noted. Blood cell velocity (Fig. 2) in arterioles (mean diameter 38.2 μm), precapillaries (11.9 μm), capillaries (6 μm), postcapillaries (14.9 μm), collecting venules (24.7 μm), and small veins (43.9 μm) decreased uniformly after 60 min of anaesthesia. Despite the increase in arterial pressure during the recovery period, blood cell velocity remained low in all of the vessel segments; blood cell velocity in arterioles and precapillaries, however, was elevated by 50% as compared to the period of surgical anaesthesia. Arterioles, precapillaries, and venules (Table 1) dilated during anaesthesia but constricted during recovery. Although MAP and CVP were reduced 15 min after induction of anaesthesia, the density of erythrocyte-per-

Table 1. Changes in the diameters of precapillaries (d_{precap}) and vanules (d_{ven}) during anaesthesia with halothane (H, n = 8) and enflurane (E, n = 7) in group I (volume replacement with 0.5 ml colloid substitution). Control: control values in awake animals; 15 min, 30 min, 60 min: values after 15 min, 30 min and 60 min of anaesthesia. Recovery: values in recovery period (mean values ± SEM)

		Control	15 min	30 min	60 min	Recovery
d_{precap}	H	11.2 ± 1.8	12.6 ± 1.9	13 ± 1.7	12.5 ± 1.4	9.6 ± 1.8
μm	E	12.6 ± 1.9	13.4 ± 1.5	14 ± 1.5	13.8 ± 1.8	10.1 ± 1.5
d_{ven}	H	27.8 ± 3.5	30.7 ± 2.6	30.1 ± 3.8	28.2 ± 2.9	19.6 ± 2.8
μm	E	28.6 ± 3	29.5 ± 2.9	30.9 ± 3.4	30.1 ± 2.9	20.4 ± 3.5

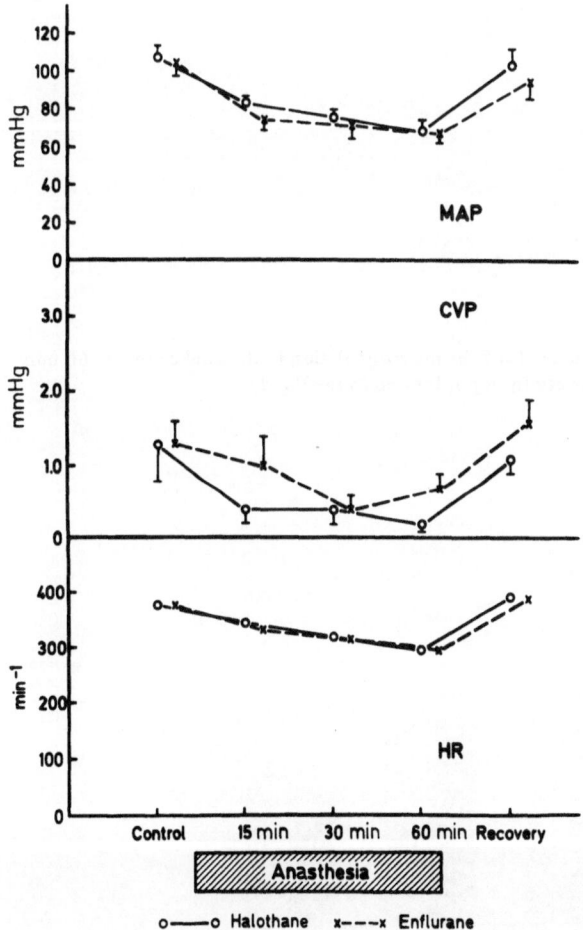

Fig. 1. Macrohaemodynamic parameters in the awake animal, during anaesthesia (halothane n = 8, enflurane n = 7 animals) and in the recovery period. Group I: 0.5 ml colloidal substitute i.v. prior to anaesthesia (mean value ± SEM). *MAP*, mean arterial pressure; *CVP*, central venous pressure; *HR*, heart rate

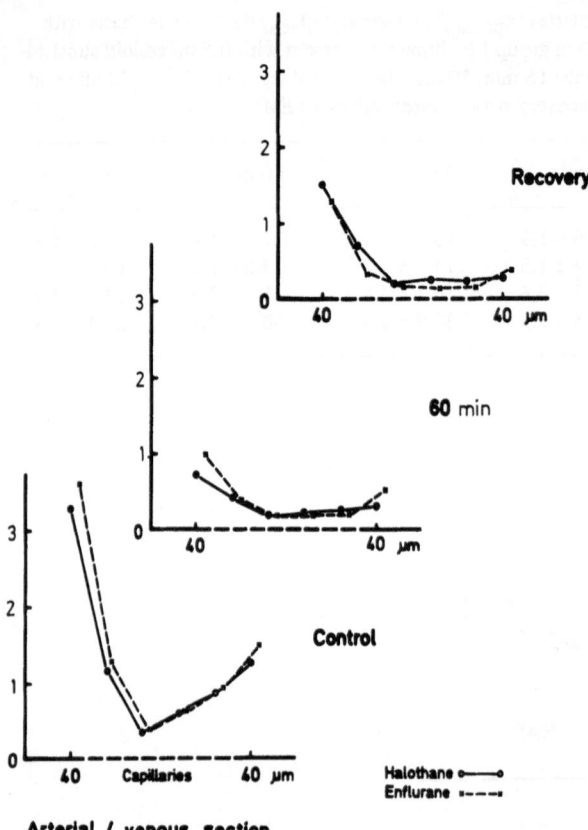

Arterial / venous section

Fig. 2. Blood cell velocity across successive segments of the microcirculation in the awake animal, 60 min after the onset of anaesthesia and during recovery (group I, for details see Fig. 1)

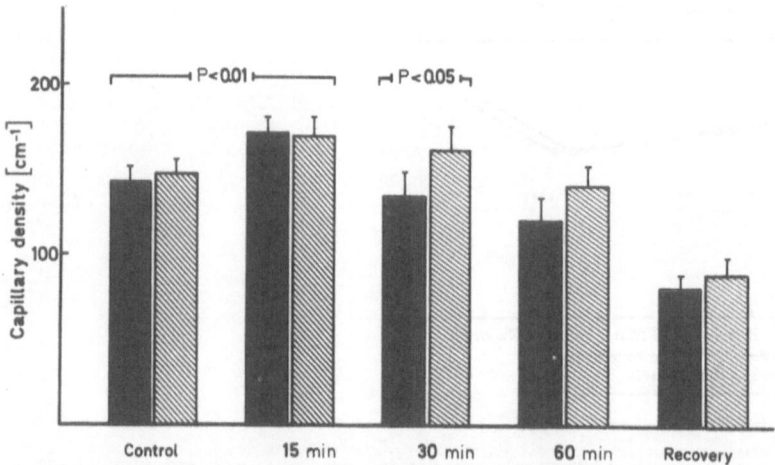

Fig. 3. Functional capillary density at control and during and after anaesthesia (group I: for details see Fig. 1)

fused capillaries (Fig. 3) was higher when compared to the values in the control period. After 30 min and 60 min of anaesthesia, functional capillary density had decreased independently of the anaesthetic employed; however, this decrease was more pronounced in the halothane group. During recovery, functional capillary density reached approximately 50% of control values only.

During anaesthesia in group II, the control value of central venous pressure was kept at its initial level by intravenous infusion of 1.2 ± 0.15 ml oxypolygelatine. Changes of MAP were observed neither during nor after anaesthesia. Heart rate fell from 380 and 390 min^{-1} respectively to 325 and 310 min^{-1} after 60 min of anaesthesia, but increased again in the recovery period. Blood cell velocity remained unchanged throughout anaesthesia in all vessel segments. Precapillaries and venules dilated from a diameter of 10.9 and 24.6 μm respectively to 12.2 and 29.4 μm after 60 min of halothane anaesthesia, and from diameters of 11.2 and 25.2 μm to 12.6 and 31.4 μm with enflurane. Vasoconstriction occurred during recovery. During this period, blood cell velocity decreased when compared to the values measured after 60 min of anaesthesia. Again, a significant difference of the macro- or microhaemodynamic response to both anaesthetics was not observed.

Functional capillary density measured in the preparation was higher than control values after 15 min of anaesthesia; it remained unchanged during anaesthesia with both drugs. However, during recovery, capillary density decreased. The histogram (Fig. 4) demonstrating the local pO_2 values on the preparation shows a normal distribution in the awake animal. After 30 min of enflurane anaesthesia, this homogeneous configuration of the histogram was preserved; however, the histogram was slightly shifted toward higher pO_2 values, with an increase in mean pO_2 from 23.6 to 29.8 mmHg.

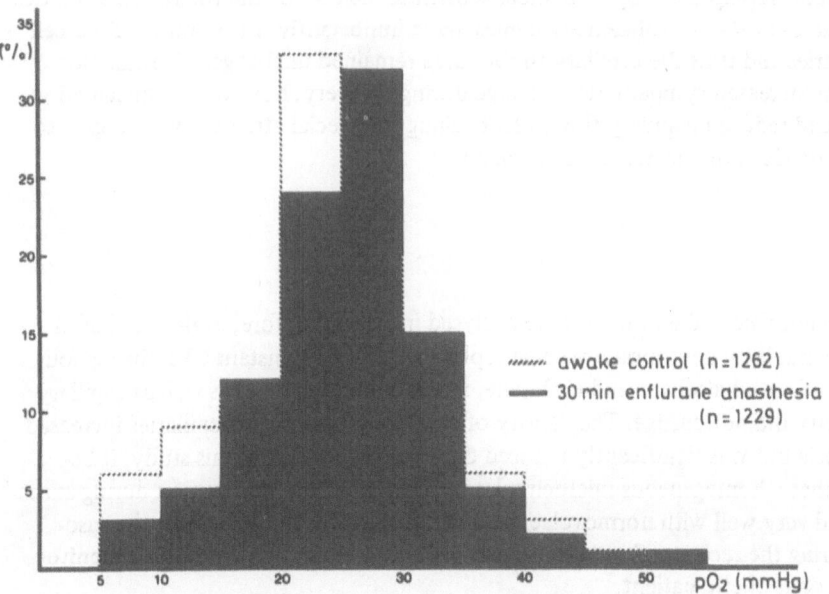

Fig. 4. Frequency distribution of local pO_2 values (arranged in gradations of 5 mmHg) before and 30 min after the onset of anaesthesia (group III, 12 animals). The histograms were computed from a total of 1262 and 1229 single pO_2 measurements respectively

Discussion

The main objective of this study was to evaluate the microcirculatory effects of halothane and enflurane anaesthesia per se. The findings obtained from the animals of group I are clearly affected by the hypovolaemia elicited by the anaesthetics despite the uniform initial volume replacement. The decrease in MAP, blood cell velocity, and functional capillary density are thus no specific effects of the anaesthetics but due to the reduction of venous return. Similar changes of the blood-pressure and capillary perfusion and distribution have been observed during hypovolaemia due to haemorrhage [2, 5, 7, 17].

Studies on microcirculatory effects of halothane and enflurane have usually been performed in pre-anaesthetized animals [1, 15, 18]. Even though in these studies a profound hypotension was consistently observed during anaesthesia, no attempts were made to correct the underlying hypovolaemia. It therefore seems appropriate to assume that the data obtained in these studies do not reflect the effects of the volatile anaesthetics per se, but reflect the results of the interaction of the basic anaesthetic, hypovolaemia-mediated changes in vascular tone, and the anaesthetic under investigation. With adequate volume replacement (group II), arterial pressure and blood cell velocity remained unchanged throughout anaesthesia. The density of erythrocyte-perfused capillaries increased and the distribution curves of surface pO_2 were shifted to the right, indicating an improved oxygen supply to tissue.

By impeding the sympathetic discharge, halothane and enflurane [1, 8] may dilate bloodvessels and depress vasomotor activity [1]. As a result, blood flow in post-arteriolar vessels will be distributed more homogeneously and more capillaries will be perfused by erythrocytes [6, 19]. This will result in enhanced functional capillary density, which in turn improves the local tissue pO_2.

If normovolaemia was provided throughout the investigations by continuous monitoring of CVP and volume replacement by a colloidal substitute, neither of the volatile anaesthetics affected the macro- or the microhaemodynamics; most importantly, the number of red cell perfused capillaries and thus the capillary surface area remained unchanged. Termination of anaesthesia with increased sympathetic discharge during recovery, however, again caused vasoconstriction and reduced capillary flow, a fact calling for special attention with regard to further volume needs in the postanaesthetic phase.

Summary

The effects of halothane and enflurane were analysed in animals before, during, and after surgical anaesthesia. With appropriate volume replacement, i.e. a constant CVP throughout the application of both halothane and enflurane, macrohaemodynamics as well as capillary blood cell velocity did not change. The density of erythrocyte-perfused capillaries increased during anaesthesia but was significantly reduced during recovery. From this study, it becomes evident that a homogeneous microcirculatory flow and flow distribution during anaesthesia correlated very well with normovolaemia and changes of CVP. Moreover, the vasoconstriction during the recovery from anaesthesia calls for a close observation and monitoring of the post-anaesthetic patient.

References

1. Akester JM, Brody MJ (1969) Mechanism of vascular resistance changes produced in skin and muscle by halothane. Pharmacol Exp Ther 170:287
2. Chien S (1967) Role of sympathetic nervous system in shock. Physiol Rev 47:214
3. Deutsch S, Linde HW, Dripps RD (1962) Circulatory and respiratory actions of halothane in normal man. Anaesthesiology 23:631
4. Endrich B, Asaishi K, Goetz A, Meßmer K (1980) Technical report. A new chamber technique for microvascular studies in unanaesthetized animals. Res Exp Med (Berl) 177:125
5. Fronek A, Witzel T (1974) Haemodynamics of terminal vascular bed in canine haemorrhagic shock. Surgery 75:408
6. Fung YC (1973) Stochastic flow in capillary blood vessels. Microvasc Res 5:34
7. Grega GJ, Schwinghammer JM, Haddy FJ (1971) Changes in forelimb weight and segmental resistances following severe haemorrhage. Circ Res 29:691
8. Hudon F, Jacques A, Dery R (1963) Respiratory and haemodynamic effects of enflurane anaesthesia. Can Anaesth Soc J 10:442
9. Intaglietta M, Tompkins WR (1973) Microvascular measurements by video image shearing and splitting. Microvasc Res 5:309
10. Intaglietta M, Silverman NR, Tompkins WR (1975) Capillary flow velocity measurements in vivo and in situ by television method. Microvasc Res 10:165
11. Kessler M, Grunewald M (1969) Possibilities of measuring oxygen pressure fields in tissue by multiwire platinum electrodes. Prog Respir Res 3:147
12. Longnecker DE, Harris PD (1972) Dilatation of small arteries and veins in the bat during halothane anaesthesia. Anaesthesiology 37:432
13. Luebbers DW (1969) Principle of construction and application of various platinum electrodes. Prog Respir Res 3:136
14. McHugh RD, Epstein RM, Longnecker DE (1979) Halothane mimics oxygen in oxygen microelectrodes. Anaesthesiology 50:47
15. Miller ED, Kistner JR, Epstein RM (1979) Distribution of blood flow with anaesthetics. Anaesthesiology 51:124
16. Schmid-Schoenbein GW, Zweifach BW, Kovalcheck S (1977) The application of stereological principles to morphometry of the microcirculation in different tissues. Microvasc Res 14:303
17. Swan H (1965) Experimental acute haemorrhage. Arch Surg 91:390
18. Yamaki T, Baez S, Feldman SM, Gootman PM, Orkin LR (1978) Microvascular responses to norepinephrine and vasopressin during halothane anaesthesia in the rat. Anaesthesiology 48:332
19. Zawicki DF, Jain RK, Schmid-Schoenbein GW, Chien S (1981) Dynamics of neovascularization in normal tissue. Microvasc Res 21:27

Distribution of EEG Frequency Bands as Revealed by Factor Analysis During Anaesthesia with Halothane and Enflurane

H. Schwilden and H. Stoeckel

Introduction

In 1950 Bickford [3] proposed a device for automatic electroencephalographic (EEG) control of general anaesthesia. Up until now this far-reaching idea has not been realized for human purposes, but it has been a starting point for many investigations [2–7, 11, 12, 15, 17–33] of the relationship between anaesthesia – especially the depth of anaesthesia – and its concomitant electroencephalographic patterns.

When EEG parameters are investigated for purposes of monitoring anaesthesia and evaluating quantitative indicators of the depth of anaesthesia, frequently a parameterization is chosen which is based on the commonly used frequency band structure (delta, theta, alpha, and beta bands; Fig. 1). One may question whether this framework is an appropriate one for the description of the EEG during anaesthesia. Factor analysis [1, 8–10, 13, 14, 16] offers a means of determining whether there exists a mathematical rationale [10, 13, 14, 16] for the clinically defined frequency bands. In essence it works as follows. The power spectrum in the range from, for instance, 0.5 to 30 Hz is divided into small frequency slices, say of 0.5 Hz, the intensities of which are treated as independent variables. Correlating each of these

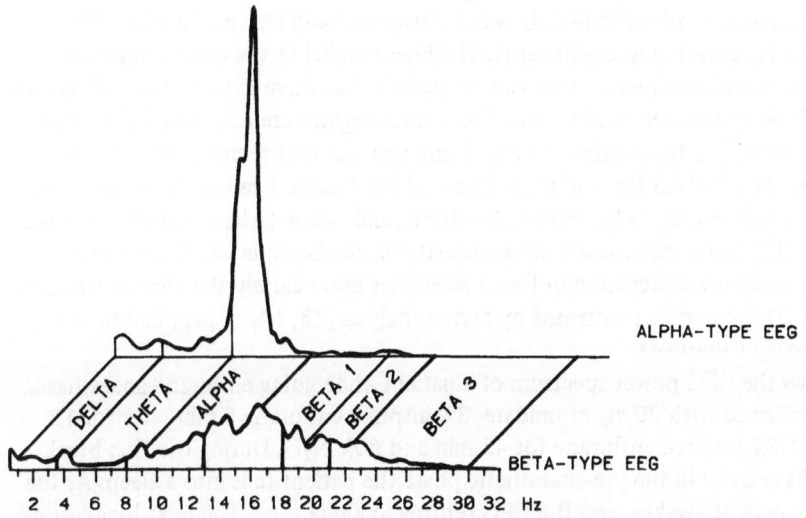

Fig. 1. Clinically defined commonly used EEG frequency bands

60 variables with each other one obtains a correlation matrix, which in turn is the basis for calculating so-called factors. These factors are artificial variables, namely linear combinations of the original variables which are defined by their correlation coefficients to the original variables. But whereas each original variable contributes only the proportion of $1/n$ (n = number of original variables) to total variance, a few factors may contribute as much as 80%–90% of total variance, while the many others represent the remainder. In this way factor analysis is a data-reducing process in so far as many variables are replaced by a few factors.

Material and Method

Using this method we investigated in a retrospective study 20 EEGs of female patients during anaesthesia with enflurane and ten EEGs of female patients during anaesthesia with halothane, of ASA classes 1 and 2 undergoing gynaecological operations. In six cases the technical circumstances did not allow factor analysis to be carried out successfully.

As leads we used C_z-O_1 and C_z-O_2 which had been stored on magnetic tape (Ampex Pr 2200). Digitalization was done with 125 Hz and 12-bit resolution. EEG epochs of 8.192 s length were the basis for calculating power spectra. Final estimates of power spectra were obtained by averaging at least four spectra and reducing frequency resolution by averaging four adjacent frequency bands of 0.122–0.488 Hz. Normalized power spectra from 0.488–30.3 Hz, i.e. 61 variables all together, were used for factor analysis.

Results

Figure 2 shows the normalized power spectrum during administration of 60% N_2O 5 min after ending a 30-min 2% enflurane administration. Factor analysis of the depicted EEG power spectrum yields the following results. Four factors were extracted, and their percentage of variance is depicted on the right-hand side of Fig. 3. As mentioned above, factors are determined by their correlation coefficients to the original variables. The abscissa scales the original variables – frequency bands of 0.488 Hz width between 0.488 Hz and 30.3 Hz. The ordinate represents the correlation coefficients. The lines parallel to the abscissa mark an r of 0.33. A first non-trivial statement which can be made is that there exist connected regions characterized by high correlation coefficients. Since these regions are connected they give rise to a band structure. For the example in Fig. 3 one may say that factor 1 exhibits bands ranging from 3–6.5 Hz, 7–10.5 Hz, and from 23.5–29 Hz. Factor 2 represents bands from 0.5–2 Hz and 11–17 Hz, factor 3 a band from 26–30 Hz, and factor 4 a band from 17–23 Hz. Compared to the EEG factor structure in deep anaesthesia, as shown in the following examples, the factor structure as depicted in Fig. 3 resembles more closely the clinical frequency band structure. This could be confirmed by factor analysis [13, 14, 16] applied to the EEG of awake, resting volunteers.

Figure 4 shows the EEG power spectrum of a patient undergoing enflurane anaesthesia. Induction was performed with 20 mg etomidate, 3% inspired enflurane 5 min later for 15 min, followed by 1.5% inspired enflurane for 45 min and 60% N_2O. During the first breakdown of high alpha activity in the pre-anaesthetic phase the patient falls into a sleep. As the nurse comes in the patient awakes, and the EEG returns to alpha type. The next long-lasting breakdown of alpha activity is caused by anaesthesia. The beam on the right margin indicates

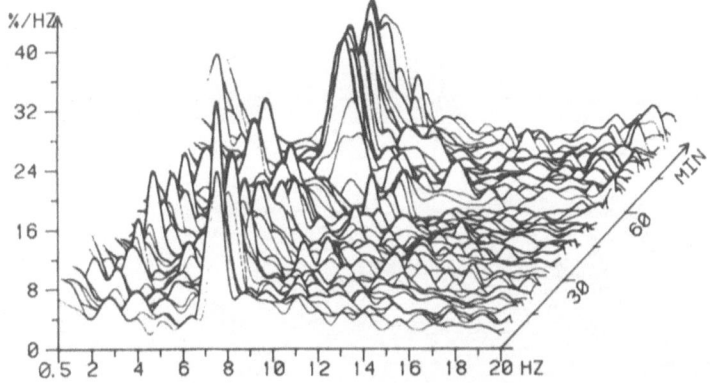

Fig. 2. Normalized EEG power spectrum during administration of 60% N_2O and 40% O_2 5 min after ending a 30-min 2% enflurane administration

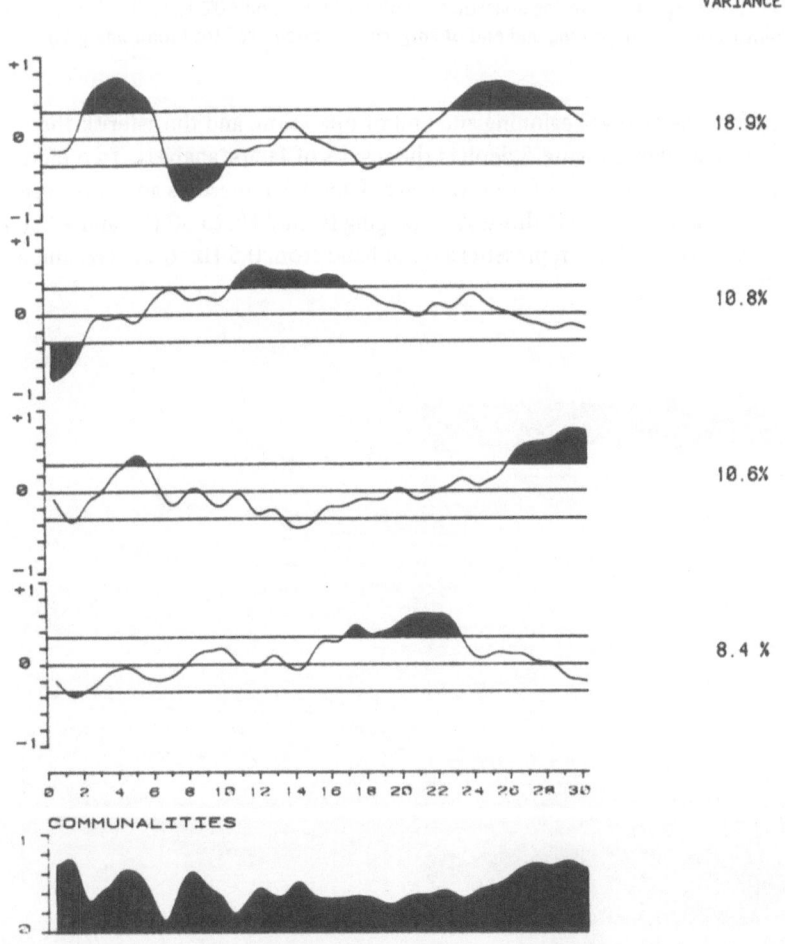

Fig. 3. Factor structure (P-technique) for the EEG power spectrum of Fig. 2. The *darkened areas* mark an $r^2 \geq 1$. The percentage of total variance is depicted on the *right margin*

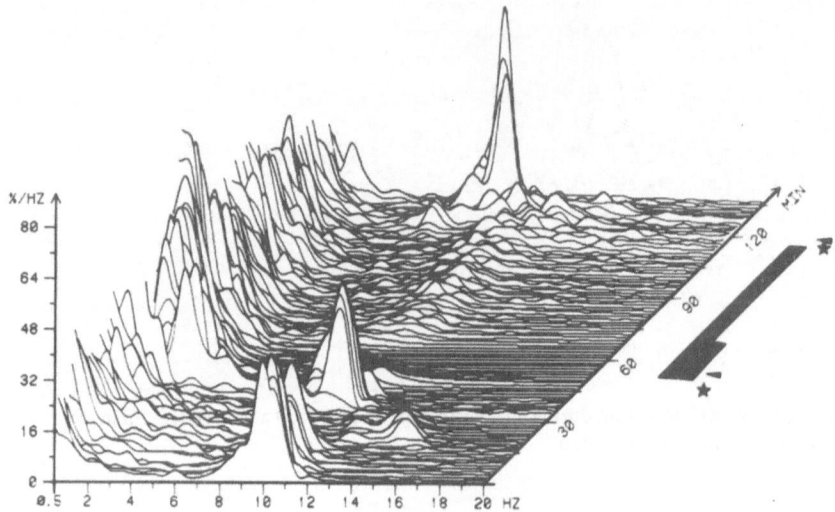

Fig. 4. Normalized EEG power spectrum during anaesthesia with enflurane and 60% N_2O. The beam symbolizes enflurane administration (▲: beginning and end of surgery; *: period used for factor analysis)

enflurane administration, the arrows beginning and end of operation, and the asterisk the period we used for factor analysis. Figure 5 depicts the results of factor analysis. Two factors were extracted representing nearly 70% of total variance. Factor 1 represents an enormously enlarged beta band − if one may name it this way − ranging from 7 Hz to 30 Hz, and a band ranging from 2 Hz to 4.5 Hz. Factor 2 represents a delta band from 0.5 Hz to 1.5 Hz, and a band from 3 Hz to 7 Hz.

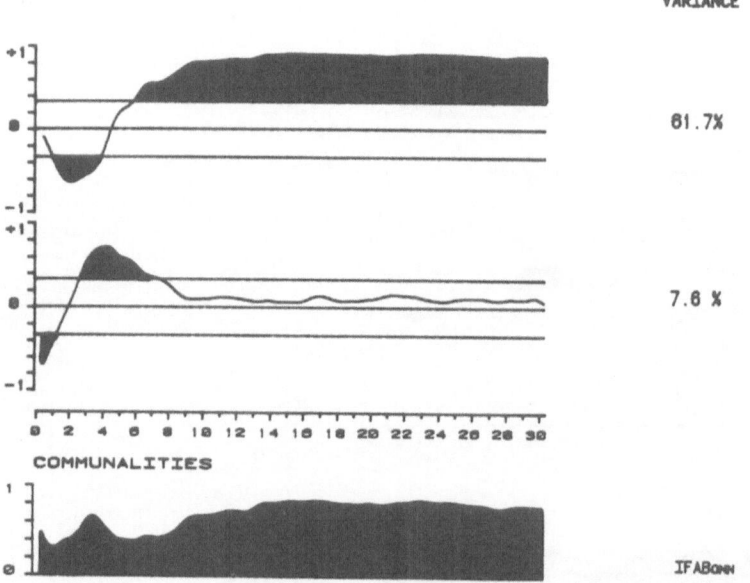

Fig. 5. Factor structure for the EEG power spectrum depicted in Fig. 4 during anaesthesia with enflurane and N_2O

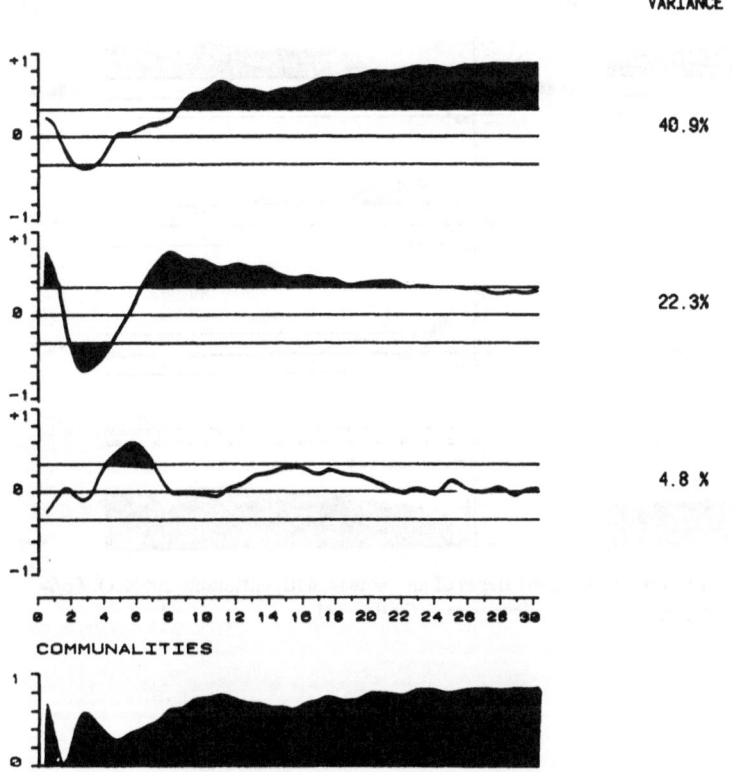

Fig. 6. Factor structure of an EEG power spectrum during anaesthesia with 2% enflurane and 60% N_2O. Merging the first and second factor would yield a factor very similar to the first factor of Fig. 5

Figure 6 shows the extracted factors for a patient's EEG during enflurane anaesthesia with 2% inspired enflurane and 60% N_2O. It is difficult to decide whether factor 1 and factor 2 define two different high-frequency bands or not, because there is no clear borderline. Merging them together one would achieve a factor similar to the first one of Fig. 5. During moderate to deep anaesthesia, we obtained in all cases factor structures like those of the last two examples: that is, a high-frequency band ranging from 30 Hz down to 7 Hz which is simply connected (type 1) or which is disconnected but with no clearly defined borderline (type 2).

Figure 7 compares the factor structure of a patient's EEG power spectrum during different stages of anaesthesia. The extracted factor structure on the right-hand side is obtained during deep anaesthesia with inspired enflurane concentrations ranging between 3% and 1.5% (the time average is 1.7%). The left-hand side shows the extracted factors during a lighter stage of anaesthesia with inspired enflurane concentrations between 1% and 0.5% with a time average of 0.75%. In both cases 60% N_2O was administered. An essential difference concerning the factor structure is the width of beta band of each factor 1, which ranges for light anaesthesia from 13 Hz to 30 Hz and for deeper anaesthetic stages down to 8 Hz. Factor 3 on the left reveals the appearence of an alpha band from 8.5 Hz to 13 Hz, which cannot be detected on the right-hand side.

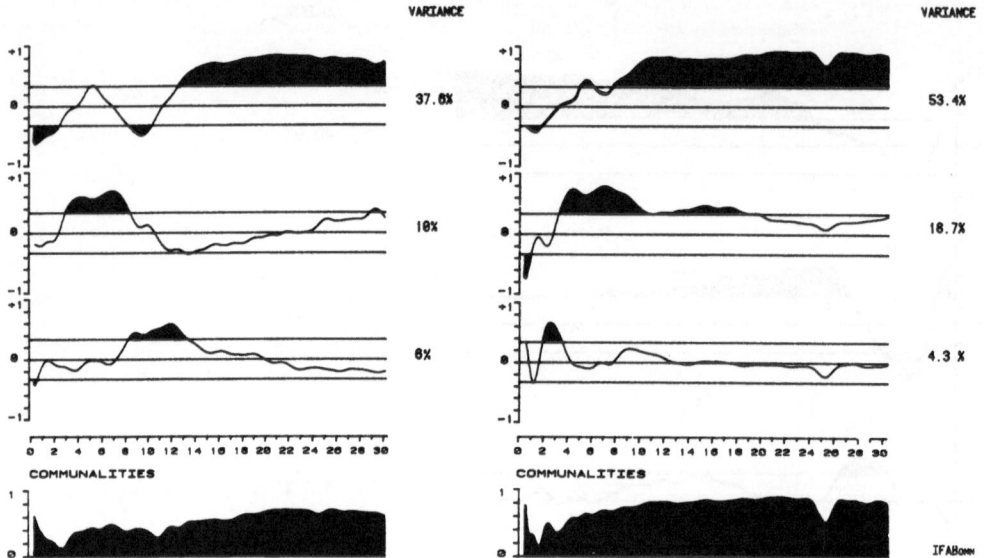

Fig. 7. Comparison of factor structure for different stages of anaesthesia with enflurane and N_2O. *Left-hand side,* light anaesthetic level; *right-hand side,* deeper anaesthetic level

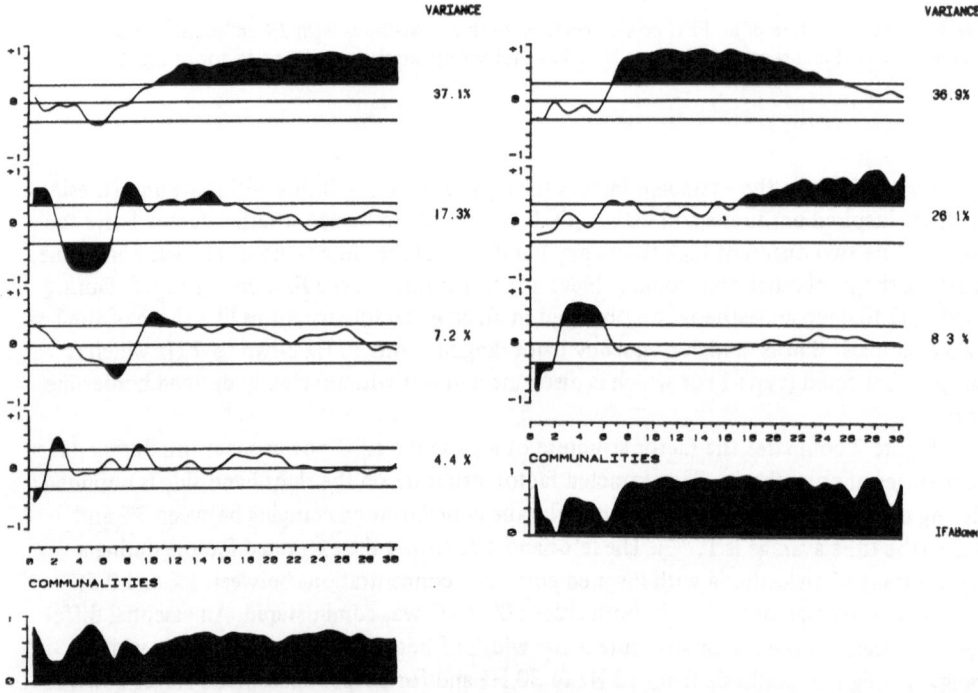

Fig. 8. Comparison of factor structure for different stages of anaesthesia with halothane and N_2O. *Left-hand side,* light anaesthetic level; *right-hand side,* deeper anaesthetic level

During halothane anaesthesia we did not find qualitative differences for the factor struc-ture in comparison to enflurane (Fig. 8). Here again two stages of anaesthesia for one patient are compared. The left-hand side figure represents a light stage with 0.5% inspired halothane and 60% N_2O, the right-hand side a deeper stage with 1.5% inspired halothane and 60% N_2O. The factors 1 and 2 on the right are very similar to the type 2 factor structure during deep anaesthesia, while the factors on the left-hand side are again characterized by a reduction of beta band (factor 1) and factor loadings in the alpha region (factor 2 and 3). To summarize, two results are remarkable: (a) factor structure changes with changing stages of anaesthesia; and (b) most prominent is the broadening of beta band in deep anaesthesia. This implies that for purposes of EEG trend monitoring during anaesthesia one should not rely on the com-monly used frequency band structure. If, for example, one would monitor alpha band acti-vity during anaesthesia one would monitor different things for different stages of anaesthe-sia: during light stages a frequency band in its own right, during deep stages part of an en-larged beta band.

In a work previously done [31] we suggested the median of the power spectrum as an appropriate parameter for trend monitoring during anaesthesia. The median is that frequen-cy which divides the area under each power spectrum into two equal parts. This parameter is, like the amplitude, totally independent of the frequency band structure. But whereas the amplitude does not contain any information about the frequency content of the EEG, the median summarizes this information in one parameter. In the same study we carried out a multi-regression analysis concerning the following list of parameters: median, mean ampli-tude, $delta_1$ (0.5–2 Hz), $delta_2$ (2–5 Hz), theta (5–8 Hz), alpha (8–13 Hz), beta (13–32 Hz), alpha/delta (the name of a band stands for its percentage of activity). We calculated for each case the correlation coefficients of all parameters to all others. The sum over all cases and parameters yielded the following list:
1. Median
2. Alpha
3. Alpha/delta
4. Beta
5. $Delta_1$
6. $Delta_2$
7. Mean amplitude
8. Theta.
The first parameter has the highest, the last one the lowest total sum. This may be interpret-ed in the following way: Assuming that the EEG is sufficiently well described by the totali-ty of all parameters except the one under discussion, the parameter with the highest total sum of correlation coefficients summarizes in the best way the EEG changes described by the others. The result that the median has the highest total sum may again reflect that for purposes of EEG trend monitoring in anaesthesia one should use parameters which are inde-pendent of the frequency band structure. The result that the mean amplitude has ranks last, but this does not necessarily imply that it is less suited for monitoring in anaesthesia — only that it does not reflect the EEG changes as described by the other parameters very well. But nevertheless, comparing median and mean amplitude in more than 80 cases, we found the median more easily interpretable than the mean amplitude, which in addition has the disad-vantage of being interindividually less stable than the median. As an example, Fig. 9 com-pares the behaviour of median and mean amplitude during anaesthesia with 2% inspired en-flurane and 60% N_2O. The sharp reduction of the median and increase of mean amplitude

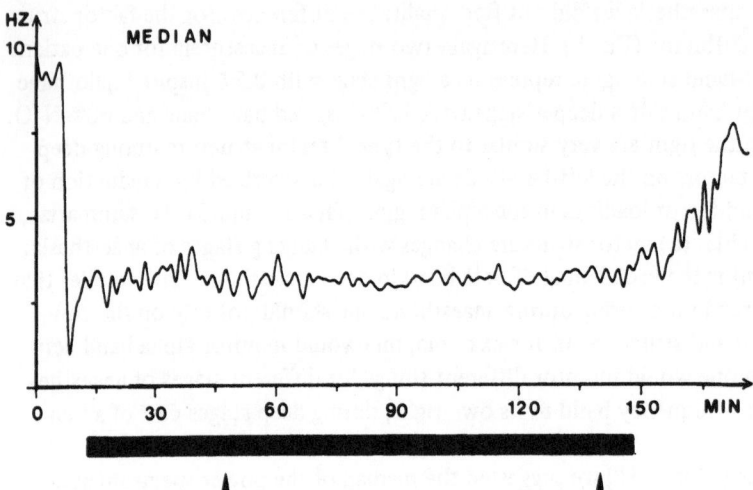

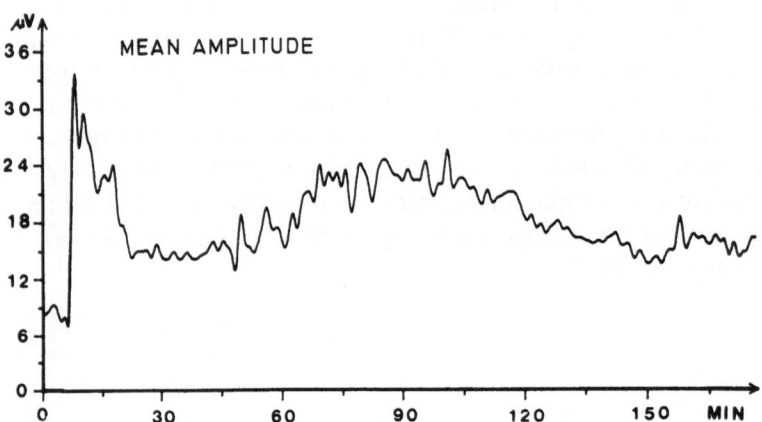

Fig. 9. Comparison of the time course of median and mean amplitude during anaesthesia with 2% enflurane and 60% N_2O. The beam indicates enflurane administration (▲: beginning and end of surgery)

in the 8th min is caused by induction with 20 mg etomidate. While the median is constant during anaesthesia, the amplitude decreases and rises astonishingly at the beginning of surgery. Assuming that rising amplitude indicates a deepening of anaesthesia, this behaviour is hard to interpret. One observes a similar behaviour at the end of enflurane administration. While the median rises as a sign of awakening, the mean amplitude remains nearly constant.

For the median we could work out a certain numerical border. In our experience a median of less than 5 Hz reflects an anaesthetic stage which is not too light. For EEG trend monitoring during anaesthesia we developed a device based on a commercially available microprocessor which depicts on line the median of the power spectrum.

Summary

Factor analysis of the EEG power spectrum during anaesthesia reveals that the frequency band structure changes with respect to EEG power spectra during normal conditions, as well as with changing stages of anaesthesia. On one hand this does suggest that for purposes of EEG trend monitoring one should use a parameterization independent of frequency band distribution. On the other hand this confirms an earlier observation of ours, according to which the median of the power spectrum was the best suited of several investigated parameters for trend monitoring during anaesthesia.

References

1. Bente D (1979) Die faktorenanalytische Verarbeitung spektraler EEG-Daten: Auswertungsstrategien mit pharmakolektroencephalographischen Anwendungsbeispielen. EEG-EMG 10:207–213
2. Berezowskyi JL, McEwen JA, Anderson GB, Jenkins LC (1976) A study of anaesthesia depth by power spectral analysis of the electroencephalogram. Can Anaesth Soc J 23:1–8
3. Bickford RG (1950) Automatic electroencephalographic control of general anaesthesia. Electroencephalogr Clin Neurophysiol 2:93–96
4. Bickford RG (1951) Use of frequency discrimination in the automatic electroencephalographic control of anaesthesia (servo anaesthesia). Electroencephalogr Clin Neurophysiol 3:83–86
5. Bostem F, Hanquet M (1976) Untersuchung des Verlaufs der Energiespektraldichte des Elektroencephalogramms unter Halothan- und Enflurane-Narkose. Anaesthesiol Wiederbeleb 99:11–16
6. Brazier MAB (1961) Some effects of anaesthesia on the brain. Br J Anaesth 33:194–204
7. Courting OF (1951) The value of continuous electroencephalographic and electrocardiographic tracings to the anaesthetist during surgery. Br J Anaesth 23:5–13
8. Defaoylle M, Dinand JP (1974) Application de l'analyse de la structure de l'E.E.G. Electroencephalogr Clin Neurophysiol 36:319–322
9. Dolce G, Decker H (1975) Application of multivariate statistical methods in analysis of spectral values of the EEG. In: Dolce G, Künkel H (eds) CEAN Computerized EEG Analysis. Gustav Fischer, Stuttgart, pp 156–171
10. Fichte U, Herrmann M, Kubicki S (1979) Mathematische Rationale für die klinischen EEG-Frequenzbänder. 3. Faktorenstruktur unter Psychopharmakabehandlung. EEG-EMG 10:31–37
11. Fleming RA, Smith NT (1979) Density modulation: A technique for the display of three dimensional variable data in patient monitoring. Anaesthesiology 50:543–546
12. Harmel MH, Klein FF, Davis DA (1978) The EEMG – a practical index of cortical activity and muscular relaxation. Acta Anaesth Scand [Suppl] 70:97–102
13. Herrmann WM, Fichte K, Kubicki S (1978) Mathematische Rationale für die klinischen EEG-Frequenzbänder. 1. Faktorenanalyse mit EEG-Powerspektralschätzung zur Definition von Frequenzbändern. EEG-EMG 9:146–154
14. Herrmann WM, Fichte K, Kubicki S (1978) Mathematische Rationale für die klinischen EEG-Frequenzbänder. 2. Stabilität der Faktorenstruktur bei zwei Länderstichproben und Meßwiederholung unter Plazebo. EEG-EMG 9:200–205
15. Kavan EM, Julien RM (1974) Central nervous systems' effects of isoflurane (Forane[R]). Can Anaesth Soc J 21:390–402
16. Kubicki S, Herrmann WM, Laudahn G (1980) Proceedings des Workshops: Faktorenanalyse und Variablenbildung aus dem Elektroencephalogramm, 15. und 16. Dec 1978, Berlin. Gustav Fischer, Stuttgart New York
17. Kugler J, Doenicke A, Laub M (1977) The EEG after etomidate. Anaesthesiol Wiederbeleb 106:31–48
18. Levy JW, Shapiro HM, Maruchak G, Meathe E (1980) Automated EEG processing for interoperative monitoring: a comparison of techniques. Anaesthesiology 53:223–236

19. Lopes da Silva FN, Smith NT, Zwart A, Nichols WW (1972) Spectral analysis of the EEG during ha-
    lothane anaesthesia input-output relations. Electroencephalogr Clin Neurophysiol 33:311–319
20. Nilson E, Ingrar DH (1967) EEG – findings in neurolept-analgesia. Acta Anaesth Scand 11:121–127
21. Oshimg E, Shingu K, Mori K (1981) E.E.G. activity during halothane anaesthesia in man. Br J
    Anaesth 53:65–72
22. Persson A, Peterson E, Wahlin A (1978) EEG-changes during general anaesthesia with enflurane
    (Ethrane^R) in comparison with ether. Acta Anaesth Scand 22:339–348
23. Pichelmayr I, Lips U (1979) Pethidin-Effekte im Elektroencephalogramm. Anaesthesist 28:433–442
24. Pichelmayr I, Lips U (1980) EEG-Effekte der Prämedikation mit Thalamonal^R. Anaesthesist 29:
    360–365
25. Prior PF (1979) Monitoring cerebral Function. Elsevier, Amsterdam
26. Pronk RAF, de Doer SJ, Cornelisson RCH, Doornbos P, Lasance UAJ, Simons AJR, van de Weide H
    (1978) Computer-assisted patient monitoring during open heart surgery with aid of the EEG. In:
    Progress Report 6. Inst. Med Phys TNO, Da Costa Kode 45, 3521 VS Utrecht, pp 85–91
27. Saunders D (1981) Anaesthesia, awareness and automation. Br J Anaesth 53:1–2
28. Schwilden H, Stoeckel H (1980) Untersuchungen über verschiedene EEG-Parameter als Indikatoren
    des Narkosezustandes. Anaesth Intensivther Notfallmed 15:279–286
29. Smith WDA, Mapleson WW, Siebold K, Hargreaves MD, Clarke GM (1974) Nitrous oxide anaesthesia
    induced at atmospheric and hyperbaric pressures. Br J Anaesth 46:3–12
30. Stoeckel H, Lange H, Burr W, Hengstmann JH, Schüttler J (1979) EEG-Spektralanalyse zur Doku-
    mentation der Narkosetiefe. Prakt Anaesth 14:227–232
31. Stoeckel H, Schwilden H, Lauven PM, Schüttler J (1981) EEG indices for evaluation of depth of
    anaesthesia. Br J Anaesth 53:P117
32. Volgyesi CA (1978) A brain function monitor for use during anaesthesia. Can Anaesth Soc J 25:
    427–430
33. Wolfson B, Siker ES, Ciccarelli HE, Gray GH jr., Jones L (1967) The electroencephalogram as a mo-
    nitor of arterial blood levels of methoxyflurane. Anaesthesiology 28:1003–1009

The Effects of Inhalational Anaesthetics on the Brain

P.A. Steen

The purpose of using inhalational anaesthetics is to depress brain function, and they do so in a dose-related fashion. Unless this effect is itself considered toxic, then respiratory or circulatory arrest with high anaesthetic concentrations should not be considered toxicity. These are only magnifications of the usual pharmacological effects in accordance with predictable dose-response curves, and are totally reversible simply by decreasing the dose [1].

Parallel to the reduction in neuronal activity, cerebral metabolic changes occur. Inhalational anaesthetics generally reduce the cerebral metabolic rate, with the possible exception of N_2O. There are some serious methodological problems inherent in the evaluation of these effects, as it is not ethically permissible to obtain control measurements without anaesthetics in animals. Thus most studies of cerebral blood flow (CBF) and metabolism ($CMRO_2$) are performed with light anaesthesia in the controls, usually 70% N_2O, assuming that this has little or no effect upon CBF or $CMRO_2$. The effects of nitrous oxide thus become important also for the evaluation of other anaesthetics, but although it is generally held that by itself it has little effect on CBF or $CMRO_2$, there are some awkward discrepancies in the literature [2]. The Philadelphia group reported in man a slight reduction in $CMRO_2$ varying from 2%–23% with no effect on CBF [3]. Theye and Michenfelder [4] showed a significant 11% increase in $CMRO_2$ in dogs, and an average 40% increase in CBF. Carlsson et al. [5] found no significant effect of 70% N_2O on CBF or $CMRO_2$ in rats, where the controls were not given anaesthetics, but had the stress-response blocked by adrenalectomy. It is possible that the great variability in results with N_2O, and thus in the control situation of many other experiments, are due to the lack of a truly anaesthetic state, with variations in cerebral function and stress-response. In dogs given N_2O, CBF can be increased by auditory stimuli, and Siesjö's group [5] showed that $CMRO_2$ doubled in unanaesthetized rats when they were paralysed and mechanically ventilated, if the stress-response was not blocked.

With this reservation about the control situation in most animal experiments, let us look at the effects of other inhalational anaesthetics on $CMRO_2$. It appears that they all, including halothane, enflurane, isoflurane, cyclopropane, and diethyl ether depress $CMRO_2$, and that they probably do so in a dose-related manner. For example, 1 MAC halothane or isoflurane reduces $CMRO_2$ by approximately 15%, 1 MAC enflurane by approximately 30%. This reduction is probably secondary to a reduced neuronal activity; there are no changes in cerebral energy stores, lactate concentrations, or L/P rations in the clinical dosage range, and the changes in metabolic rate correlate well the changes in electroencephalogram (EEG) [1].

Cerebral metabolic rate is gradually reduced with increasing doses of halothane, enflurane, and isoflurane in dogs as reported by Stullken et al. [6], but the most dramatic reduction occurs when the EEG changes from an awake to an anaesthetized pattern. It should also be noted that this occurs at concentrations below 1 MAC. In contrast to barbiturates, where the correlation between cerebral function and metabolic rate is complete in that $CMRO_2$ no longer changes when EEG is flat, it continues to fall with further increase in dose in the case of at least one inhalational anaesthetic, halothane. The reason for this is uncertain, but it could well be a sign of toxicity. Thus when dogs are exposed to halothane concentrations in steady state from 2.3%–9%, we see a dose-related decrease in cerebral ATP and PCr concentrations, and an increase in the lactate concentration and the L/P ratio. This is observed despite maintenance of adequate O_2 delivery to the brain, and is in direct contradistinction to the lack of such detrimental effects when high doses of barbiturates are used. Thus at concentrations above 3 MAC halothane can be shown to have direct toxic effects upon brain metabolism in vivo, significantly interfering with oxidative phosphorylation. These metabolic changes were shown to be fully reversible when the halothane concentration was decreased, and two dogs that were allowed to recover showed no gross alterations in neurological function [7]. Such effects have not been investigated for other inhalational agents; for enflurane $CMRO_2$ was no different at 2.2% than at 4.2%.

It is tempting to correlate these in vivo findings with the results of Cohen and Marshall [9] in liver mitochondria in vitro. Halothane produced a dose-related inhibition of respiration by blocking the oxidation of NADH, and with concentrations above 2% there was an increasing failure of recovery. The same effect has been described for methoxyflurane, enflurane, and diethyl ether, but in another study Rosenberg and Haugaard [10] failed to find a similar effect on central nervous system (CNS) mitochondria.

In regional cerebral ischaemia, Smith et al. [11] found that a high concentration of halothane (1.9%) was clearly detrimental. While barbiturates reduced the neurological deficit in comparison to the controls, halothane 0.6% was without effect and 1.9% increased the neurological deficit significantly. It is therefore again apparent that halothane at around 3 MAC has untoward cerebral effects. This could be due to the toxic effects suggested above, or possibly to haemodynamic effects.

A puzzling observation over the years has been that all inhalational anaesthetics, again with the possible exception of N_2O, disrupt the normally close relationship between cerebral metabolism and blood flow. Smith and Wollman's article [3] shows the ratio of CBF to $CMRO_2$ as a function of anaesthetic depth for a variety of anaesthetics. It is apparent that the ratio increases during anaesthesia, and it does so in a dose-related fashion. This might be viewed as beneficial, since O_2 delivery to the brain is increased relative to the O_2 needs. Alternatively, one might conclude that for reasons unknown the brain requires a higher O_2 tension in the presence of volatile anaesthetics, which is not reflected in the levels of cerebral metabolites, however.

In connection with this, inhalational anaesthetics modify the autoregulation curve. Under control conditions CBF is constant for perfusion pressures from 60 to 150 mmHg. This control is gradually reduced with increased doses of volatile anaesthetics, so that CBF is finally totally dependent upon the cerebral perfusion pressure. The two bends on the curve also move towards lower pressures with increasing doses, with a higher CBF for the same perfusion pressure. Thus it is likely that the brain can tolerate lower perfusion pressures during inhalational than during intravenous anaesthesia, at least in the absence of areas with rigid stenosis. This effect can be explained by a direct vasodilation caused by the anaesthetics or by an effect upon the CO_2 response. Volatile anaesthetics thus also modify this by potentiating the effects of CO_2 upon the CBF within the outer limits of this effect, but these limits seem to be unchanged. The concequences of these haemodynamic effects are discussed in the following paper, and are therefore not dealt with here.

Most inhalational anaesthetics have been reported to cause convulsions. Until the introduction of enflurane, convulsions were most frequently observed with diethyl ether, while halothane rarely if ever produces convulsions. Enflurane is the most thoroughly investigated anaesthetic in this regard. I think all investigators agree that by using relatively high concentrations (up to 3.5%) where there is hypocapnia, seizures can be induced spontaneously or by sudden auditory stimuli. Electroencephalic changes have been seen with concentrations as low as 1%; the incidence of muscle twitching has been reported to be approximately 7%, accompanied by occasional spiking activity. This EEG activity is reversible with reductions in anaesthetic concentrations and avoidance of hypocapnia [1]. Both in man and dogs the seizures increase $CMRO_2$ to or above control levels obtained before the anaesthesia, but in the dogs CBF increased simultaneously; thus O_2 delivery remained adequate and there has been no evidence of cerebral hypoxia during the seizures [8].

In an extensive study in dogs Joas et al. [12] examined a number of anaesthetics for their potential to induce seizures in the presence of hypocapnia. Diethyl and divinyl ether produced spontaneous seizures and enflurane and fluroxene seizures after auditory stimuli, while isoflurane only caused spiking, and halothane, chloroform, and cyclopropane failed to elicit seizures.

Chronic exposure to trace amounts of inhalational agents has not been established as a cause of neurological damage. A possible exception is the recent report by Cohen et al. [13] which is discussed elsewhere in this symposium and indicates numbness and muscle weakness in dental workers exposed to N_2O. This effect also seemed dose-dependent. The only other evidence for CNS effects in man is possible behavioural changes during or immediately after a few hours of exposure, as reported by Bruce and Bach [14] for 500 ppm N_2O combined with either halothane or enflurane. Three other independent groups have not been able to reproduce these results, however [1].

Stevens et al. [15] found no consistent brain injury after chronic exposure to subanaesthetic doses of halothane, isoflurane, or diethyl ether in rats, mice, or guinea-pigs, while Chang et al. [16] reported on pathological changes in brain cells after chronic exposure to trace amounts of halothane in rats and in the offspring after exposure during gestation. It should be noted that the validity of this work has been challenged.

In conclusion it seems that there are no serious CNS effects of normal concentrations of inhalational anaesthetics that deter from their use in most clinical situations.

References

1. Steen PA, Michenfelder JD (1979) Neurotoxicity of anaesthetics. 50:437–453
2. Siesjö BK (1978) Brain energy metabolism. John Wiley & Sons, Chichester New York Brisbane Toronto
3. Smith AL, Wollman H (1972) Cerebral blood flow and metabolism: Effects of anaesthetic drugs and techniques. Anaesthesiology 36:378–400
4. Theye RA, Michenfelder JD (1968) The effect of nitrous oxide on canine cerebral metabolism. Anaesthesiology 29:1119–1124
5. Carlsson C, Hägerdal M, Siesjö BK (1976) The effect of nitrous oxide on oxygen consumption and blood flow in the cerebral cortex of the rat. Acta Anaesth Scand 20:91–95

6. Stullken EH, Milde JH, Michenfelder JD, Tinker JH (1977) The nonlinear response of cerebral meta-
    bolism to low concentrations of halothane, enflurane, isoflurane and thiopental. Anaesthesiology
    46:28–34
7. Michenfelder JD, Theye RA (1975) In vivo toxic effects of halothane on canine cerebral metabolic
    pathways. Am J Physiol 229:1050–1055
8. Michenfelder JD, Cucchiara RF (1974) Canine cerebral oxygen consumption during enflurane anaes-
    thesia and its modification during induced seizures. Anaesthesiology 40:575–580
9. Cohen PJ, Marshall BE (1968) Effects of halothane on respiratory control and oxygen consumption
    of rat liver mitochondria. In: Fink BR (ed) Toxicity of anaesthetics. Williams & Wilkins, Baltimore,
    pp 24–36
10. Rosenberg H, Haugaard N (1973) The effects of halothane on metabolism and calcium uptake in
    mitochondria of the rat liver and brain. Anaesthesiology 39:44–52
11. Smith AL, Hoff JT, Nielsen SL, et al. (1974) Barbiturate protection in acute focal ischaemia. Stroke
    5:1–7
12. Joas TA, Stevens WC, Eger EI II (1971) Electroencephalic seizure activity in dogs during anaesthesia.
    Br J Anaesth 43:739–745
13. Cohen EN, Brown BW, Wu MC, et al. (1980) Occupational disease in dentistry and chronic exposure
    to trace anaesthetic gases. J Am Dent Ass 101:21–31
14. Bruce DL, Bach MJ (1975) Physiological studies of human performance as affected by traces of en-
    flurane and nitrous oxide. Anaesthesiology 42:194–196
15. Stevens WC, Eger EI II, White A, et al. (1975) Comparative toxicities of halothane, isoflurane and
    diethyl ether at subanaesthetic concentrations in laboratory animals. Anaesthesiology 42:408–419
16. Chang LW, Dudley AW Jr, Katz J (1976) Pathological changes in the nervous system following in
    utero exposure to halothane. Environ Res 11:40–51

The Effects of Inhalation Anaesthetics on Intracranial Pressure

G. Cunitz

Intracranial pressure (ICP) is built up by the components brain tissue, blood-vessels (including cerebral volume), and cerebrospinal fluid. If one of them increases its volume, pressure within the skull will rise, for there is no room for rapid compensation. A pressure increase or decrease under the influence of anaesthetics is mainly caused by changes in cerebral blood flow, or rather blood volume. Recently it was shown that the brain tissue itself can in this context contribute to a pressure increase during anaesthesia. Modern inhalation anaesthetics, such as halothane, enflurane, or methoxyflurane, are well known to increase ICP. Since the investigations of McDowall et al. [6], Marx et al. [5], Jennett et al. [4], and others, we know that halothane increases ICP, that this effect is dosage-dependent, and that the increase will be greater the higher the pre-existing pressure level is.

Enflurane also elevates ICP, but to a lower degree when compared with halothane on the basis of MAC values. We administered halothane and enflurane alternately to ten neurosurgical patients who had already received a basic anaesthesia consisting of a neurolept analgesia (NLA). An NLA, in its steady state, leaves ICP unchanged. Our results showed that halothane (1%–1.7%) increased ICP by 13 torr, whereas enflurane (1.5%–2.5%) did so by only 4 torr in mean [2].

Figure 1 gives a practical example of our results. A 63-year-old woman suffering from a syringomyelia was alternately given ethrane, penthrane, and halothane. All increased ICP, but enflurane, used in a dosage comparable with halothane, did so to a clearly lower degree. Blood-pressure fell after all anaesthetics in a remarkable manner; PCO_2 remained nearly the same during the measurements, an important prior condition. But in our investigations pre-existing ICP level was in the range of only 0–20 torr. With higher ICP values enflurane can also markedly elevate ICP, as Schulte am Esch and co-workers [10] were able to show. Nevertheless, they observed too that the effect of enflurane often seemed to be somewhat slighter than that of halothane.

Halogenated inhalation anaesthetics increase ICP. How far this increase involves a danger for the patient remains a question for later discussion. But what about nitrous oxide? For quite a long time nitrous oxide had been regarded as an inert gas without any real practical influence on body function. In 1973 Hendriksen and Jörgensen [3] described an ICP increase after nitrous oxide. Twelve patients were given 66% nitrous oxide in oxygen through a face mask. Intracranial pressure rose to a remarkably high level. The pressure increase was 27 torr (in mean). PCO_2 remained the same during their investigation. The authors concluded that nitrous oxide should not be used for induction of anaesthesia in intracranial pathology. Figure 2 gives an example of the ICP-elevating effect of nitrous oxide. It is taken from a paper by Schulte am Esch and co-workers [10]. Eight patients suffering from head injury, re-

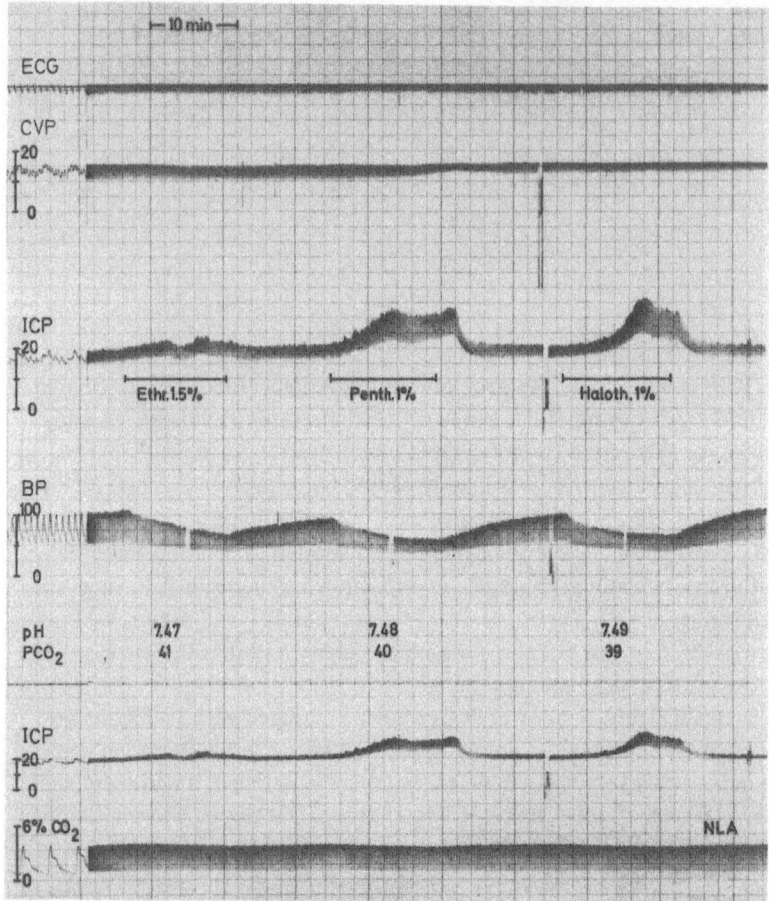

Fig. 1. Effect of Ethrane, Penthrane, and halothane on central venous pressure (*CVP*), intracranial pressure (*ICP*), and blood-pressure (*BP*). *ECG*, electrocardiogram. The patient has a basic neurolept analgesia

laxed by pancuronium, received 66% nitrous oxide in oxygen. A clear ICP increase can be seen. Pressure dropped while the gas was still being administered. Blood-pressure fell by 16%. Cerebral perfusion pressure also dropped. This is quite an interesting effect of the so-called innocent nitrous oxide.

The situation is, however, not as clear as it might seem after these examples and statements. The question arises why the effect of nitrous oxide on ICP was detected so late, and why, until today, so few conclusions have been drawn from these findings. Figure 3 might contribute to an answer. A 24-year-old woman suffering from an hydrocephalus internus was given 66% nitrous oxide during an NLA. When the volatile anaesthetic was removed, nothing happened. Intracranial pressure remained unaffected, ranging between 8 and 10 torr.

Now, nitrous oxide elevates the pressure within the skull. But this effect is neutralized by various agents used in anaesthesia, among them i.v. anaesthetics and the drugs used in an NLA [7]. The pressure-increasing effect of halothane and enflurane can also be counterbalanced by i.v. anaesthetics, and sometimes by hyperventilation [1]. By these techniques the

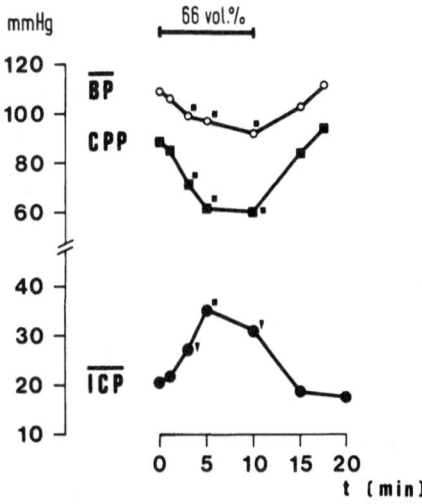

Fig. 2. Influence of 66% nitrous oxide in oxygen on blood-pressure (*BP*), cerebral perfusion pressure (*CCP*), and intracranial pressure (*ICP*). The patients with head injury (n = 8) are relaxed and ventilated. ▲ = $p < 0.05$, ■ = $p < 0.01$. Schulte am Esch [10]

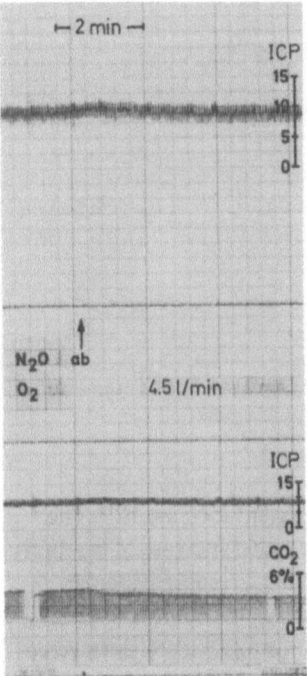

Fig. 3. Behaviour of intracranial pressure (*ICP*) after removal of nitrous oxide (66% in oxygen). The patient has received a basic sedation

pressure increase can be diminished but often not eliminated. Figure 4 presents some results obtained from a 37-year-old man with a Lindau tumour. The patient was given etomidate 15 mg, whereafter a decrease in pressure occurred. It rose again to reach its previous level, but after injection of 150 mg thiopental 15 min later, fell once more. The patient then received 1% halothane. The intracranial pressure now clearly rose in an expected manner. By the injection of 4 ml althesine this pressure increase was able to be promptly neutralized.

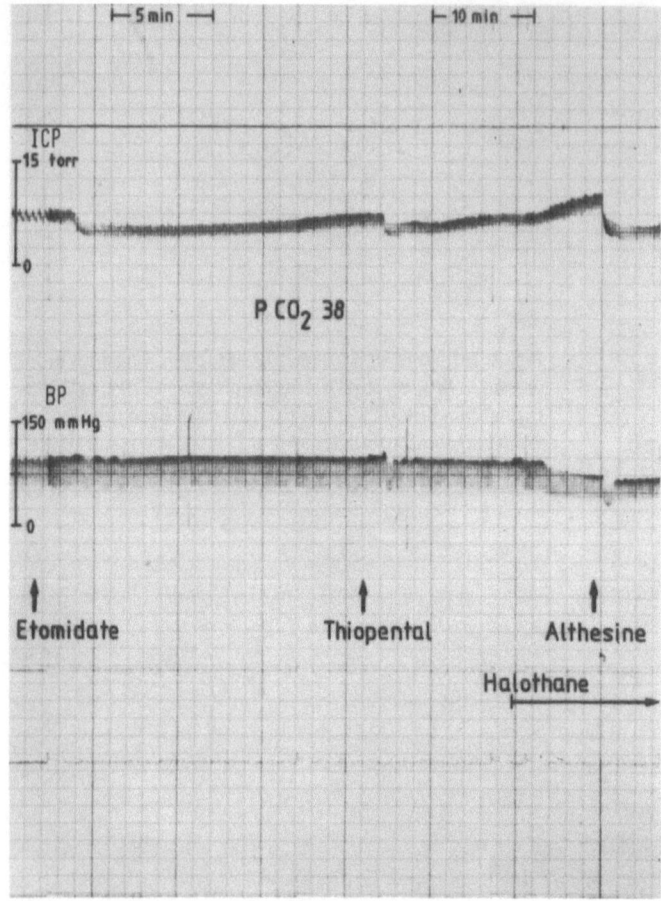

Fig. 4. Changes of intracranial pressure (*ICP*) and blood-pressure (*BP*) after administration of etomidate, thiopenthal, halothane, and althesine. The patient has been given a neurolept analgesia

It is clear that volatile anaesthetic drugs to a greater or lesser extent increase ICP. The result is, as we know, effected by a cerebral vascular dilatation, or rather increase in cerebral blood volume. Any attempts to neutralize this effect aim at achieving a cerebral vascular constriction, for example by hyperventilation or injection of i.v. anaesthetics. A new point of view has been brought into the discussion by the results of Schettini [9]. They discovered a real augmentation in brain stiffness and elastance under the influence of modern, strong-acting inhalation anaesthetics, the effect of which was independent of the cerebral vascular system. They even speak of a metabolic oedema produced by halothane. Figure 5 shows their main results. Recorded are surface brain pressure and electrical impedance. The latter reflects the state of fluid and electrolyte accumulation in the brain tissue. The results were obtained from dogs under thiopental and hyperventilation. It can be seen that enflurane, isoflurane, and above all halothane produce increased surface pressure and electrical impedance, in comparison to those of control animals. A thiopental anaesthesia by itself did not produce such changes.

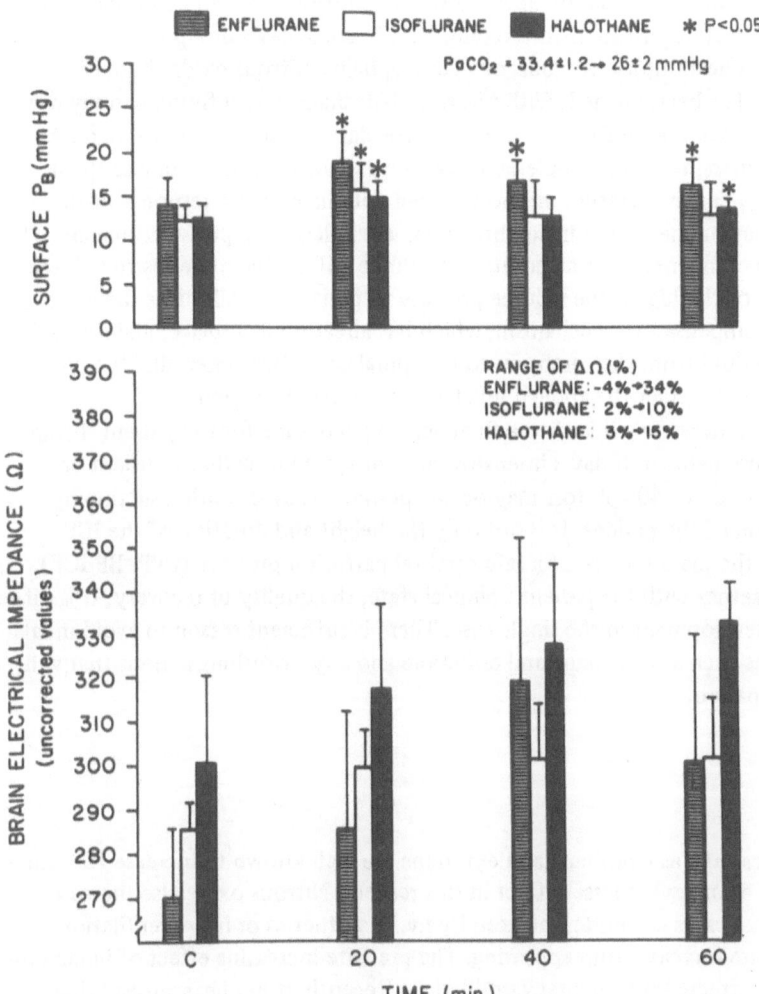

Fig. 5. Augmentation of surface brain pressure and brain electrical impedance after application of enflurane, isoflurane, and halothane in dogs (n = 9; x ± SD). Schettini et al. [9]

These new and somewhat exciting results lead us to the conclusion that halogenated inhalation anaesthetics increase ICP not by cerebral vasodilation alone, but by a real augmentation of brain tissue itself. Schettini and Furniss [8] supported their arguments by the additional findings that it was the water and electrolyte content in the brain tissue that increased in the course of halothane anaesthesia. Hyperventilation and injection of thiopental were not able to counterbalance these effects.

The changes observed by the workers cited were small. The question arises whether these findings have or will have practical consequences for anaesthesia. The answer is not clear at the moment. In critical situations with regard to ICP and cerebral oedema, however, these potentially harmful effects of halothane and probably of enflurane should be borne in mind.

Is there any indication for inhalation anaesthetics in neurosurgery and neurological diagnostic investigation? With regard to nitrous oxide: Yes. In some cases of a pre-existing high ICP, however, in severe head injury, tumour, or hydrocephalus, nitrous oxide should be witheld until the skull has been opened. With regard to halothane and enflurane, in my opinion, there is no conclusive reason for their use in the special situations discussed here. An NLA or a barbiturate drip-infusion, completed by an analgaesic, are able to replace them. It depends on the compliance, or rather on the so-called volume-pressure response of the brain to what extent an augmentation in cerebral volume will lead to a pressure increase. The ability of the brain to compensate for an additional volume will be the more restricted, the lower the compliance or the higher the volume-pressure response. In reality it is the underlying illness and the compensatory mechanism, which has already taken place, mainly by shifting cerebrospinal fluid from the cerebrum to the spinal cord, that determine the pressure increase which occurs under the applied inhalational anaesthetic agents.

Not every pressure increase will lead to a final negative outcome for the patient. From continuous ICP measurements in today's intensive care units, we know that transient pressure elevations reaching up to 40–60 torr may occur spontaneously or during suctioning, coughing, or intubation of the patient. It is not only the height and duration of the ICP peaks, but even more the maintenance of a safe cerebral perfusion pressure (CPP=BP-ICP), which determines, together with the patient's clinical state, the quality of recovery. It is difficult to predict the development in the single case. There is sufficient reason to avoid inhalation anaesthetic agents such as halothane and enflurane and any disturbing actions that will increase the ICP of a patient.

Summary

Inhalation anaesthetics such as halothane and enflurane are well known to increase ICP. Enflurane seems to have a somewhat lesser effect in this respect. Nitrous oxide also increases ICP. This effect in most cases is counterbalanced by i.v. anaesthetics or hyperventilation, thus preventing pressure increase from appearing. The pressure-increasing effect of inhalation anaesthetics is mainly effected by cerebral vasodilation. Recently it has been proved that strong-acting inhalation anaesthetics augment cerebral tissue itself, thus producing more stiffness and elastance in the tissue. There exist enough reasons to avoid halothane and enflurane in the presence of high ICP, or where there is the danger of ICP elevation.

References

1. Adams RW, Gronert GA, Sundt TM, Michenfelder JD (1972) Halothane, hypocapnia and cerebrospinal fluid pressure in neurosurgery. In: Brock M, Dietz H (eds) Intracranial pressure. Springer, Berlin Heidelberg New York, pp
2. Cunitz G, Danhauser I, Gruß P (1976) Die Wirkung von Enflurane (Ethrane) im Vergleich zu Halothan auf den intracraniellen Druck. Anaesthesist 25:323–330
3. Henriksen HT, Jörgensen PB (1973) The effect of nitrous oxide on intracranial pressure in patients with intracranial disorders. Br J Anaesth 45:486–492
4. Jennett WB, Barker J, Fitch W, McDowall DG (1969) Effect of anaesthesia on intracranial pressure in patients with space-occupying lesions. Lancet I:61–68

5. Marx GF, Andrews IC, Orkin LR (1962) Cerebrospinal fluid pressures during halothane anaesthesia. Can Anaesth Soc J 9:239–245
6. McDowall DG, Jennett WB, Barker J (1968) The effects of halothane and trichloroethylene on cerebral perfusion and metabolism and on intracranial pressure. Prog Brain Res 30:
7. Phirman JR, Shapiro HM (1977) Modification of nitrous oxideinduced intracranial hypertension by prior induction of anaesthesia. Anaesthesiology 46:150–151
8. Schettini A, Furniss WW (1979) Brain water and electrolyte distribution during the inhalation of halothane. Br J Anaesth 51:1117–1124
9. Schettini A (1980) Incompatiblity of halogenated anaesthetics with brain surgery. In: Shulmann K, Marmarou A, Miller JD, Becker DP, Hochwald GW, Brock M (eds) Intracranial pressure, vol 4. Springer, Berlin Heidelberg New York, pp
10. Schulte am Esch J, Thiemig I, Pfeifer G, Entzian W (1979) Die Wirkung einiger Inhalationsanaesthetika auf den intracraniellen Druck unter besonderer Berücksichtigung des Stickoxydul. Anaesthesist 28:136–141

The Effects of Inhalation Anaesthetic Agents on Liver Blood Flow and Hepatic Oxygen Consumption

W. Fitch, R.L. Hughes, I. Thomson, and D. Campbell

Introduction

Recent years have witnessed the introduction and development of new techniques in hepato-biliary surgery such as those now employed in the elective management of high bile duct strictures and the solitary metastatic lesion of the liver. In addition, definitive treatment of primary hepatic tumours and bile duct neoplasms can be attempted.

However, although technical expertise has advanced steadily, it must be accepted that knowledge of the physiological control of liver haemodynamics has not progressed as rapidly. Moreover, even less is known about how the basic physiological processes are modified by the administration of anaesthetic drugs and the application of techniques of anaesthesia such as intermittent positive pressure ventilation, positive end-expiratory pressure, and induced hypotension. In addition, disorders of liver function are encountered not infrequently in intensive care areas, often as a component of multiple organ failure. Unfortunately, we must admit our inability to reverse such disorders − largely because we lack insight into the alterations in normal function which have taken place and do not know whether prolonged mechanical ventilation, for instance, adds to or lessens the physiological trespass.

An animal model was developed to permit the investigation of the basic responses of the intact hepatic circulation to alterations in physiological variables such as carbon dioxide tension, oxygen tension, and metabolic balance. The effects of certain anaesthetic agents such as halothane, enflurane, and nitrous oxide have been assessed and are considered further in this presentation.

Materials and Methods

Anaesthesia

Anaesthesia was induced in greyhounds (25−35 kg) with thiopentone (20 mg $\cdot$ kg^{-1} i.v.) and maintained with pentobarbitone (initial dose 30 mg $\cdot$ kg^{-1} i.v. plus supplements of 2 mg $\cdot$ kg^{-1} i.v. when required). Following endotracheal intubation the lungs were ventilated artificially with a mixture of nitrogen 75% in oxygen. The minute volume of ventilation and the inspired oxygen concentration were adjusted as necessary to maintain stable physiological tensions of carbon dioxide and oxygen in arterial blood. Pancuronium (0.15 mg $\cdot$ kg^{-1} i.v.) was administered to produce and maintain neuromuscular blockade.

Surgical Procedure

The operative procedure has been detailed previously [2]; it is summarized here. Following laparotomy, hepatic arterial and portal venous blood flows were measured using Statham SP 2202 electromagnetic flowmeters with appropriate probes. Cannulae placed into the portal vein and the hepatic vein permitted measurement of the pressures in the portal and hepatic veins, and the withdrawal of blood for the determination of oxygen content. Systemic arterial pressure was monitored continuously and cardiac output (thermodilution technique) determined at intervals. Hepatic arterial resistance and hepatic oxygen consumption were calculated using the following equations:

Hepatic arterial resistance =

$$\frac{\text{Mean arterial pressure} - \text{hepatic venous pressure (mmHg)}}{\text{hepatic arterial blood flow (ml} \cdot \text{min}^{-1}).}$$

Hepatic oxygen consumption (ml $\cdot$ min^{-1})

$$= \left[\frac{\text{portal venous blood flow}}{100} \times (\text{portal venous} - \text{hepatic venous O}_2 \text{ content}) \right]$$
$$+ \left(\frac{\text{hepatic arterial blood flow}}{100} \times \text{hepatic arterial} - \text{hepatic venous O}_2 \text{ content} \right)$$

where portal venous and hepatic arterial blood flows are expressed in ml $\cdot$ min^{-1}. Arterial blood gas tensions and the acid-base status of the animals were measured using a Corning 165 blood gas/pH analyser. The haematocrit was measured hourly to ensure that it remained greater than 40%. The liver was removed and weighed at the end of each investigation.

Experimental Programme

Nitrous Oxide

Baseline values were obtained in seven animals and nitrous oxide in a concentration of 30% was administered. The remainder of the inspired gas mixture was made up of oxygen and nitrogen adjusted as necessary to maintain a PaO$_2$ of 100 mmHg. Measurements were obtained and blood samples withdrawn after 30 min at 30% nitrous oxide. The animals were ventilated without nitrous oxide for 30 min and further measurements obtained. This procedure was repeated with nitrous oxide concentrations of 50% and 70%.

Halothane

Six animals were prepared as described above and after the determination of baseline values halothane was added to the inspired gas mixture in concentrations of 0.5%, 1%, 1.5%, and 2%. Each concentration was administered for 30 min and measurements of hepatic arterial blood flow, portal venous blood flow, and mean arterial pressure noted. The concentration of halothane was increased and further measurements obtained (the preparation was not returned to baseline between each halothane concentration).

Enflurane

A further group of six greyhounds received enflurane in concentrations of 1%, 1.5%, 2% and 3%. Measurements were obtained and blood samples withdrawn as in the halothane group.

Results

The administration of nitrous oxide induced stepwise decreases in hepatic arterial blood flow and portal venous blood flow, which were reflected in similar decreases in total liver blood flow (Table 1). Systemic vascular resistance was increased during the administration of nitrous oxide 50% and 70%, and hepatic arterial resistance increased significantly at all the concentrations studied.

Portal venous blood flow decreased significantly with each concentration of halothane to a minimum value of about 45% of the baseline with halothane 2% (Table 2). The decrease in hepatic arterial blood flow was greater, reaching 35% of the baseline during the administration of halothane 2%. Hepatic arterial resistance did not change significantly.

The administration of enflurane significantly decreased portal venous blood flow at each step increase in concentration, and hepatic arterial blood flow at 3% enflurane. Hepatic arterial resistance decreased significantly with enflurane 1.5% and 3%.

Discussion

A reciprocity of response has been shown under a variety of conditions between portal venous and hepatic arterial blood flows [1], such that there is a concomitant decrease in hepatic arterial resistance (increase in hepatic arterial flow) as portal venous blood flow is decreased. In this way the oxygen supply to the liver is protected. In the present study, halothane induced a decrease in portal venous blood flow and an increase in hepatic arterial resistance. The administration of enflurane induced decreases in portal venous blood flow similar to those produced by equipotent concentrations of halothane, but since hepatic arterial resistance decreased significantly, hepatic arterial blood flow was decreased less during enflurane. Millar and Biscoe [3] have shown that halothane increased post-ganglionic sympathetic activity in the rabbit, and this could be a mechanism by which vasodilatation in the hepatic arterioles is prevented during the administration of halothane.

The investigations described here were undertaken in an intact animal model with normal liver function. Nevertheless, they set the foundation for further studies in man under conditions of normal and abnormal liver function using appropriate techniques of blood flow measurement.

Acknowledgements. These investigations were supported by a grant from the Scottish Hospital Endowment Research Trust and were undertaken at the Wellcome Surgical Institute, University of Glasgow. The assistance of Miss Diane E. McCorkindale in typing the manuscript is noted with appreciation.

Table 1. Effects (mean ± SEM) of nitrous oxide on portal venous, hepatic, and total liver bloods flows and hepatic arterial resistance

Nitrous oxide	Baseline	30%	Baseline	50%	Baseline	70%
Portal venous blood flow (ml · 100 g · min⁻¹)	102 ± 14	91 ± 14[b]	95 ± 17	87 ± 18[b]	96 ± 15	82 ± 13[b]
Hepatic arterial blood flow (ml · 100 g · min⁻¹)	44 ± 6	39 ± 6[b]	44 ± 7	37 ± 6[b]	37 ± 6	29 ± 6[b]
Total liver blood flow (ml · 100 g · min⁻¹)	147 ± 18	130 ± 18[c]	139 ± 22	123 ± 21[c]	134 ± 15	111 ± 13[b]
Hepatic arterial resistance (units)	0.65 ± 11	0.85 ± 18[a]	0.70 ± 0.14	1.06 ± 0.3[a]	0.77 ± 0.13	1.07 ± 0.21[b]

[a] $p < 0.05$; [b] $p < 0.01$; [c] $p < 0.001$

Table 2. Effects (mean ± SEM) of equipotent concentrations of halothane and enflurane on portal venous and hepatic arterial blood flows, and hepatic arterial resistance

	Portal venous blood flow (% baseline)	Hepatic arterial blood flow (% baseline)	Hepatic arterial resistance (% baseline)
Halothane (n = 6)			
0.5%	74 ± 7[b]	76 ± 6[a]	95 ± 5
1%	72 ± 6[a]	60 ± 5[a]	110 ± 7
1.5%	55 ± 6[c]	37 ± 4[a]	125 ± 12
2%	45 ± 5[c]	35 ± 4[b]	94 ± 5
Enflurane (n = 6)			
1%	75 ± 108[b]	80 ± 10	75 ± 7
1.5%	65 ± 5[b]	75 ± 11	65 ± 4[a]
2%	65 ± 5[b]	74 ± 12	63 ± 12
3%	44 ± 6[b]	55 ± 7[a]	50 ± 10[a]

[a] $p < 0.05$; [b] $p < 0.01$; [c] $p < 0.001$

References

1. Hanson KM, Johnson PC (1966) Local control of hepatic arterial and portal venous flow in the dog. Am J Physiol 211:712
2. Hughes RL, Mathie RT, Campbell D, Fitch W (1979) The effect of hypercarbia on hepatic blood flow and oxygen consumption in the greyhound. Br J Anaesth 51:289
3. Millar RA, Biscoe TJ (1966) Postganglionic sympathetic discharge and the effect of inhalational anaesthetics. Br J Anaesth 38:92

Total Effect of Repeated Anaesthetics on Liver Function

J.P.H. Fee, G.W. Black, and J.W. Dundee

Halothane and enflurane are the only widely used potent inhalational agents, and the latter is often substituted for halothane when repeated administrations are required, although there has been no clear evidence that it is a safe alternative which would reduce the possibility of hepatitis. Comprehensive prospective studies were clearly needed to obtain data on the repeated use of anaesthetics, and it was decided to carry out a trial to try to determine (a) the extent of the relationship between repeated administrations of halothane and enflurane and the onset of hepatic dysfunction, and (b) which patients are liable to develop liver damage after repeated anaesthesia.

The agents were studied in two groups of patients who were broadly comparable as regards age, sex, and physical characteristics. Sixty-three patients received two or more administrations of halothane, and 66 had two or more enflurane anaesthetics. The main emphasis of the study centred on liver function tests. Blood was withdrawn for analysis before anaesthesia and again on the 4th and 14th post-operative days. A large number of laboratory tests were carried out on the samples, but the most useful data came from the determinations of alanine aminotransferase (ALT) and gamma glutamyl transpepidase (GGT). A significant number of patients who received halothane repeatedly had abnormal levels of GGT and ALT, and this trend became more pronounced as the number of administrations increased. This was not the case with enflurane, little alteration in liver function tests being noted with repeated anaesthesia.

The vast majority of abnormal liver function tests occurred in obese subjects who had received repeated halothane anaesthetics. Repeated halothane anaesthesia lead to disturbed hepatic function in 48% of obese patients and in only 10% of non-obese. In the case of enflurane there was little difference between the obese patients and those of normal build. Indeed, if the data relating to obese patients were excluded there would be little difference between the two agents as regards altered enzymatic activity. Such findings may be accounted for by the lower fat solubility and reduced storage of enflurane in the body. The incidence of disturbed liver function was more pronounced when anaesthesia was given repeatedly within a 6-week period, an observation which supports the findings of earlier reports.

It seems reasonable to assumethat the changes in serum enzyme concentrations which often accompany repeated anaesthesia reflect some degree of hepatic damage. When halothane was introduced into clinical practice some 25 years ago, it was assumed that it was inert substance eliminated from the body in an unchanged state. We now know that the majority of inhalational anaesthetics are metabolized in the body, and concern has been expressed that their biotransformation products may exert toxic effects on organs such as the liver and kidneys.

It is difficult to know why there should be such a high incidence of disorder of liver function after repeated halothane anaesthesia, and yet the incidence of massive hepatitis be mercifully low. It may be that substantial increases in halothane metabolism are necessary before clinical evidence of liver damage occurs. It seems reasonable to assume that the relatively minor changes in liver function tests noted in this study should not be ignored. When associated with other factors a sequence of events may take place which could lead to the onset of a fatal hepatitis.

The Effect of Inhalation Anaesthetics on Pulmonary Ventilation and Perfusion

L.J. Bjertnæs

During the last 2 decades, a number of investigators have demonstrated that general anaesthesia tends to impair pulmonary gas exchange [15, 16, 17]. Unless this tendency is counteracted by enhancing the oxygen concentration of the anaesthetic gas mixture, arterial hypoxaemia may develop. Although this condition is well documented, the pathophysiological mechanisms involved have been unsettled untill the last few years.

General anaesthesia has been shown to give rise to changes in pulmonary ventilation mechanics. Laws [13] found a fall in functional residual capacity upon induction of anaesthesia. At the beginning of the last decade, investigators [7, 10, 11, 12] demonstrated that the reduction in functional residual capacity in certain subjects contributes to the closure of peripheral dependent airways. On the basis of direct roentgenographic observations, Froese and Bryan [9] suggested that changes in ventilation mechanisms of this type are mainly due to a cephalad displacement of the diaphragm during anaesthesia. They further found that most of the lung movements during inflation occur in the non-dependent regions. The high blood solubility of anaesthetic gases in comparison to air facilitates absorption of gas trapped behind closed airways. These changes promote hypoventilation and/or atelectasis, especially in the dependent regions where initial volumes are small. If it should happen that regional perfusion is unchanged or even increased in such hypoventilated or atelectatic lung areas, arterial hypoxaemia will result.

In the awake state vasoconstriction within poorly ventilated regions of the lungs acts to divert local blood flow to better ventilated areas [22]. A possible explanation of the development of arterial hypoxaemia during anaesthesia therefore could be that this beneficial mechanism for redistribution of blood flow is hampered by anaesthetic agents. Already in 1972 and 1973, Sykes and co-workers [18, 19], using different models of isolated dog lungs, published results in support of such an idea.

At the Institute of Physiology, University of Oslo, we started to work on this hypothesis in 1974. Our experimental model was a preparation of isolated rat lungs perfused with blood at constant flow and constant outflow pressure. Pulmonary vasoconstrictor responses were then reflected as increments in inflow pressure – so-called pressor responses. Such responses were elicited by ventilating the lungs for standardized periods with a hypoxic – alternating with a normoxic gas mixture. When hypoxic pressor responses of a slightly increasing or equal magnitude were obtained, the anaesthetic agent to be tested was added either to the ventilation gas or to the blood reservoir. Figure 1 shows eight succeeding pressor responses to ventilation hypoxia. When diethyl ether was added to the ventilation gas at 103 and 135 min respectively from start of perfusion, the responses were almost completely abolished.

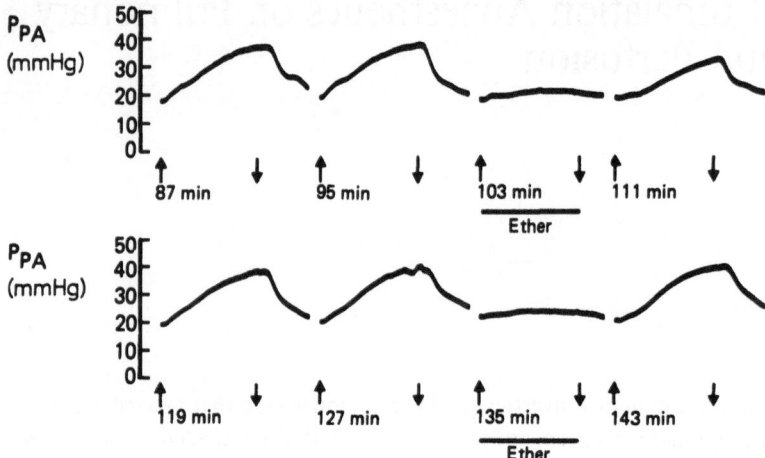

Fig. 1. Pulmonary arterial (*PA*) pressor responses to constant periods of ventilation hypoxia (↑ ↓). At 103 and 135 min respectively from start of perfusion, ether was administered together with the hypoxic gas mixture. [From Acta Anaesth Scand 21:139 (1977)]

In all the experiments with ether, the striking observation was a stepwise reduction of the pressor response with increasing concentration of the anaesthetic (Fig. 2). Such dose-response curves between reduction of response and blood concentration of inhalation anaesthetic were additionally obtained with halothane, methoxyflurane, and enflurane [2, 4]. Confirmatory evidence of a reducing effect of diethyl ether has also been reported by Sykes and co-workers [20], on the basis of observations on dogs exposed to unilateral hypoxia. In contrast, when the effects of halothane [21] and methoxyflurane [14] were evaluated by means of the same model, no change in response could be found.

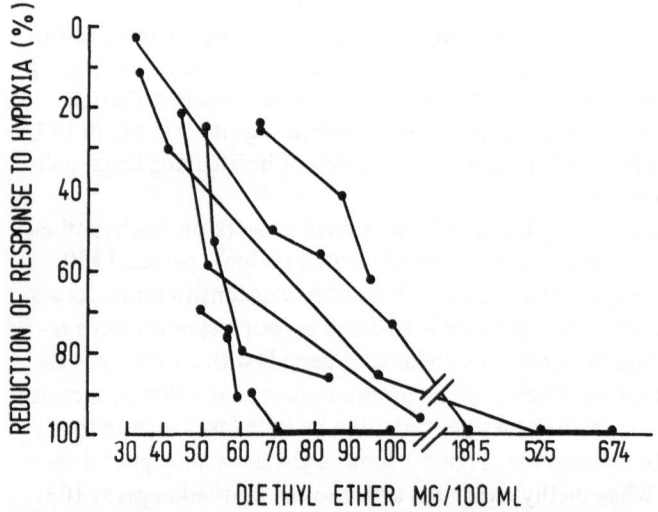

Fig. 2. Reduction of pulmonary arterial pressor responses to ventilation hypoxia caused by increasing concentrations of ether. [From Acta Anaesth Scand 21:139 (1977)]

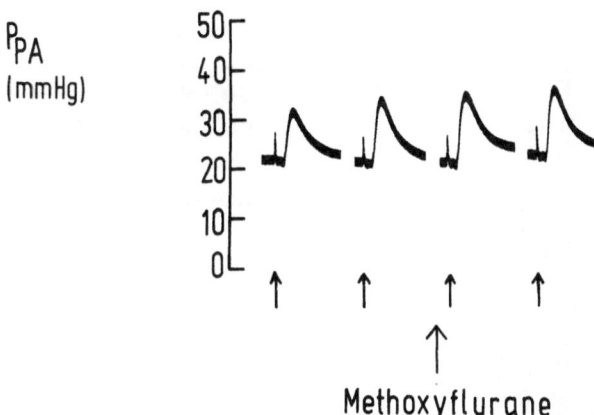

Fig. 3. Pressor responses to pulmonary arterial injection of a standardized dose of bradykinin (*small arrows*). The two last responses were obtained during administration of methoxyflurane (starts at *large arrow*) in a concentration which completely blocked any pressor response to ventilation hypoxia. [From Acta Anaesth Scand 21:143 (1977)]

Even when the inhalation anaesthetics ether, halothane, and methoxyflurane were administered in concentrations which completely abolished the pressor response to hypoxia, pressor responses to other stimuli such as bradykinin and kallidin remained unaltered. Figure 3 shows pressor responses to a standardized dose of bradykinin injected into the pulmonary artery (small arrows) before and during administration of methoxyflurane. The large arrow indicates start of methoxyflurane administration. The latter observation is in agreement with the hypothesis that the pressor response to hypoxia is controlled by a specific mechanism. This mechanism, however, can be pharmacologically blocked maintainig complete integrity of vascular smooth muscles. In contrast to the volatile inhalation anaesthetics, nitrous oxide and several anaesthetics for intravenous use, including fentanyl and the barbiturates, had no damping effect on the pressor response to hypoxia [2].

The observation that the hypoxic vasoconstriction in isolated rat lungs was inhibited by inhalation anaesthetics was a challenge to test ether and halothane for the same effect in man. The subjects, 17 young men, were anaesthetized with thiopental and curarized with pancuronium bromide. Repeated doses of fentanyl and thiopental were given intravenously for maintainance of anaesthesia. A cuffed Carléns double lumen tube was inserted, thus allowing independent ventilation of the lungs. One lung, the test lung, was ventilated with nitrogen, the other received pure oxygen. $PaCO_2$ was kept normal and constant within ± 0.5 kPa.

Figure 4 shows the arterial oxygen tension of some of the subjects plotted against time. The points to the extreme left indicate oxygen tensions before induction of anaesthesia. The points starting the uninterrupted lines represent arterial oxygen tensions shortly after induction of intravenous anaesthesia and start of unilateral hypoxia. When hypoxic vasoconstriction started, pulmonary blood flow was diverted to the oxygenated lung. A gradual increase in PaO_2 therefore occurred for the next 20–30 min. When a maximal hypoxia-induced vasoconstriction could be expected in the test lung, as judged by the arterial PO_2, a dose of ^{99}Tc human serum albumin macroaggregates was injected intravenously. This technique allowed determination of pulmonary blood flow distribution by means of scintigraphy after the operation. Halothane or ether administered to the hypoxic lung brought about a rapid decline in PaO_2. When no further fall in PaO_2 occurred, a second isotope, ^{131}I human serum albu-

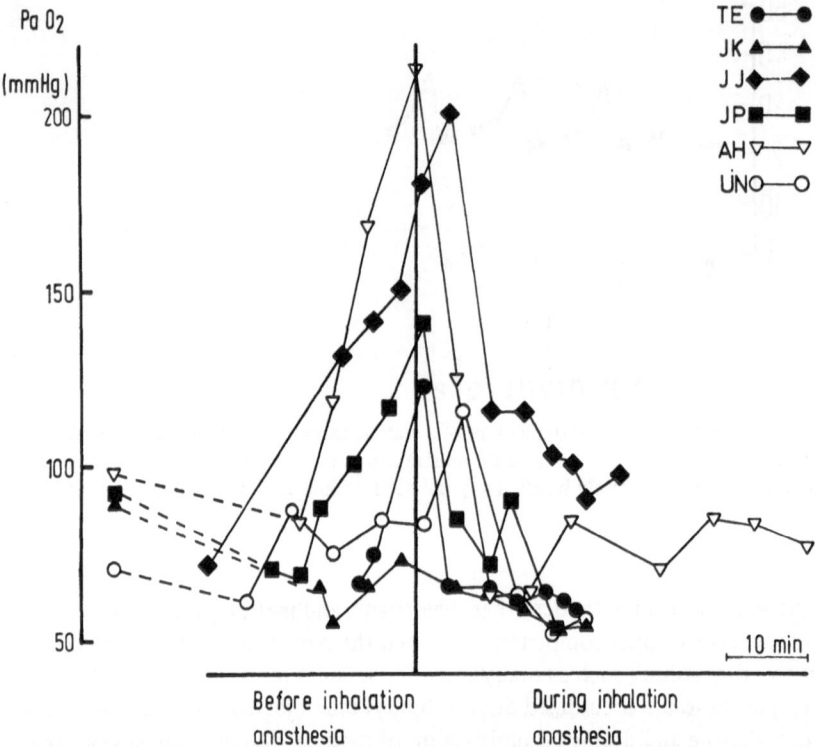

Fig. 4. Arterial oxygen tension (PaO$_2$) in six subjects prior to (*points to the extreme left*) and during unilateral hypoxia (*uninterupted lines*). In the first sequence of unilateral hypoxia the subjects were anaesthetized with intravenous anaesthetics. In the second sequence one of the inhalation anaesthetics halothane (*closed symbols*) or diethyl ether (*open symbols*) was administered via the hypoxic lung resulting in a reduction of PaO$_2$ within 10 min. [From Acta Physiol Scand 96:284 (1976)]

min macroaggregates was injected intravenously. The blood flow distribution thus obtained was compared with the normal distribution obtained by scintigraphy 2 days post-operatively.

Figure 5 shows three typical scintigrams from the examination of a 31-year-old man. The blood flow to the test lung (right lung) was reduced from 50% of the total pulmonary blood flow during air breathing (top) to 28% during unilateral hypoxia (middle). Following ipsilateral administration of diethyl ether, it increased to 48% indicating that hypoxic vasoconstriction is almost abolished (bottom). The upper and middle scintigrams were obtained with ^{99m}Tc, the lower one with ^{131}I.

The median distribution of blood flow to the test lung in this group was 50% (range 40%–64%) in the control situation, 26% (range 19%–46%) during unilateral hypoxia, and 37% (range 28%–49.4%) when one of the inhalation anaesthetics ether or halothane was superimposed on unilateral hypoxia. These findings clearly demonstrate that hypoxic vasoconstriction is severely impaired by ether and halothane, even in man [3].

In the above experiments we have studied hypoxic vasoconstriction in ventilated lungs. In many types of lung disease, atelectasis is a prominent feature. The atelectatic process may be local, for example limited to a lobe, or scattered throughout the lungs. Patients with atelectasis, as judged from chest radiograms, in many cases are surprisingly well oxygenated due

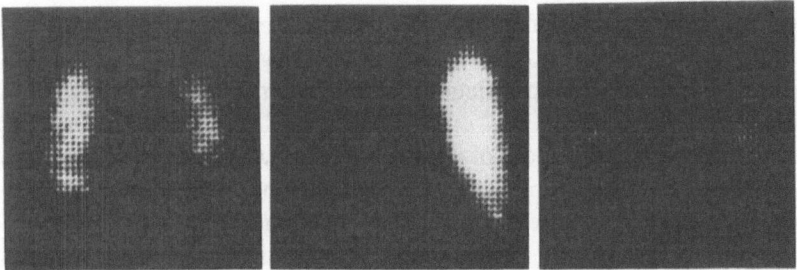

Fig. 5. Scintigrams of UN. The blood flow to the test lung was reduced from 50% of the total pulmonary blood flow during air breathing (*on the left*) to 28% during unilateral hypoxia (*middle*). Ipsilateral administration of ether brought about an increase to 48% (*on the right*). The upper and the middle scintigrams are taken with ^{99m}Tc, the lower one with ^{131}I

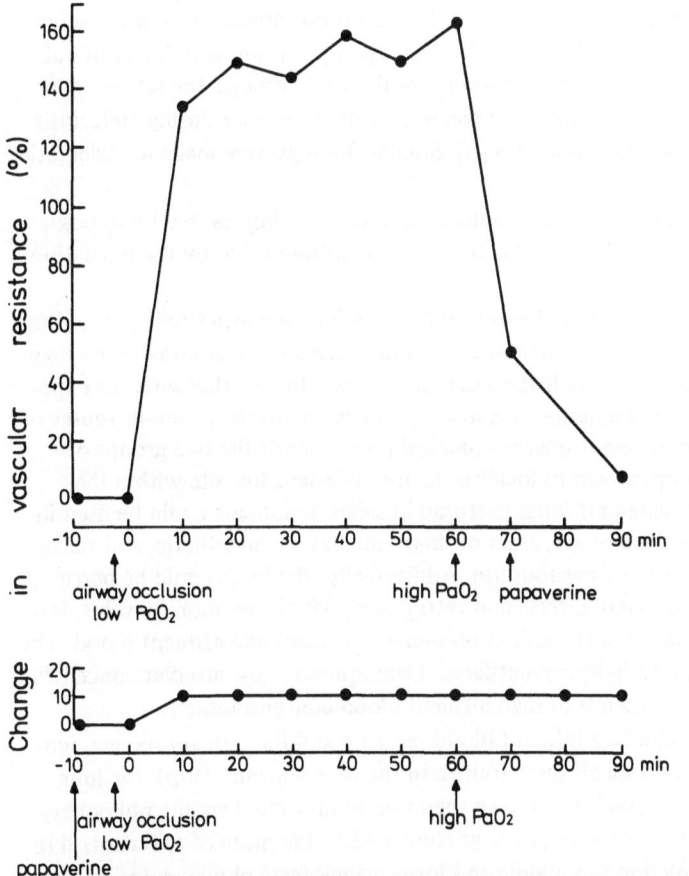

Fig. 6. Relative contribution of mechanical obstruction to the total rise in vascular resistance in atelectatic rat lungs. In one group consisting of ten preparations in which vascular reactivity was intact (*upper curve*), vascular resistance increased with 163% (median) above baseline during airway occlusion and perfusion with low perfusate PaO_2. The *arrows* indicate change to high perfusate PaO_2 and injection of papaverine respectively. In another group consisting of seven preparations (*lower curve*), papaverine was given prior to airway occlusion and perfusion with low perfusate PaO_2. In the latter group vascular reactivity increased with 10% (median) above baseline and no reduction was observed upon perfusion with high arterial PO_2

to diversion of blood to ventilated areas of the lungs. There is, however, no general agreement on whether the increased vascular resistance in atelectatic lungs is mainly caused by
mechanical obstruction or by active vasoconstriction, for example induced by low PO_2 of
mixed venous blood.

In order to settle this question, two pairs of isolated rat lungs were perfused in series.
In every experiment, one of the preparations was made atelectatic by airway occlusion. Simultaneously the other preparation was ventilated with a hypoxic gas mixture to give low
pulmonary arterial ("mixed venous") PO_2 in the atelectatic lung pair. Two groups were studied to determine the relative contribution of mechanical obstruction and active vasoconstriction to the total rise in vascular resistance during 1 h atelectasis. In one group (ten experiments) vascular reactivity was intact; in the other group (seven experiments) the vasculature
was paralysed by papaverine before airway occlusion (Fig. 6). In the first group, vascular
resistance increased with a median of 163% above baseline. High arterial PO_2 and papaverine
returned the median increase to 50% and 7% respectively. In the second group, papaverine
was added to the perfusate before airway occlusion. In this group vascular resistance increased with a median of 10% and no reduction was observed upon perfusion with high arterial
PO_2. If we compare the increase in vascular resistance in the latter groups, the relative contribution of mechanical obstruction to the total rise in vascular resistance during atelectasis
would at most have been 10/163, i.e. about 6% [6]. Similar findings were made in atelectatic
dog lung lobes by Benumof [1].

Since the increased vascular resistance in atelectatic lungs is mainly caused by hypoxic
vasoconstriction, it was not surprising to find a dose-dependent inhibition by the inhalation
anaesthetics ether, halothane, and enflurane.

In the first series of experiments [2], it was found that inhalation anaesthetics including
halothane reduced the hypoxia response in a dose-dependent fashion. In contrast, even high
doses of anaesthetics for intravenous use had no damping effect. In a further series of experiments [5], we wanted to find out whether this discrepancy is due to the different routes of
administration, rather than to different pharmacological properties of the two groups of
anaesthetics. An additional purpose was to localize the hypoxia-sensitive site within the
lungs. By using two pairs of isolated rat lungs perfused in series, halothane could be used in
the same preparation both via the airways, as an ordinary inhalation anaesthefic, and via the
bloodstream as an anaesthetic for intravenous use. Additionally, the lungs could be perfused
both anterogradely via the pulmonary artery, and retrogradely via the pulmonary veins. Halothane concentrations were determined both in pulmonary influent and effluent blood. The
lung preparations were continuously hyperventilated. Consequently, low alveolar concentrations could be expected in the presence of high influent blood concentrations.

Figure 7 demonstrates pulmonary influent blood-pressure and the effluent oxygen tension. Halothane was administered via all three routes. In the first sequence (top), the lung
preparation was retrogradely perfused. Halothane then was administered via the pulmonary
veins resulting in a 9% reduction of the response as compared to the mean of two control responses. The sequences presented in the middle and lower panels were obtained during normal anterograde perfusion. Administration via the pulmonary artery (middle) resulted in
43% reduction despite the influent blood halothane concentration was less. Following administration via the airways, the response was reduced by 93%.

In six preparations halothane was introduced via all three routes. Figure 8 presents the
relationship between reduction of the response as a percentage along the ordinate, and
blood concentrations of halothane along the abcissa. Reductions of the response caused by

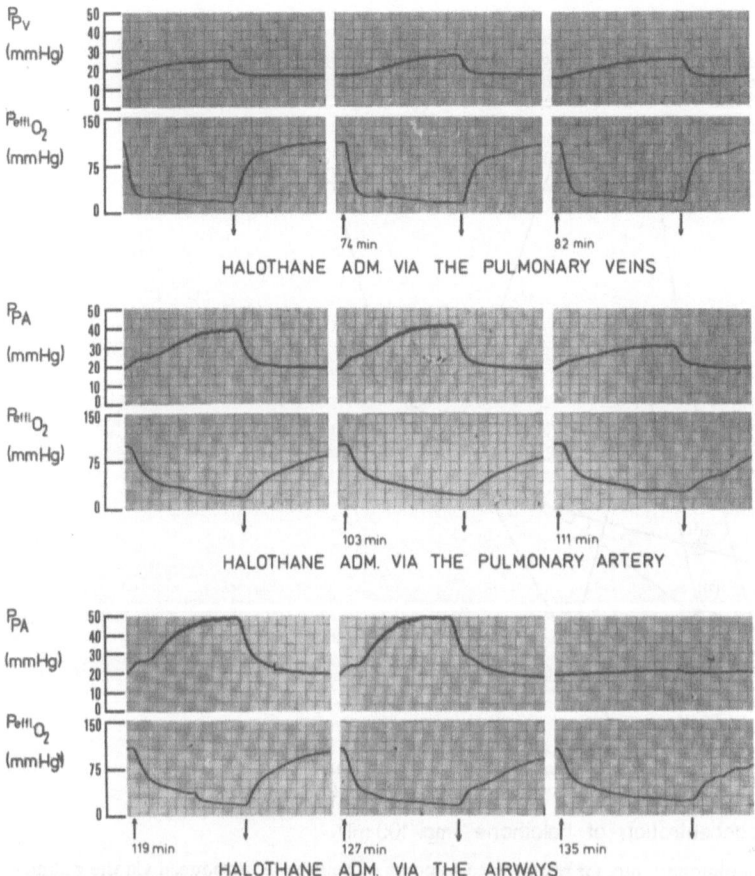

Fig. 7. Pulmonary pressor responses to hypoxia in one pair of isolated rat lungs before and during administration of halothane via the pulmonary veins (*upper panel*), the pulmonary artery (*middle panel*), and the airways (*lower panel*). Concomitant reductions in effluent PO_2 are shown below the pressure recordings. *Arrows* indicate start and termination of hypoxic periods. Time from start of perfusion is given. Flow was kept constant regardless of flow direction

venous administration (semi-closed circles) and arterial administration (closed circles) are plotted against the halothane concentration in pulmonary influent blood. Simultaneously determined concentrations in effluent blood are shown in parenthesis. Reductions caused by airway administration (open circles) are plotted against the resulting concentrations in effluent blood. The lines connect tests performed on the same preparations. In each preparation, three levels of response reduction was found, depending on whether halothane was given via the veins, the artery, or the airways. The response was always most effectively inhibited when halothane was administered via the airways, less when introduced via the pulmonary artery, and least when introduced via the pulmonary veins. In quantitative terms, equimolar concentrations of halothane reduced the response about six times as effectively when introduced via the airways, and 2.5 times as effectively when introduced via the pulmonary artery, compared with administration via the pulmonary veins.

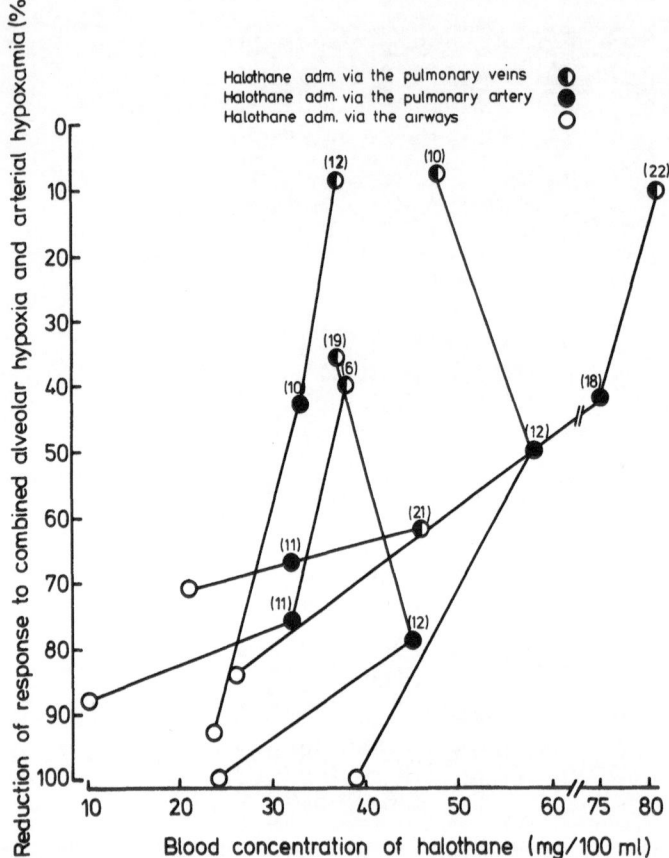

Fig. 8. Reduction of the pulmonary pressor response to hypoxia of halothane introduced via the pulmonary veins and artery plotted against influent blood concentrations, and via the airways plotted against effluent concentrations of the anaesthetic. *Lines* connect tests within the same rat lung preparation. *Numbers in parentheses* indicate effluent blood concentrations during administration via blood

Figure 9 shows hypothetical curves for the changes in halothane tension along the pulmonary vasculature during administration of halothane via the airways [1], the pulmonary artery [2] and the pulmonary veins [3]. Below is a schematic model of the lung. Since the response is damped by halothane in a dose-dependent fashion, the concentration at the hypoxia-sensitive site (circles) would be expected to be least during pulmonary venous administration and sequentially higher during pulmonary arterial and airway administration respectively. The model suggests that the hypoxia-sensitive site is localized extravascularly on the arterial side, functionally closer to the airways than to the responding vessels.

In conclusion, general anaesthesia promotes the development of hypoventilation and atelectasis. The present experiments have shown that volatile inhalation anaesthetics in contrast to intravenous anaesthetics, inhibit the pulmonary vasoconstrictor response to hypoxia even in man. Suggestedly this inhibition takes place at a receptor site on the arterial side of the vasculature, but closer to the airways than to the constricting vessels. The practical implication of these findings is that volatile inhalation anaesthetics should be given with some caution to patients suffering from lung disease.

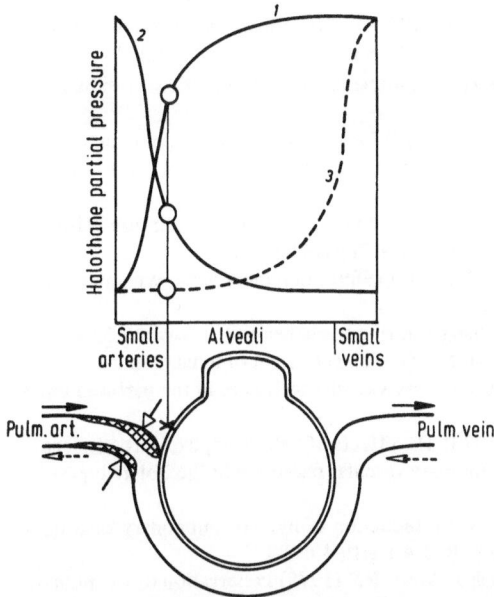

Fig. 9. Schematic lung model with the proposed hypoxia-sensitive site (*x*) on the arterial side of the vasculature. The *upper panel* shows hypothetical halothane partial pressure curves along the pulmonary vasculature during administration via the airways (*1*), the pulmonary artery (*2*), and the pulmonary veins (*3*). *Open circles* symbolize the projection of the hypoxia-sensitive site on the halothane partial pressure curves, thereby indicating the postulated relation between the halothane partial pressures at this site during administration via different routes. *Continuous* and *broken arrows* indicate flow direction, whereas *small arrows* indicate the proposed vasoconstrictor site. Fig. 8 should be studied simultaneously

References

1. Benumof JL (1979) Mechanism of decreased blood flow to atelectatic lung. J Appl Physiol 46:1047
2. Bjertnæs L (1977) Hypoxia-induced vasoconstriction in isolated perfused lungs exposed to injectable or inhalation anesthetics. Acta Anaesth Scand 21:133
3. Bjertnæs L (1978) Hypoxia-induced pulmonary vasoconstriction in man: inhibition due to diethyl ether and halothane anesthesia. Acta Anaesth Scand 22:570
4. Bjertnæs L, Mundal R (1980) The pulmonary vasoconstrictor response to hypoxia during enflurane anesthesia. Acta Anaesth Scand 24:252
5. Bjertnæs L, Hauge A, Torgrimsen T (1980) The pulmonary vasoconstrictor response to hypoxia. The hypoxia-sensitive site studied with a volatile inhibitor. Acta Physiol Scand 109:447
6. Bjertnæs L, Mundal R, Hauge A, Nicolaysen A (1980) Vascular resistance in atelectatic lungs: Effects of inhalation anesthetics. Acta Anaesth Scand 24:109
7. Don HF, Wahba WM, Craig DB (1972) Airway closure, gas trapping, and the functional residual capacity during anesthesia. Anesthesiology 36:533
8. Don HF, Wahba M, Cuadrado L, Kelkar K (1979) The effects of anesthesia and 100 per cent oxygen on the functional residual capacity of the lungs. Anesthesiology 32:521
9. Froese AB, Bryan AC (1974) Effects of anesthesia and paralysis on diaphragmatic mechanisms in man. Anesthesiology 41:242
10. Gilmour I, Burnham M, Craig DB (1976) Closing capacity measurement during general anesthesia. Anesthesiology 45:477
11. Hedenstierna G, Santesson J, Norlander OP (1976) Airway closure and distribution of inspired gas in the extremely obese, breathing spontaneously and during anesthesia with intermittent positive pressure ventilation. Acta Anaesth Scand 20:334

12. Hickey RF, Visick WD, Fairly HB, Fourcade HE (1973) Effects of halothane anesthesia on functional residual capacity and alveolararterial oxygen tension difference. Anesthesiology 38:20

13. Laws AK (1968) Effects of induction of anaesthesia and muscle paralysis on functional residual capacity of the lungs. Can Anaesth Soc J 15:325

14. Marin JLB, Carruthers B, Chakrabarti MK, Sykes MK (1979) Preservation of the hypoxic pulmonary vasoconstrictor response to alveolar hypoxia during administration of halothane in dogs. Br J Anaesth 50:1185

15. Marshall BE, Cohen PJ, Klingenmaier CH, Aukberg S (1969) Pulmonary venous admixture before, during and after halothane: oxygen anesthesia in man. J Appl Physiol 27:653

16. Price HL, Cooperman LH, Warden JC, Morris JJ, Smith TC (1969) Pulmonary hemodynamics during general anesthesia in man. Anesthesiology 30:629

17. Stark DCC, Smith H (1960) Pulmonary vascular changes during anaesthesia. Br J Anaesth 32:460

18. Sykes MK, Loh L, Seed RF, Kafer ER, Chackrabarti MK (1972) The effect of inhalational anaesthetics on hypoxic pulmonary vasoconstriction and pulmonary vascular resistance in the perfused lungs of the dog and cat. Br J Anaesth 44:776

19. Sykes MK, Davies DM, Chakrabarti MK, Loh L (1973) The effects of halothane, trichloroethylene and ether on the hypoxic pressor response and pulmonary vascular resistance in the isolated, perfused cat lung. Br J Anaesth 45:655

20. Sykes MK, Hurtig JB, Tait AR, Chakrabarti MK (1977) Reduction of hypoxic pulmonary vasoconstriction during diethyl ether anaesthesia in the dog. Br J Anaesth 49:293

21. Sykes MK, Gibbs JM, Loh L, Marin JLB, Obdrzalek J, Arnot RN (1978) Preservation of the pulmonary vasoconstrictor response to alveolar hypoxia during administration of halothane in dogs. Br J Anaesth 50:1185

22. Von Euler US, Liljestrand G (1946) Observations on the pulmonary arterial blood pressure in the cat. Acta Physiol Scand 12:301

Effects of Inhalation Anaesthetics on Renal Function A Brief Review with Special Reference to Renal Handling of Fluoride Ions

P.O. Järnberg

General Effects of Anaesthetics on Renal Function

General anaesthesia produced by inhalation anaesthetics and neurolept anaesthesia is associated with profound changes in renal function [1–3]. Renal blood flow, glomerular filtration rate, electrolyte and water excretion are all depressed (Tables 1 and 2). The mechanisms responsible for these changes include: decreases of cardiac output and arterial blood pressure, increased sympatho-adrenal activity, release of antidiuretic hormone (ADH), and possibly an aldosterone effect on the tubules secondary to the activation of the renin-angiotensin system. However, renal function is usually restored within a few hours after termination of anaesthesia and surgery, with the exception of free water excretion, which is often impaired for several days, probably due to remaining high ADH activity [4].

In some cases renal function becomes impaired after anaesthesia and surgery, so that the kidneys cannot vary urine volume and content according to homeostatic requirements. Such post-operative renal failures vary in severity from lighter passing disturbances to more serious

Table 1. Inter-operative changes from control (%) of inulin clearance (C_{In}) and P-aminohippuric acid (PAH) clearance (C_{PAH}) during anaesthesia with various types of general anaesthetic

	C_{In}	C_{PAH}
Halothane	−19	−38
Enflurane	−22	−45
Isoflurane	−37	−49
Neurolept anaesthesia	−24	−45

Table 2. Inter-operative changes from control (%) of urine flow rate (UF), sodium clearance (C_{Na}), osmolar clearance (C_{Osm}), and free water clearance (C_{H_2O}) during anaesthesia with various types of general anaesthetic

	UF	C_{Na}	C_{Osm}	C_{H_2O}
Halothane	−91	−67	−53	free water reabsorption
Enflurane	−82	−59	−15	free water reabsorption
Neurolept anaesthesia	−74	−65	−28	free water reabsorption

polyuric or anuric conditions. Apart from those cases associated with methoxyflurane anaesthesia, the development of post-operative renal failure is not due only to the choice of anaesthetic, but to a combination of factors of which the anaesthetic agent is usually a minor one. Other more important factors comprise: type and duration of surgical procedure, pre-operatively existing renal and/or cardiovascular disease, management of electrolyte and fluid balance pre-, per-, and post-operatively, and administration of nephrotoxic substances.

Methoxyflurane

Modern inhalational anaesthetics are either halogenated ethanes or ethers. They are metabolized to a varying extent and the metabolites are eliminated principally by renal excretion [5]. These metabolites may be potentially nephrotoxic. There are convincing data that the metabolism of methoxyflurane, with production of fluoride ions, is aetiologically associated with its dose-related nephrotoxicity [6]. The well-known clinical picture is vasopressin-resistant polyuria, Hypernatraemia, hyperosmolality, and increasing serum creatinine. The nephrotoxic threshold is believed to be about 50 μM F^- in man [6], although a transient decrease in concentrating ability after anaesthesia has been found at levels around 35 μM [7].

Halothane

The fluoride ion is the only known metabolite of modern inhalation anaesthetics that with certainity has nephrotoxic properties. As halothane metabolism results in significant fluoride formation only under hypoxic conditions [5], the risk of specific renal function impairment in connection with halothane anaesthesia is very slight.

Enflurane

The biotransformation of enflurane during and after anaesthesia and the resulting plasma levels of fluoride are well documented [8–10]. In clinical practice plasma levels mostly range between 15 and 25 μM, which is well below the nephrotoxic threshold. Occasionally values in the toxic range have been measured. In man clinical polyuric renal failure after enflurane anaesthesia has been described only in a few patients, all of whom had impairment of renal function prior to anaesthesia [11–13]. Therefore it seems wise to avoid enflurane as an anaesthetic in patients with pre-operatively known reduction of renal function.

Fluoride Excretion

Renal handling of fluoride is characterized by glomerular filtration and a varying degree of tubular reabsorption. Normally 40%–60% of fluoride is excreted in the urine and the rest is accumulated in calcified tissues [14]. Normal renal clearance of fluoride (C_F) in healthy volunteers ranges between a third and two-thirds of the actual glomerular filtration rate (GFR) [14]. During enflurane anaesthesia C_F is decreased to approximately a thenth of the actual GFR [10]. After termination of anaesthesia C_F increases, and this increase seems to be relat-

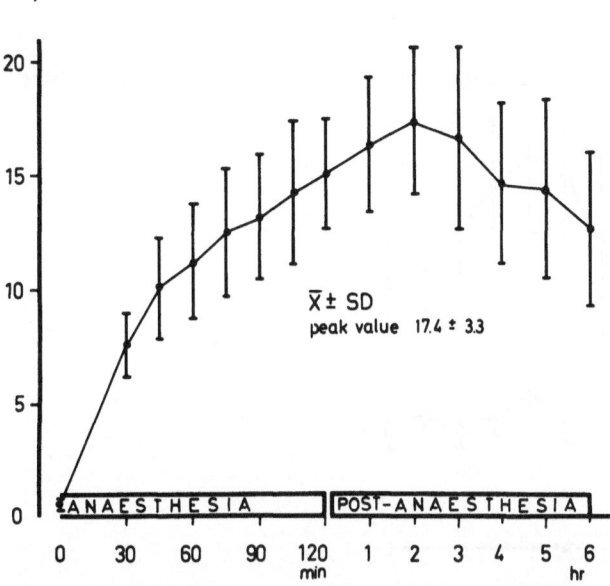

Fig. 1. Plasma inorganic fluoride (F⁻) concentrations in seven patients before, during, and after enflurane anaesthesia (mean ± SD)

ed to urinary pH. There is an almost perfect correlation between an increase in urinary pH post-operatively and the increase in C_F [15]. The probable explanation is that fluoride is reabsorbed by non-ionic diffusion as hydrogen fluoride (HF) from the renal tubules under acid urinary conditions. The uncharged HF molecules penetrate the tubular epithelium more easi-

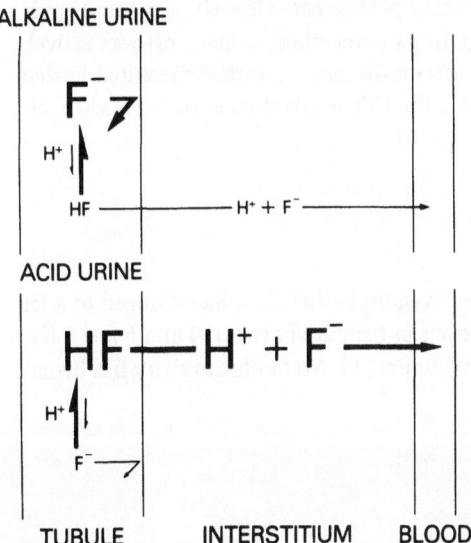

Fig. 2. Proposed mechanism of fluoride renal reabsorption. The process occurs by non-ionic diffusion of hydrogen fluoride from the tubules. In the peritubular fluid, where pH is higher HF is dissociated, and the fluoride ions are returned to the systemic circulation via the peritubular capillaries

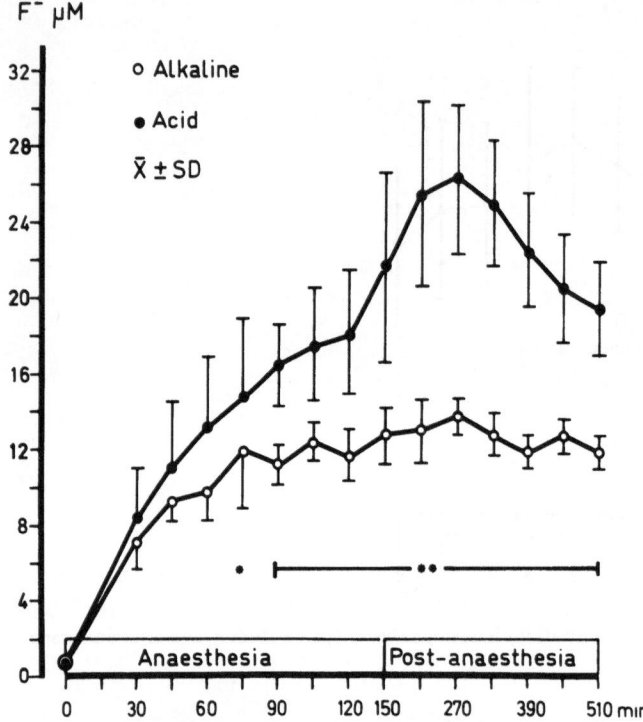

Fig. 3. Plasma fluoride levels before, during, and after enflurane anaesthesia in two groups of patients with pre-operatively induced alkaline and acidic urinary conditions (mean ± SD)

ly than do the freely charged fluoride ions. As urinary pH increases less HF is created, and the excretion of F^- increases accordingly (Fig. 2). In patients where urinary pH was actively manipulated, acid urinary conditions during and after enflurane anaesthesia resulted in significantly lower fluoride excretion and higher plasma fluoride levels than in patients with alkaline urine [16] (Fig. 3).

Isoflurane

Isoflurane, like enflurane, is a pentafluorinated methylethyl ether. It is metabolized to a lesser extent than enflurane. Peak plasma fluoride levels in man are between 4 and 5 μM 6 h after anaesthesia with a mean dose of 3.1 ± 1.3 MAC-hours [1]. No nephrotoxicity has been demonstrated.

References

1. Mazze RI, Cousins MJ, Barr GA (1974) Renal effects and metabolism of isoflurane in man. Anesthesiology 40:536–542
2. Deutsch S (1975) Effects of anesthetics on the kidney. Surg Clin North Am 55:775–786

3. Järnberg P-O, Santesson J, Eklund J (1978) Renal function during neurolept anaesthesia. Acta Anaesth Scand 22:167–172
4. Moran WH, Miltenberger FW, Shuayb WI et al. (1964) The relationship of antidiuretic hormone secretion to surgical stress. Surgery 56:205–210
5. Cohen EN, Van Dyke RA (1977) Metabolism of volatile anesthetics. Implications for toxicity. Addison-Wesley Reading, pp 63–125
6. Mazze RI, Shue GL, Jackson SH (1971) Renal dysfunction associated with methoxyflurane anesthesia: a randomized, prospective clinical evaluation. JAMA 216:278–288
7. Mazze RI, Calverley RK, Smith NT (1977) Inorganic fluoride nephrotoxicity: Prolonged enflurane and halothane anesthesia in volunteers. Anesthesiology 46:265–272
8. Maduska AL (1974) Serum inorganic fluoride levels in patients receiving enflurane anesthesia. Anesth Analg (Cleve) 53:351–353
9. Cousins MJ, Greenstein LR, Hitt BA et al. (1976) Metabolism and renal effects of enflurane in man. Anesthesiology 44:44–53
10. Järnberg P-O, Ekstrand J, Irestedt L et al. (1979) Renal function, fluoride formation and excretion during enflurane anaesthesia. Acta Anaesth Scand 23:444–453
11. Hartnett MN, Lane W, Bennett WM (1974) Nonoliguric renal failure and enflurane. Ann Intern Med 81:560
12. Loehning RE, Mazze RI (1974) Possible nephrotoxicity from enflurane in a patient with severe renal disease. Anesthesiology 40:203–205
13. Eichhorn JH, Hedley-Whyte J, Steinman TI et al. (1976) Renal failure following enflurane anesthesia. Anesthesiology 45:557–560
14. Carlson CH, Armstrong WD, Singer L (1960) Distribution and excretion of radio-fluoride in the human. Proc Soc Exp Biol Med 104:235–239
15. Järnberg P-O, Ekstrand J, Irestedt L et al. (1980) Renal fluoride excretion during and after enflurane anaesthesia: dependency on spontaneous urinary pH-variations. Acta Anaesth Scand 24:129–134
16. Järnberg P-O, Ekstrand J, Irestedt L (1981) Renal fluoride excretion and plasma fluoride levels during and after enflurane anesthesia are dependent on urinary pH. Anesthesiology 54:48–52

The Effect of Inhalation Anaesthetics on Skeletal and Smooth Muscle

J.F. Crul

The classic indication of anaesthesia depth in different stages and planes is best understood in terms of a progressive depression of certain groups of striated and smooth muscles. This scheme was primarily based on the symptoms of progressive depth of ether anaesthesia, and was later found to be the same for other inhalation anaesthetics. First the muscles of eyes, head, and neck, later of the extremities, were paralysed, followed by the muscles of the trunk and abdomen, and finally the intercostal muscles and those of the diaphragm. At around the same level also smooth muscles of vessels, intestine, pupil, and bronchi started to relax, and finally the heart muscle also failed. The depth of inhalation anaesthesia was regulated by the degree and sites of muscle relaxation required for certain operations. Later, the need for muscle relaxation was fulfilled by peripherally acting muscle relaxants, and the need for deep inhalation anaesthesia no longer existed. This progressive muscle relaxation differed considerably in degree from one inhalation anaesthetics to the other, but the sequence of relaxation was always the same. This points primarily to a central origin of the muscle paralysis caused by inhalation anaesthetics, which is confirmed by the experiments.

Internuncial and motor neurons in the brain-stem and spinal cord are progressively depressed by inhalation anaesthetics. As a result of this the oligosynaptic H.reflexes are depressed to a degree corresponding to the observed muscle relaxation. Only in deeper levels of anaesthesia are peripheral effects on normal neuromuscular transmission also noticed. The post-synaptic depolarization is particularly diminished and slowed down by reduced Na conductance after stimulation. One MAC equivalent of an anaesthetic depresses the depolarization of the post-junctional membrane by 20%–40% depending on the type of anaesthetic. This becomes visible in a depression of muscle contraction when at least a 50% depression of the depolarization is already present [1]. With enflurane this occurs at a concentration of 2.5%–3%. This leads to a reduced margin of safety of neuromuscular transmission which is only detected when other factors affect the same mechanism. It is therefore not surprising that inhalation anaesthetics strongly enhance the effects of non-depolarizing muscle relaxants. The dose-response curves of all these agents shift to the left in a dose-dependent way.

Foldes demonstrated that halothane potentiated the effect of gallamine [2]. Katz demonstrated the potentiating effect of halothane on d-tubocurarine and hexafluorenium [3], which has been confirmed by others [4, 5]. The potentiating effect of halothane has been shown to be concentration-dependent [6], but not related to the duration of exposure [7]. With enflurane, the potentiating effect has proved to be dependent on both concentration and duration of administration [8]. Enflurane potentiates non-depolarizing relaxants more strongly than halothane [1, 9, 10]. The new inhalational anaesthetic, isoflurane, which was recently released on the American market, will probably become available in Europe in a few years. In 1971 it was shown to influence the pharmacodynamics of non-depolarizing muscle relaxants to at least the same extent as halothane does [11]. This was later confirmed in an experimental set-up [12, 13].

The pharmacokinetics of d-tubocurarine in man are not significantly altered by halothane or enflurane [8, 14]; half-life times, volume of distribution, and total plasma clearance are the same. There is, however, a significant difference in the plasma concentration at which 50% depression of the twitch contraction is present, indicating an increased sensitivity of the receptor to d-tubocurarine. This receptor sensitivity for relaxants depends on the anaesthetic used and its concentration. At equipotent concentrations, enflurane, in in vitro studies, decreased the EC_{50} (concentrations at which 50% depression of the twitch height occurs) to one-third of the control, ether and fluroxene to half of the control, and halothane, methoxyflurane, and isoflurane to two-thirds of the control values [13]. Studies in man confirmed these results [9, 15]. In contrast to halothane [7, 14], with enflurane the increase in receptor sensitivity in man was also dependent on the duration of exposure to the anaesthetic [8]. No explanations are at present available for this dependency on duration for enflurane.

In contrast to d-tubocurarine, there is a clear difference in the pharmacokinetics of pancuronium in cats under halothane or enflurane anaesthesia, compared to thiopental anaesthesia. The half-life time in the elimination phase ($t\frac{1}{2}\beta$) is prolonged and the total plasma clearance low [20]. Because of the species differences in the pharmacokinetics, it is not certain whether these results can be extrapolated to man. Halothane and enflurane increase the receptor sensitivity for pancuronium, both in cats [20] and in man [9, 11]. Since halothane and enflurane have no effect on the relaxant-receptor complex dissociation rate constants for d-tubocurarine and pancuronium [16], it must be concluded that the increased receptor sensitivity is not a real increase in receptor sensitivity, but a reflection of the decreased margin of safety of the neuromuscular transmission. Thus, in our opinion, halothane and enflurane block some acetylcholine receptors, and less relaxant is therefore needed to block the remaining receptors.

From the discussion of the factors mentioned, it should be clear that the influence of the volatile anaesthetics on the post-junctional membrane is likely to be clinically the most important factor in the interaction between volatile anaesthetics and the non-depolarizing muscle relaxants.

Recently, it has been demonstrated that muscle relaxants also influence the depth of anaesthesia caused by inhalation anaesthetics. The MAC value of halothane is significantly decreased by pancuronium [17]. Possible explanations for this effect are:
1. Muscle relaxation abolishes a great number of afferent impulses from muscle spindles, retrodromally from motor neuron and from the Renshaw cells. Cerebral arousal and therefore wakefulness depend to a large extent on impulses of such a large muscle mass.
2. Muscle relaxants pass the blood-brain barrier in measurable amounts, as has been demonstrated for d-tubocurarine [18] and pancuronium (P. Waser, personal communication).
They may thus occupy central acetylcholine receptors, and thereby influence the cerebral activity. Support for this theory may be found in the observation that intravenous gallamine and d-tubocurarine elevate the seizure threshold of lidocaine in monkeys [19].

If this reverse action of muscle relaxants is of any importance for the depth of inhalation anaesthesia, it would be logical also to reduce the concentration of inhalation anaesthetics when combined with muscle relaxants. It even may be beneficial to use muscle relaxants not as a possible substitute for good clinical anaesthesia-as we always taught our students — but as an integral part of balanced anaesthesia. Of course, airways and ventilation should be safely guarded at all times. Clinical impressions of recent origin have substantiated this state-ment but extensive experimental and clinical studies should still be done before this can be accepted as a standard routine. It certainly ought to change the whole conduct of inhalation anaesthesia dramatically.

In conclusion, volatile anaesthetics do potentiate the effect and the duration of action of the non-depolarizing muscle relaxants, and the dosage of these compounds should be rela-ted to the type and concentration of the anaesthetic used. When halothane or isoflurane are administered, the dosage of the relaxants may be reduced to two-thirds of what has to be administered in nitrous oxide-narcotic anaesthesia to obtain the same blockade. During en-flurane anaesthesia, one-third of the amount of relaxant is sufficient; we should also keep in mind the influence of the duration of administration of enflurane. Small amounts of muscle relaxants potentiate and facilitate inhalation anaesthesia, and should probably become an in-tegral part of its balanced use.

Far less is known about the effect of inhalation anaesthetics on smooth muscle. In vitro, halothane is shown to reduce smooth muscle tone of the bronchi of asthmatic guinea-pigs, and can also prevent the histamine challenge response of pre-sensitized guinea-pig trachea [21]. In vivo experiments in dogs showed the same effects: after vagal stimulation broncho-constriction was abolished by 0.5% halothane [22]. Smooth muscle tone of the rat colon is also reduced by halothane and diethyl ether [23]. In clinical circumstances only the effect of halothane on bronchial smooth muscle is used to advantage. None of the other effects on smooth muscle seem to be of clinical importance.

References

1. Waud BE, Waud DR (1979) Effects of volatile anesthetics on directly and indirectly stimulated skeletal muscle. Anesthesiology 50:103
2. Foldes FF, Sokoll M, Wolfson B (1961) Combined use of halothane and neuromuscular blocking agents for the production of surgical relaxation. Anesth Analg (Cleve) 40:629
3. Katz RL, Gissen AJ (1967) Neuromuscular and electromyographic effects of halothane and its inter-actions with d-tubocurarine in man. Anesthesiology 28:564
4. Baraka A (1968) Effects of halothane on tubocurarine and suxamethonium block in man. Br J Anaesth 40:602
5. Walts LF, Dillon JB (1970) The influence of the anesthetic agents on the action of curare in man. Anesth Analg (Cleve) 49:17
6. Bonta IL, Goorissen EM, Derkx FH (1968) Pharmacological interaction between pancuronium bromide and anesthetics. Eur J Pharmacol 4:83
7. Miller RD, Crigue M, Eger EI II (1976) Duration of halothane anesthesia and neuromuscular block-ade with d-tubocurarine. Anesthesiology 44:206
8. Stanski DR, Ham J, Miller RD, Sheiner LB (1980) Time-dependent increase in sensitivity to d-tubo-curarine during enflurane anesthesia in man. Anesthesiology 50:483
9. Fogdall RP, Miller RD (1975) Neuromuscular effects of enflurane, alone and combined with d-tubo-curarine, pancuronium and succinylcholine in man. Anesthesiology 42:173
10. Lambo R (1977) Action of enflurane (Ethrane[R]) on the neuromuscular block induced by AH 8165D. Acta Anaesthesiol Belg 28:13
11. Miller RD, Eger EI II, Way WL, Stevens WC, Dolan WM (1971) Comparative neuromuscular effects of forane and halothane alone and in combination with d-tubocurarine in man. Anesthesiology 35:38
12. Vitez TS, Miller RD, Eger EI II, van Nijhuis LS, Way WL (1974) Comparison in vitro of isoflurane and halothane potentiation of d-tubocurarine and succinylcholine neuromuscular blockades. Anesthesiology 41:53

13. Waud BE (1979) Decrease in dose requirement of d-tubocurarine by volatile anesthetics. Anesthesiology 51:298
14. Stanski DR, Ham J, Miller RD, Sheiner LB (1979) Pharmacokinetics and pharmacodynamics of d-tubocurarine during nitrous-oxyde-narcotic and halothane anesthesia in man. Anesthesiology 51:235
15. Miller RD, Way WL, Donlon WH, Stevens WC, Eger EI II (1971) Comparative neuromuscular effects of pancuronium, gallamine and succinylcholine during forane and halothane anesthesia in man. Anesthesiology 35:509
16. Waud BE, Cheng MC, Waud DR (1973) Comparison of drugreceptor dissociation constants at the mammalian neuromuscular junction in the presence and absence of halothane. J Pharmacol Exp Ther 187:40
17. Forbes AR, Cohen NH, Eger EI II (1979) Pancuronium reduces halothane requirement in man. Anesth Analg (Cleve) 58:497
18. Matteo RS, Pua EK, Khambatta HJ, Spector RS (1977) Cerebrospinal fluid levels of d-tubocurarine in man. Anesthesiology 46:396
19. Munson ES, Wagman IH (1973) Elevation of lidocaine seizure threshold by gallamine. Arch Neurol 28:329
20. Miller RD, Agoston S, van der Pol F, Booij LHDJ, Crul JF (1979) Effect of different anesthetics on the pharmacokinetics and pharmacodynamics of pancuronium in the cat. Acta Anaesth Scand 23:285
21. Cabanas A, Souhrada JF, Aldrete JA (1980) Effects of ketamine and halothane on normal and asthmatic smooth muscle of the airway in guinea pigs. Can Anaesth Soc J 27:47
22. Jones JG, Graf PD, Lemen R (1978) The influence of bronchial smooth muscle tone on critical narrowing of dependent airways. Br J Anaesth 50:735
23. Clanachan AS, Muir TC (1978) Effects of end-tidal concentrations of cyclopropane, halothane and diethyl ether on peripheral autonomic neuroeffector systems in the rat. Br J Pharmacol 62:259

Inhalation Anaesthesia and Endocrine Disease

St. Jeretin

Introduction

The number of surgical patients with endocrine disease is increasing. There are more and more patients being admitted for surgery on the endocrine glands, and even more patients with accompanying endocrine disorders or receiving hormonal therapy unconnected with the planned surgical procedure [20].

Generally, anaesthesia affects the normal endocrine system and triggers off a series of reactions which are commonly described as reactions to stress and known as a normal endocrine response to anaesthesia, trauma, or surgery. In patients with endocrine disease this response is altered, first, by the changed function of the endocrine glands and, secondly, by the surgical procedure, i.e. removal of the gland with consecutive total or partial hypo- or afunction.

Anaesthesia in Patients with Disease of the Pituitary Gland and Hypophysectomy

The pituitary controls the secretion of many endocrine glands. Its action is controlled by the level of circulating hormones secreted by the target glands and by the action of several parts of the central nervous system (CNS). Secretions of the pituitary, the deficiency or excess of which may threaten the patient's life and are therefore of importance in anaesthesia, are: adrenocorticotropin (ACTH), human growth hormone (HGH), thyroid-stimulating hormone (TSH), and antidiuretic hormone (ADH).

Pathophysiology

Adrenocorticotropin (ACTH)

Adrenocorticotropin stimulates secretion of cortisol and androgens by adrenal glands. Deficiency results in a diminished secretion of cortisol. In these patients we may find anaemia associated with endocrine abnormalities such as hypothyroidism and hypoparathyroidism, and frequently moniliasis. In severe untreated cases the common findings are a low serum sodium and elevated serum potassium. The effects of vasopressors in these patients are not always positive. Hypersecretion of ACTH results in hypersecretion of cortisol. Typical for this condition are arterial hypertension, high or normal serum sodium, and low to normal serum potassium levels.

Human Growth Hormone (HGH)

Human growth hormone mobilizes free fatty acids and raises the level of blood sugar; it stimulates nitrogen retention and causes growth of long bones and soft tissues. In adults deficiency does not give rise to any clinical symptoms; in children it results in growth failure. Hyperproduction of HGH before puberty causes gigantism, whereas after puberty, when the growth centres are closed, it results in acromegaly. Basic metabolic rate is elevated by up to 50%. In about 75% of cases, kyphosis and enlargement of organs and muscle mass lead to terminal heart failure. Diabetes mellitus is encountered in 40% of patients.

Thyroid-Stimulating Hormone (TSH)

Thyroid-stimulating hormone governs secretion of thyroxine and triiodothyronine by the thyroid gland. Deficiency results in production of inadequate thyroxine and leads to hypothyroidism (secondary hypothyroidism). In these patients TSH increases ^{131}I uptake, contrary to the case in patients with primary hypothyroidism. Serum cholesterol of patients with secondary hypothyroidism is frequently normal. (It is elevated in primary hypothyroidism.) Patients with hypothyroidism are very susceptible to stress, and the risks attending anaesthesia and surgery are increased. Excess of TSH does not cause any known clinical syndrome. Graves' disease results from the extra-pituitary TSH.

Antidiuretic Hormone (ADH)

Antidiuretic hormone, or vasopressin, regulates the reabsorption of free water in the kidneys. Free water is reabsorbed along a concentration gradient, and a concentrated urine can be excreted. Deficiency leads to the development of diabetes insipidus resulting in large water losses (5–10 l urine/day). Patients become hypovolaemic and hypernatraemic, and have elevated blood urea nitrogen. Oliguria and vascular collapse are the pre-terminal features. Excess of ADH is characterized by low serum sodium, low blood urea nitrogen, and water retention. Water loads are very poorly tolerated and lead to convulsions and death. Urinary osmolarity is high.

Panhypopituitarism (Simmonds' Disease, Sheehan's Syndrome)

Panhypopituitarism is caused by severe damage to the anterior pituitary, resulting from thrombosis, necrosis, or tumour. Clinical symptoms depend on the degree of secondary losses of the adrenal, thyroid, and gonad functions. Typical symptoms of acute failure are hypotension, bradycardia, hypoglycaemia, hypometabolism, and hypothermia. In acute pituitary deficiency due to thrombosis involving the pituitary gland (anterior), as seen in septic shock or with disseminated intravascular coagulation (DIC), the haemodynamics do not readily respond to vasopressors and cortisone. Partial necrosis can result in a more insidious type of panhypopituitarism. The pituitary function in these patients may be sufficient for a relatively normal life. Symptoms develop if the condition is not identified before anaesthesia and surgery.

Indications for Pituitary Surgery and Surgical Approach

Hypophysectomy has been used in treatment of pituitary tumours, such as pituitary adenomas and craniopharyngioma. As a palliative procedure in selected patients it has been utilized in mammary cancer, prostatic cancer, haemorrhagic diabetic retinopathy, and incurable pain syndromes, as well as in treatment of acromegaly and Cushing's disease (pituitary). There are two possible means of surgical approach to the pituitary gland: by craniotomy and through the sphenoid.

Pre-Anaesthetic Evaluation and Planning

After a specific anaesthesia-oriented case history has been obtained and the endocrinologist's report reviewed, the patient's overall condition is first considered. This involves his general health; nutritional status; cardiorespiratory function; oxygen-carrying capacity of blood; metabolism of water, electrolytes and carbohydrates; renal function; CNS function; etc.

If necessary, specific diagnostic tests and laboratory study are reviewed or carried out to confirm the diagnosis and estimate the extent of metabolic and functional derangement. The therapeutic regimen is reviewed. In patients to undergo hypophysectomy for pituitary tumours, space-occupying problems and intracranial pressure variations during and after anaesthesia might be important. Hypophysectomy also permanently interrupts the pituitary function. Pre-existing alterations of the cardiocirculatory function and electrolyte metabolism may affect the capacity for rapid haemodynamic adjustments. Any rapid change of blood-pressure secondary to haemorrhage, anaesthetic agent, etc., may be deleterious. This applies to patients with Simmonds' disease and Sheehan's syndrome who are subjected to any kind of surgery without proper pre-operative hormone substitution [17]. Intubation problems can show up in acromegalic patients. Inhalation anaesthetics and anaesthetic agents may frequently cause haemodynamic changes during induction and maintenance of anaesthesia. Inhalation anaesthetics such as halothane, enflurane, and methoxyflurane are suitable agents, and make it easy for the anaesthesist to adjust the plane of anaesthesia to the patient's needs [18].

Preparation of the Patient and Premedication

Functions of vital organs, blood volume, electrolytes, etc. should be corrected to reach the best possible condition. Time to carry out corrections (therapy) depends on the surgical diagnosis. Treatment for accompanying disease should be given in time to permit improvement, and is part of the pre-anaesthetic preparation. Additional corticosteroid administration is necessary. Patients not receiving cortisone are given 100 mg cortisone i.m. on the morning before surgery and an equal dose of cortisone i.m. in the evening. On the day of operation 100 mg of cortisone is given i.v. 2 h before anaesthesia [19]. Insulin preparations are withdrawn 1 day before surgery and blood sugar is controlled by regular insulin. Flunitrazepam 2 mg is given orally the evening before, and in the morning on the day of operation, when the drug may be injected together with atropine.

Monitoring Requirements and Special Equipment

Continuous monitoring should include electrocardiogram (ECG), temperature, and end-tidal CO_2. Mechanical ventilation is essential and a hypothermia unit should be available.

Anaesthesia

The patient is put on the thermoblanket and prepared in the usual way. An intravenous cannula is put in place and a 5% glucose in water slow drip is started. The ECG electrodes are
attached. Induction can be started either with barbiturates, flunitrazepam, etc., or inhalation.
Major blood-pressure changes during induction and intubation of the airways should be
avoided by using adequate doses and proper timing. Fluothane, enflurane, and methoxyflurane
can be given smoothly thanks to non-irritant vapours and well-tolerated higher concentrations during induction. Intubation is facilitated by the use of muscle relaxants. Pancuronium
is recommended, but some anaesthesists prefer to use succinylcholine chloride for intubation.
As usual, in neurosurgical anaesthesia non-kinking tubes should be used and ventilation (mechanical) should be managed carefully. End-tidal CO_2 monitoring makes it possible to maintain a constant level of moderate hyperventilation. The patient having been anaesthetized,
a second intravenous line (either a central venous pressure (CVP) catheter or a gauge 14 i.v.
canula) is inserted. An urinary catheter is introduced, the bladder emptied, and the catheter
connected to a urine-collecting system.

The patient is next positioned for surgery. During repositioning and positioning procedure, blood-pressure must be closely observed. Rapid changes of position should be avoided.
If necessary, urea or mannitol are now administered. The most probable cause of intra-operative hypotension is blood loss. Replacement must be prompt and adequate. Administration
of cortisol, usually 200 mg by intravenous infusion, is necessary.

Post-anaesthetic Management

The hypophysectomized patient or any patient with hypopituitarism subjected to surgery
(not involving the pituitary gland) should be transferred to the intensive care unit. Haemodynamic monitoring is essential for at least 24 h. The patient should be intubated and ventilated mechanically until adequate respiratory function and level of consciousness are stated.
Fluid and electrolyte balance should be carefully adjusted on a 6-hour basis.

Cortisone (100 mg) is normally given i.m. or i.v. immediately after surgery. Later on it
should be administered according to the schedule in Table 1.

Antibiotics should be given for several days after the frontal or sphenoidal sinuses have
been opened. Even better is the regular prophylactic use of a 1% silver sulphadiazine solution. Twice a day 50 ml of a 1% solution is instilled through the urinary catheter. All punc-
ture sites of i.v. catheters and cannulas are covered with a 1% cream. Intra-operative local

Table 1. Post-operative administration of cortisone. Oyama T [19]

Post-op. day	Medication	Dose
1st	Cortisol	50 mg × 4 im.
2nd–4th	Cortisol	50 mg × 4 im.
5th–6th	Cortisol	50 mg × 3 im.
7th	Cortisol	50 mg × 2 im.
8th–10th	Dexamethasone	0.5 mg × 4 orally
11th–13th	Dexamethasone	0.5 mg × 3 orally
14th onwards	Dexamethasone	0.5 mg × 2 orally

application of 1% silver sulphadiazine into the frontal or sphenoidal sinus could also be useful [13]. In the immediate post-operative period regular insulin is used. Diabetic patients require higher doses.

Anaesthesia and Adrenal Disease

The adrenal cortex produces hormones with a common nucleus – the cyclopentanoperhydrophenantren structure. These hormones can functionally be divided into five groups, of which only three are of importance for anaesthesia: (a) glucocorticoids – cortisol and corticosterone; (b) mineralocorticoids – aldosterone and deoxycorticosterone; (c) androgens. The overall activity of the adrenal cortex is under the control of the pituitary hormone ACTH. This is released under the influence of a specific corticotropin-releasing factor (CRF) formed in the hypothalamus. The CRF release is inhibited by plasma corticosteroids. Secretion of all adrenal corticoids is increased by ACTH, but the aldosterone secretion is much less dependent than the other steroids and is mainly regulated by the angiotensin-renin system.

Pathophysiology

Glucocorticoids

Glucocorticoids form about 85% of the total steroid production of the adrenal. Their main action is stimulation of gluconeogenesis by increased protein catabolism, inhibition of protein synthesis, inhibition of tissue carbohydrate turnover, impaired glucose tolerance, etc. The two adrenals together secrete about 30 mg cortisol per day. Under stress, this amount can be increased to 300 mg per day.

Prolonged and excessive exposure to glucocorticoids results in the characteristic clinical picture of Cushing's syndrome. It makes no difference whether the excessive cortisol is endogenous or exogenous, cortisone or a similar synthetic compound. The typical features of the condition are a round face, thin skin, pink abdominal striae, easy bruisability, arterial hypertension, impaired glucose tolerance, osteoporosis, supraclavicular fat pads, posterior nuchal buffalo hump, muscle weakness, centripedal obesity, and impaired growth (in children). Cushing's disease is caused by:
1. Bilateral adrenal cortical hyperplasia – increased pituitary ACTH secretion
2. Primary adrenal adenoma (carcinoma) – unilateral
3. ACTH-producing extra-pituitary source (tumours of lung, thymus, pancreas, bronchi)
4. Excessive administration of glucocorticoids or ACTH – iatrogenic.

Cortisol deficiency can be caused by destruction of the adrenal glands, pituitary ACTH deficiency, and exogenous corticosteroids (iatrogenic), and leads to the clinical entity of Addison's disease. Clinical features of adrenocortical insufficiency are weakness and fatigue, weight loss, hyperpigmentation, gastro-intestinal symptoms, hypotension, syncope, CNS symptoms (e.g. apathy), hypoglycaemia, etc.

Aldosterone

Aldosterone is the principal mineralocorticoid secreted by the adrenal cortex. Aldosterone increases sodium reabsorption in the distal renal convoluted tubule in exchange for hydrogen and potassium. Secretion of aldosterone is primarily regulated by the renin-angiotensin system, plasma sodium levels, serum potassium, and ACTH being of secondary importance. Aldosterone hypersecretion is caused either by aldosterone-producing adenoma or, in rare cases, bilateral nodular hyperplasia (primary aldosteronism). Secondary aldosteronism is caused by renal artery stenosis or malignant nephrosclerosis. The clinical picture of aldosteronism (chronic hypersecretion of aldosterone) was first described by Conn. The main symptoms are hypertension, expanded extra-cellular fluid volume not associated with oedema, hypokalaemia, alkalosis, low serum magnesium, and high serum sodium. Aldosterone deficiency is an accompanying phenomenon of chronic adrenocortical insufficiency.

Androgens

Adrenal androgens may cause clinical symptoms described as adrenogenital syndromes. In the congenital adrenogenital syndrome, partial or complete absence of enzymes required for production of cortisol results in a shortage of cortisol. Due to deficient supply of cortisol, the ACTH secretion is not inhibited and this causes hypertrophy of the adrenal cortex. Typical is accumulation of androgens and cortisol only high enough to sustain life. In adrenogenital syndrome associated with adrenal tumours producing excessive amounts of androgen, the clinical appearance (masculinization, hirsutism) is similar to that in the congenital form, but there is no deficiency of cortisol. Tumours often produce mixed effects with combined masculinization and Cushing's syndrome.

Indications for Adrenal Surgery and Surgical Approach

Unilateral or bilateral adrenocortical tumours must be removed. Adrenalectomy is probably the most reliable method. In ACTH-stimulated cortical adrenal hyperplasia, adrenalectomy does not stop ACTH secretion. In patients with mild Cushing's disease, irradiation of the pituitary is indicated rather than adrenalectomy. Usually bilateral adrenalectomy is performed 6–12 months after irradiation of the pituitary. In cases with metastatic carcinoma of the adrenal cortex, in poor-risk patients, and in patients with ectopic ACTH-producing tumours, medical treatment with inhibitors of cortisol synthesis is indicated. The surgical approach is either anterior, through the abdomen, or posterior, through a subcostal incision.

Pre-anaesthetic Evaluation and Planning

A specific anaesthesia-oriented case history is taken, and the surgical report and the endocrinologist's report are reviewed. The general condition of the patient is considered next. This involves the physical status of the patient and assessment of his cardiocirculatory and respiratory function, determination of the oxygen-carrying capacity, blood volume (if necessary), electrolyte and acid-base status, renal function, etc. Specific diagnostic tests and laboratory study are performed if necessary. Especially in patients with endocrine disease accompanying the surgical condition, it is important to know the characteristic features of metabolic and functional derangement. The therapeutic regimen is reviewed.

    In patients with hypersecretion of corticosteroids to undergo surgical procedures not involving the endocrine glands, it must be kept in mind that the problems likely to arise are related to diabetes, hypokalaemia, arterial hypertension, and osteoporosis. In Cushing's disease the most serious problems are hypertension (leading to death if untreated) and low potassium stores. Potassium deficit together with increased protein catabolism may result in muscle weakness. Potassium balance and glucose tolerance studies are essential. Increased respiratory work due to fat tissue distribution, muscle weakness, and kyphosis may cause serious problems. Patients are very susceptible to infection. In iatrogenic Cushing's disease the hypothalamic-pituitary-adrenal axis is suppressed and the patients become addisonian if the supply of exogen cortisol is interrupted.

In aldosteronism, hypokalaemia may result in muscle weakness leading to respiratory embarrassment and atrial and ventricular arrhythmias. After unilateral adrenalectomy, glucocorticoid secretion is usually adequate. In adrenogenital syndrome, only congenital adrenal hyperplasia is of importance for anaesthesia, because these patients can not produce adequate amounts of cortisol. In all cases of bilateral adrenalectomy surgery results in a complete interruption of cortisol production. Therefore these patients should be treated as addisonian immediately after both adrenals have been removed. In unilateral tumours (hypersecreting adenoma) the contralateral adrenal gland is suppressed and is unable to respond to ACTH.

Patients with Addison's disease, especially if not treated, can be in a very poor pre-operative condition. If not managed before surgery, hyponatraemia, hyperkalaemia, low blood volume, dehydration, and arterial hypotension, combined with position on the operating table, mechanical ventilation, blood loss and cardiovascular effects of anaesthesia agents, will greatly increase the risk involved in operation.

Pharmacological properties of anaesthetic agents affecting cardiovascular dynamics are important. Interestingly, several inhalation anaesthetics such as halothane, enflurane, and particularly methoxyfluorane raise the plasma cortisol level [16]. The effect might be useful in anaesthesia for surgery not involving the adrenals. In adrenalectomized patients all these effects are lost.

Preparation of the Patient and Premedication

In Cushing's disease, pre-operative treatment should consist of blood-pressure reduction, correction of potassium depletion by low sodium diet (if there is time), and oral or intravenous administration of potassium. Diuretics, preferably with digitalis, should also be applied to treat congestive heart failure. Diabetes should be controlled. All potential sources of intercurrent infection, e.g. infections of oral cavity, teeth, or genito-urinary tract, should be treated before surgery. Local application of silver sulphadiazine preparations are very useful. Pre-operative cortisol administration is not necessary. Corticosteroids are given on the day of surgery and post-operatively.

In aldosteronism hypertension is usually benign, but should be treated if present simultaneously with congestive heart failure. If necessary, potassium chloride up to 200 mval should be given intravenously. Corticosteroids are not necessary as preparation for surgery. Only when bilateral adrenalectomy is performed are corticosteroids given as shown in the schedule. Patients with Addison's disease should have their blood volume corrected before surgery. In chronic advanced hypoadrenocorticism, sodium, water, and glucose should be given intravenously in sufficient amounts. As part of pre-operative preparation ACTH is not effective in patients with iatrogenic addisonism. Cortisol should be given to all patients with Addison's disease, as well as patients given corticosteroids for more than 4 days during the last 6 months. The usual schedule for steroid therapy as used by Fox [16] is given in Table 3.

Table 2. Schedule for corticosteroid treatment of patients with Cushing's syndrome and adrenalectomy. After Oyama T [19]

Pre-operative days	None
Day of operation	Cortisol 100 mg (i.v.) during op.
	Cortisol 50 mg × 2 (i.m.) post-op.

Post-operative day	
2th–4th	Cortisol 50 mg × 4 (i.m.)
5th–6th	Cortisol 50 mg × 3 (i.m.)
7th	Cortisol 50 mg × 2 (i.m.)
8th–10th	Dexamethasone 0.5 mg × 4 oral
11th–13th	Dexamethasone 0.5 mg × 3 oral
14th onwards	Dexamethasone 0.5 mg × 2 oral

Table 3. Peri-operative steroid therapy in adrenal disease

Evening before operation	Cortisone acetate 100 mg i.m. at 9 PM
Anaesthesia	Cortisol 100 mg i.v. in bolus before induction
	Cortisol 100 mg i.v. during surgery

Post-operatively	
Day of surgery	Cortisol 50 mg i.v. or i.m./6-hourly
1st day	Cortisol 50 mg i.m./6-hourly
2nd day	Cortisol 50 mg i.m./8-hourly
3rd day	Cortisol 30 mg i.m./8-hourly
4th day	Cortisol i.m. or orally 40 mg + 20 mg
5th day	Cortisol i.m. or orally 30 mg + 10 mg
6th day	Cortisol i.m. or orally 20 mg + 10 mg

Premedication on the evening before surgery should ensure a good sleep. Diazepam 2–5 mg or flunitrazepam 1–2 mg orally, or barbiturates, yield good results. In patients with Addison's disease lower doses are recommended. On the morning of operation premedication is given. Morphine, short-acting barbiturates, Demerol (meperidine), as well as diazepam and flunitrazepam together with atropine have been used.

Monitoring Requirements and Special Equipment

Continuous monitoring of ECG and temperature is essential. Cardiovascular pressure and blood-pressure monitoring equipment should be available. Mechanical ventilation is obligatory. Electric transfusion pump/blood warmer/filter unit (Jeretin) should be available.

Anaesthesia

An intravenous drip of 5% glucose in water solution is started if the patient had no intravenous line on arrival at the operating-room. Monitoring of ECG, etc. is started. Usually anaesthesia is induced with thiopentone, but inhalation anaesthetics can also be used safely. Halothane, enflurane, and methoxyflurane have been used for many years with excellent results. The effects of inhalation anaesthetics on the adrenocortical function are not uniform [19]. Many studies were performed to determine the stimulating or depressing effect of anaesthetics on the corticopituitary axis. However, there is as yet no agreement as to whether it is better to use an agent depressing the adrenocortical function or to employ an anaesthetic method which stimulates adrenal function. In patients with adrenocortical disease undergoing surgery not involving the endocrine glands, it may be of benefit to use anaesthetics with stimulating effects on the adrenals. However, the maximum rise in cortisol secretion normally appears post-operatively, and is caused by and in proportion to the magnitude of surgical trauma and the wound [1]. In patients to undergo bilateral adrenalectomy, stimulating or depressive effects, at least from the moment of removal on, are irrelevant.

Much more important are the pharmacological effects of the anaesthetics used in relation to specific conditions caused by the endocrine disease (low blood volume, poor control of vascular tonus, hyper-hypokalaemia, etc.). Especially in Addison's disease it is important to be able to control serious blood-pressure falls by rapid transfusion of whole blood and appropriate use of cortisol 100–200 mg i.v. Therefore a large calibre (14 gauge) cannula is placed into an arm vein before surgery.

Muscle relaxants should be used to facilitate intubation of the trachea and to provide good muscular relaxation during the operation. In some patients (i.e. in aldosteronism,) succinylcholine is preferable to d-tubocurarine. The effect of d-tubocurarine may be prolonged in these patients. If non-depolarizing muscle relaxants are used, smaller doses and careful titration should be employed.

Post-anaesthetic Management

All adrenalectomized patients and all patients with adrenal disease should be monitored carefully. Mechanical ventilation should be continued in all cases with muscle weakness or respiratory problems for as long as necessary to establish sufficient respiratory function. Water and electrolyte balance should be adjusted on a 4–6-h basis. Intensive monitoring of cardiocirculatory function is essential in addisonians to detect causes of hypotension and initiate appropriate treatment. Cortisol should be given in boluses of 100 mg i.v. whenever the cause of hypotension is obscure. All patients after adrenal surgery or prolonged adrenocortical supression should receive cortisol post-operatively, as shown in the schedule.

Anaesthesia and Phaeochromocytoma

Phaeochromocytomas are functioning tumours of the chromaffin tissue. They are usually benign but cause hypertension through the production of epinephrine and norepinephrine. Most tumours are found in the adrenal medulla but they can also develop from aberrant tissue along the aortic bifurcation or the sympathetic chain.

Pathophysiology

The related signs and symptoms are the effects of epinephrine and norepinephrine released by the tumour. These two adrenergic amines cause rapid elevations of arterial blood-pressure (systolic and diastolic), increased oxygen consumption, free fatty acid mobilization from adipose tissue, and elevation of blood glucose level. These effects can be persistent or episodic in tumours secreting intermittently. The main symptoms are headache, hypertension, palpitations, excessive perspiration, blurred vision, and heat intolerance. Phaeochromocytomas are found in general to secrete adrenaline 15% and noradrenaline 85%, which is a reversal of the normal secretion ratio of the adrenal medulla.

Pre-anaesthetic Evaluation and Planning

Patients with established diagnosis of phaeochromocytoma should be evaluated before anaesthesia in the usual way. A specific anaesthesia-oriented history, physical status, laboratory findings, and the functions of vitally important organ systems are the basis of planning. If there is no other disease accompanying phaeochromocytoma, the main problems are hypertension, with its effects on blood volume; ventricular arrhythmias; and, after the removal of the tumour, hypotension. The most important factor in phaeochromocytoma and associated hypertension is the decreased blood volume. During anaesthesia, through the effects of anaesthetic agents on the cardiac output or vascular tone, blood-pressure may fall, and the decrease in blood volume becomes evident. Additionally, post-operative blood cathecholamine level may fall immediately due to the very short half-lives of adrenaline and noradrenaline. In the presence of a significantly decreased blood volume this can create a very serious situation.

Ventricular arrhythmias commonly observed include bigeminy, multi-focal ventricular premature contractions, and ventricular tachycardia. Some inhalation anaesthetics, such as halothane, potentiate arrhythmias but, on the other side, during halothane anaesthesia the sympatho-adrenal system is not elicited [4, 25]. As long as diastolic pressure is within physiological levels, direct myocardial depression seems to be beneficial [25].

Methoxyflurane does not sensitize the myocardium in man. Enflurane has a minimal effect on cardiac output but may produce a marked hypotension with increasing depth of anaesthesia. Halothane [2, 15, 22], methoxyflurane [23], and enflurane [12] have been used successfully for anaesthesia during the removal of phaeochromocytoma [6]. Of greater importance than the anaesthetic agent is the pre-operative preparation of patients with alpha- and beta-blockers, and replacement of blood volume. An even more serious risk are patients with phaeochromocytoma discovered during surgery or labour.

Probably muscle relaxants with histamine-liberating effects should not be used because of the possibility of a histamine-like effect, but clinical experience shows that d-tubocurarine can be used safely [4, 7]. Recently, pancuronium is mostly utilized [6].

Preparation of the Patient and Premedication

It is necessary to neutralize the effects of circulating catecholamines before anaesthesia. Propranolol and Dibenzyline (phenoxybenzamine) have been the most useful drugs. Treatment is usually started 1 week before surgery with 10–20 mg of phenoxybenzamine orally two to three times a day. Propranolol is used only in frequent episodes of arrhythmias. Propranolol 10–40 mg is given orally three times a day. If there are signs of congestive heart failure induced by the use of propranolol, treatment with digitalis should be considered.

On the evening before anaesthesia and surgery, diazepam 2–5 mg or Nembutal (pentobarbital) 100 mg orally will give a good rest. In the morning either barbiturates, such as phenobarbital 100 mg, diazepam 2–5 mg, or flunitrazepam 1–2 mg orally or i.m., with or without narcotics, are used. Atropine is contra-indicated [11].

Monitoring Requirements and Special Equipment

Continuous monitoring of ECG and arterial blood-pressure is essential. Monitoring of tempe-rature, end tidal CO_2 and CVP is optimal. Mechanical ventilation is obligatory. Electric blood transfusion pump/blood warmer/filter unit should be available.

Anaesthesia

An intravenous 5% glucose in water drip is started if the patient had no i.v. line on arrival at the operating-room. Preferably a central venous catheter is introduced. A large gauge 12 or 14 intravenous cannula is introduced into a peripheral vein (cephalic or basilic) and con-nected to the blood transfusion pump set. Monitoring is started.

Induction of anaesthesia with thiopentone 250–300 mg or flunitrazepam 2 mg i.v. is followed by succinylcholine chloride administration to facilitate the orotracheal intubation. Accurate timing is important to ensure a smooth induction free from reactions caused by ca-techolamines.

Inhalation anaesthesia is started with the agent chosen in sufficient concentration to prevent reactions to pain. However, it should be kept in mind that the patient has been re-ceiving propranolol.

Pancuronium 2–4 mg is usually used to achieve muscular relaxation. Mechanical ventila-tion is adjusted to maintain an end-tidal CO_2 of 4%–5%. When surgery is started, drugs to control hypertensive episodes, i.e. phentolamine in a 0.01% solution or sodium nitroprusside 0.02% solution in a slow intravenous drip, can be used. In the case of arrhythmias proprano-lol 1 mg i.v. in repeated doses, if necessary, or Xylocaine (lidocaine) 50–100 mg in a bolus given i.v. can be used. To treat hypotension vasopressors have been used, but rapid transfu-sion of blood in excess of the measured blood loss have proved very effective. Central venous pressure must be monitored using this technique.

Postanaesthetic Management

Continuous and careful blood-pressure monitoring should be continued for up to 36 h. Hy-potension is the most common cause of death in the post-operative period. Vasopressors should be available close to the patient. After adrenalectomy, cortisol 100 mg every 6 h may be useful. Its use is justified even if adrenalectomy was not done, to maintain blood-pressure with an unadequate response to volume substitution and vasopressors.

Anaesthesia and Disease of the Thyroid Gland

The thyroid gland is concerned with the concentration and metabolism of iodine in order to produce the thyroid hormones thyroxine (T4) and triiodothyronine (T3). The secretion is regulated through a negative feedback mechanism. The hypothalamus, perceiving excess or deficit of circulating thyroid hormone, decreases or increases TSH secretion [8].

Pathophysiology

Thyroxine and triiodothyronine are the two physiologically active thyroid hormones. The *most important* functions of these two hormones are their influence on the rate of metabolism and their calorigenic effect. Released into circulation, T4 and T3 are transported bound to plasma proteins. On reaching the cells, they regulate the energy transfer [5].

Hyperthyroidism is characterized by excessive secretion of thyroid hormones, hyperplasia of the thyroid parenchyma, increased metabolic rate, and sometimes by exophthalmos. The clinical signs typical of this condition are weight loss, tachycardia, diarrhoea, warm moist skin, muscle weakness, nervousness, and heat intolerance. Excessive thyroid hormone production can be caused by toxic adenoma nodule and diffuse toxic goitre.

Hypothyroidism is a condition due to a deficient secretion of the thyroid hormones. The clinical symptoms indicate a general decrease of all bodily functions, including a decline in cerebration, constipation, dry skin, bradycardia, and intolerance of cold.

Indications for Surgery and Surgical Approach

Hyperthyroidism may be effectivly treated by antithyroid drugs like propylthiouracil (PTU), radioactive iodine (^{131}I), and surgery. Subtotal thyroidectomy gives a faster control of the disease and lower incidence of hypothyroidism as compared to the radioiodine therapy. Surgery is recommended in the presence of a large goitre or a thyroid nodule that may be cancer, as well as in treatment of pregnant patients or patients unable to maintain a long-term follow-up. As a rule, 3–10 g of the thyroid are removed, the parathyroid glands being spared.

Pre-anaesthetic Evaluation and Planning

After a specific anaesthesia-oriented case history has been obtained and a physical examination performed, the reports of the surgeons and endocrinologists are reviewed. The function of vital organ systems is evaluated. The therapeutic regimen is reviewed and its effectiveness evaluated. Patients with hyper- or hypothyroidism are a greater anaesthetic risk than euthyroid patients. Therefore, if possible, they should undergo pre-anaesthetic management.

In the case of emergency surgery, however, it is impossible to treat the patient pre-operatively. In hyperthyroid patients the degree of hypermetabolism will affect the dose of drugs used for sedation. Regional anaesthesia is a reasonable technique in emergency surgery, if feasible. As in hyperthyroid patients cardiac work is increased; arrhythmias during anaesthesia may lead to heart failure. Tachycardia and arrhythmias can be effectively controlled with lidocaine and propranolol. Oxygen consumption is elevated; therefore short interruptions of ventilation (during intubation, manipulation of the patient's system, changes of position, etc.) can cause rapid falls in arterial oxygen tension. Adequate ventilation during anaesthesia should assure a moderate degree of hyperventilation. The proportion of N_2O to O_2 should be, if possible, 1:1, and never below 2:1 l/min. Heat production in these patients is increased. Sweating is a physiological mechanism to regulate body temperature, but adequate intravenous fluids and electrolytes should be provided during anaesthesia. Atropine should be avoided.

Undiagnosed hypothyroid patients are at great risk. They do not need large doses of sedatives and hypnotics. Cardiovascular collapse may occur during anaesthesia. Cardiac output and tissue perfusion are delayed; therefore induction of anaesthetics and elimination are slow.

Preparation for Anaesthesia and Premedication

Pre-operative therapy is necessary in all patients with hyper- or hypothyroidism. In hyperthyroid patients treatment is usually started with PTU 100 mg four times a day for 6–7 weeks. When the patient is euthyroid, iodine is added (Lugol's solution 10 drops orally three times a day for 10 days) to reduce the vascularity of the gland.

Hypothyroid patients should also be made euthyroid. Thyroxine or triiodothyronine should be given over a period of 4 weeks. Premedication is given on the evening before surgery. Usually the hyperthyroid patient requires a heavier premedication to prevent an increase in the metabolic rate due to apprehension. Barbiturates (short-acting) are the drug of choice. In the morning the barbiturate is repeated and narcotics can be added. However, the use of atropine is to be avoided and one should be careful with phenothiazines, since they have the tendency to increase heart rate.

Monitoring Requirements and Special Equipment

In the euthyroid patient there are no special requirements, with exception of anaesthesia for emergency surgery, which requires ECG and body temperature monitoring. A thermoblanket should also be available, and anti-arrhythmic drugs and cortisone at hand.

Anaesthesia

Most of the anaesthetic techniques and agents have been used in euthyroid patients for subtotal thyroidectomy. In the hyperthyroid patient either regional analgesia or general anaesthesia can be used safely. Inhalation anaesthetics such as halothane, methoxyflurane [19], and enflurane [9] have been used successfully. After induction with thiopentone and succinylcholine chloride it is important to use a non-kinking (armed) tube, especially in retrosternal struma. The tube should be inserted far enough to extend past the area of tracheal compression. Care must be taken not to enter the bronchus. When positioning the patient for surgery (over-extended head position), gentle handling of the patients head is important to avoid reflex activity. Cardiac arrests may follow rough and sudden hyperextension of the neck in cases with retrosternal struma (S. Jeretin, 1965, personal observations).

Cardiac arrhythmias during anaesthesia of hyperthyroid patients can be treated with propranolol 1 mg given slowly i.v., or with lidocaine. The hypothyroid patient is more prone to develop cardiovascular collapse during anaesthesia. Low cardiac output typical for these patients slows down induction and elimination of anaesthetics.

Post-anaesthetic Care

Respiratory obstruction is the most common complication of the immediate post-operative period. Therefore patients should be watched closely, and instruments necessary to inspect and open the wound and for intubation of the trachea should be available at the bedside. Thyrotoxic crisis is a very serious complication. Its typical features are high fever (above 40 °C), agitation, delirium, tachycardia, atrial fibrillation, vomiting, diarrhea, dehydration, and vascular collapse. Therapy consists of sedation with barbiturates, large doses of PTU, sodium iodide 2–3 g i.v. every 6 h, hydrocortisone i.v., and infusion of glucose in water and electrolytes. Propranolol and guanethidine can be used to control the sympathetic hyperfunction.

Anaesthesia and Diabetes Mellitus

Diabetes is a chronic disease caused by insulin deficiency. The severe form, if not treated, leads to the fully developed form of keto-acidosis. A serious complication or consequence of diabetes is the degeneration of small blood-vessels. In juvenile diabetes, insulin deficiency is the major factor. The adult form of diabetes is associated with a significant insulin secretion as shown by quite frequently observed high plasma insulin levels, but there are other factors antagonizing the insulin action.

Pathophysiology

There is no universally accepted explanation for the cause of diabetes. Insulin deficiency is surely the most important factor in juvenile diabetes. In diabetes appearing in the adult, however, other mechanisms must be involved. It seems that somatostatin [26] and glucagon secretion [21] play a definite role in forms where blood insulin is not low. Somatostatin ameliorates diabetes through reduction of carbohydrate absorption from the gastro-intestinal tract, and inhibits secretion of HGH, insulin, and glucagon.

Insulin deficit causes several metabolic changes affecting not only carbohydrate, but also fat and protein. Insulin deprivation causes a rise in blood sugar, the utilization of glucose in peripheral tissues is decreased, and release of hepatic glucose — gluconeogenesis — is increased. Protein breakdown is increased and the enhanced fat hydrolysis causes a rise in the serum-free fatty acids. The fatty acids, when oxidized to supply energy, partially replacing glucose, are broken down to ketone bodies. Utilization of ketone bodies in the periphery is impaired in the absence of insulin, a fact contributing to the development of keto-acidosis. Relative shortage of carnitine slows down the rate of resynthesis of ketone bodies into fatty acids as well as oxygenation of ketone bodies and fatty acids by impairing the transfer of fatty acids through the mitochondrial membrane [10, 14].

Additional pathways of glucose metabolism in the diabetic hyperglycaemic patient are the pentose pathway and the glucuronic acid cycle, which are involved in the development of such complications as cataract, cerebral oedema, involvement of peripheral nerves, and capillary basement membrane thickening [3].

Clinically, diabetes can be staged into seven groups:
1. Prediabetes: positive family history, obesity, etc.
2. Stress diabetes: infection, injury, cortisone treatment may be the predisposing factor
3. Asymptomatic diabetes: normal fasting and elevated post-prandial blood sugar, no ketosis, abnormal glucose tolerance test
4. Manifest diabetes: increased fasting and post-prandial blood sugar, typical clinical triad of polyuria, polydipsia, polyphagia is evident.

Stages 5—7 are based on the presence and degree of keto-acidosis. Ketonuria unassociated with significant accumulation of ketone bodies in plasma is typical of stage 5. Diabetic keto-acidosis with a plasma ketone body high enough to lower the serum bicarbonate for about 2—10 mval/l is usually recognized as stage 6, whereas stage 7 is characterized severe diabetic keto-acidosis and coma.

Pre-anaesthetic Evaluation and Planning

A specific anaesthesia-oriented case history, physical examination, review of the surgical and endocrinological report, together with specific tests to assess the functioning of the vital organs, and a review of the effectiveness of the treatment received are the basis for evaluation and planning. At this point, it is also important to know the magnitude of the surgical stress to be expected. The latter, together with anaesthesia, initiate the so-called post-aggression metabolism [24]. Typical of these post-traumatic changes of intermediary metabolism is increased lipolysis, elevated serum-free fatty acids, and decreased resynthesis of fatty acids, together with impaired glucose utilization in the periphery. Gluconeogenesis is increased. This in a way normal response to aggression, added to metabolic derangements due to diabetes, even in the absence of other complications (infection, shock, cardiorespiratory difficulties), creates a serious situation, especially with manifest diabetes. It is also clear that surgery is contra-indicated in patients with keto-acidosis.

Inhalation anaesthetics do affect the blood sugar level and cause increased secretion of ACTH, ADH, etc., but obviously the most important factor involved is the stress induced by operation, and not a specific effect of an anaesthetic. Therefore the choice of anaesthetic agent will be much more dependent on the function of the vital organ systems than the possibility of blood glucose elevation due to the chosen anaesthetic agent.

Preparation of the Patient and Premedication

Patients on oral drugs should continue to take them until 24 h before operation (48 h with long-acting chlorpropamide). In adult patients with mild diabetes (blood sugar below 150 mg%), it is possible not to use insulin at all. Minor surgery under regional analgesia and of short duration can be handled with 75% of the patient's usual drugs (oral diabetic drugs or insulin).

One of the recomended ways of preparing patients for elective (major) surgery is to give the patient half of his daily insulin requirement in the morning, subcutaneously, as regular insulin immediately after a 5% glucose in water (G5W) infusion is started. This infusion is continued throughout anaesthesia and about 2000 ml G5W is given. If surgery is scheduled for later, one-third of the insulin is given s.c. in the morning, 5% glucose in water is continued, and 1000 ml is given before anaesthesia. Urine glucose and ketone are monitored, frequency depending on the severity of diabetes and derangement. If necessary, blood glucose level is monitored.

In emergency surgical procedures in untreated diabetics, severe keto-acidosis is contra-indication for surgery. Patients must be treated with insulin: 10—20 units of regular insulin given i.m. or i.v. at frequent intervals is mostly very effective. Water and electrolyte deficiency should be corrected. Glucose solutions, hypotonic solutions, dextrans, and lactate should be avoided in the initial phase. After several hours, with good renal function hypokalaemia may develop. At this point 5% glucose in water and KCl up to 40 mEq is given by bottle and can be repeated until deficit is corrected. Blood volume should be restored with blood, plasma, or substitutes. Blood sugar, ketone, acid-base status, blood gases, electrolytes, blood urea nitrogen, etc. should be taken at the beginning of treatment and repeated after 2—4 h. Urine glucose should be frequently controlled. If possible, pre-operative blood sugar should be about 200 mg%.

Premedication must be given with care, because diabetic patients are very sensitive to medication. Narcotics may cause nausea and vomiting likely to complicate the situation. Atropine is used routinely, barbiturates in 50%–75% of usual dosage.

Special Requirements and Monitoring

Usual monitoring of ECG and end-tidal CO_2 is optimal. In long-lasting surgery (2–8 h) an indwelling urinary catheter is essential, and urine glucose and ketone as well as blood glucose should be determined at appropriate intervals. In acidosis mechanical ventilation is essential.

Anaesthesia

Intravenous infusion of G5W is continued. Induction is started with barbiturates and succinylcholine chloride. After intubation of the trachea, anaesthesia is maintained with the anaesthetic agent of choice. There are no special indications for any anaesthetic agent. All newer inhalation anaesthetics such as halothane, methoxyflurane, and enflurane have been shown to give good results. No insulin should be given during anaesthesia unless blood sugar is controlled. Patients should wake up as quickly as possible to allow identification of hypoglycaemia.

Post-anaesthetic Care

Post-operatively, the patient should be monitored and observed according to the requirements defined by the surgical procedure, patient's condition, and function of vital organs. Blood sugar, urine glucose, etc. should be monitored. In severe cases of diabetes, fluid and electrolyte balance studies should be done on a 2–4-h basis. Insulin treatment should be continued until patient resumes oral feeding and metabolism returns to normal. Intravenous alimentation should supply sufficient amounts of glucose, amino-acids, and electrolytes at constant concentration, composition of infused solutions, and rate of infusion, to reduce insulin requirements (S. Jeretin, 1981, Parenterale Ernährung von Beatmungspatienten, unpublished work).

References

1. Brown PS, Clark CG, Crooks J, Elston RC, Parbrook ED, Torburn AR (1964) Thyroid and adrenocortical responses to surgical operation. Clin Sci 27:447–452
2. Cecat P, Proye C, Sonnenfeld H et al. (1979) Haemodynamic aspects of pheochromocytomas during operative period in patients under alpha adrenergic block. Lille Chir 34:8–12
3. Clements RS (1972) The role of hyperglycaemia in the development of diabetic complications. Pfizer Laboratories Division Publications
4. Cooperman LH, Engelman K, Mann PEG (1967) Anaesthetic management of pheochromocytoma employing halothane and adrenergic blockade. Anaesthesiology 28:575–581
5. De Groot LJ (1965) Current views on formation of thyroid hormones. N Engl J Med 272:243–248
6. Desmonds JM, Le Hoveleur J, Remond P, Duvaldestin P (1977) Anaesthetic management of patients with pheochromocytoma, a review of 102 cases. Br J Anaesth 49:991–998
7. Engelbrecht ER, Hugill JT, Graves HB (1966) Anaesthetic management of pheochromocytoma. Can Anaesth Soc J 13:598–603

8. Goldman L, Greenspan FS (1965) Applied physiology of the thyroid and parathyroid glands. Surg Clin N Am 45:313–318
9. Goichoechea JM (1975) Anaesthesia and reanimation in thyroid and parathyroid surgery. In: Aris A et al. Excerpta medica. American Elsevier, Amsterdam Oxford New York, pp 339–343
10. Gravina E, Gravina Sanvitale G (1969) Effect of carnitine on blood acetoacetate in fasting children. Clin Chim Acta 23:376–377
11. Humble RM (1967) Pheochromocytoma, neurofibromatosis and pregnancy. Anaesthesia 22:296–299
12. Janeczko GF, Ivankovich AD, Glisson SN et al. (1977) Enflurane anaesthesia for surgical removal of pheochromocytoma. Curr Res Anaesth Analg 51/1:62–77
13. Jeretin S (1979) Erfahrungen mit Silbersulfadiazine in der Vorbeugung und Therapie von Infektionen in der Intensivtherapie. Hyg Med 4:24–25
14. Jeretin S, Music B (1980) The role of carnitine in total parenteral nutrition. Abstr 7th World Congr Anaesthesiologists, Hamburg 1980, Abstr No. 458, 238
15. Katano K, Morisawa N, Obi M et al. (1978) The anaesthesia for pheochromocytoma. J Saitama Med School 4/3:443–446
16. Katz J, Kadis LB (1973) Anaesthesia and uncommon disease. Saunders, Philadelphia London Toronto
17. Lavine MH, Stopjack JC, Jerrold TL (1968) An adrenal crisis secondary to extraction of a tooth in a patient with panhypopituitarism. J Am Dent Assoc 76:354–356
18. Oyama T (1971) Plasma levels of antidiuretic hormone in man during halothane anaesthesia and surgery. The year book of anaesthesia 1971. Year Book Medical Publishers, Chicago, pp 50–52
19. Oyama T (1973) Anaesthetic management of endocrine disease. Springer, Berlin Heidelberg New York
20. Pender JW, Fox M, Basso LV (1973) Diseases of the endocrine system. In: Katz RL, Kadis LB (eds) Anaesthesia in incommon disease. Saunders, Philadelphia London Toronto, pp 121–127
21. Raskin P, Unger R (1978) Hypoglycaemia and its suppression. N Engl J Med 299:433–436
22. Rollason WN (1964) Halothane and pheochromocytoma. Br J Anaesth 36:251–255
23. Stringel G, Ein SH, Creighton R et al. (1980) Pheochromocytoma in children – an update. J Pediatr Surg 15/4:496–500
24. Schultis K (1976) Postagressionsstoffwechsel als Adaptation und Krankheit. In: Heberer G, Schultis K, Hoffmann K (eds) Postaggressionsstoffwechsel, vol 3. Schattauer, Stuttgart New York
25. Shimasoto S (1978) Altered cardiac performance to general volatile anaesthetics in health and disease. In: Haemodynamic changes in anaesthesia, tome 2,5th European congress of anaesthesiology, Paris 1978. Excerpta medica, Amsterdam Oxford, pp 1019–1036
26. Wahren J, Felig P (1976) Influence of somatostatin on carbohydrate disposal and absorption in diabetes mellitus. Lancet 1213–1216

Concept in Patients with Hypertension and Coronary Heart Disease - Clinical and Experimental Aspects

K. van Ackern, U. Mittmann, U.B. Brückner, H.O. Vetter, Ch. Madler and H. Victor

In patients with coronary artery disease, heart function depends on the balance between myocardial oxygen consumption and oxygen supply. Therefore for such patients a type of anaesthesia must be chosen which presents no increase in myocardial oxygen consumption. Intra- and post-operative hypertension, which is frequently observed in patients with coronary artery disease [2], should be strictly avoided.

In the first study presented here, 12 patients undergoing coronary bypass surgery with hypertensive reactions were investigated [7]. Patients were anaesthetized with a modified neurolept anaesthesia. When during surgery systolic blood-pressure exceeded 150 mmHg, 0.5 mg of fentanyl was initially administered to ensure sufficient analgesia. If blood-pressure did not fall in response to this therapy, enflurane was added at a concentration of 1.2−1.8 vol.% in the inspired gas. The administration of enflurane was continued until systolic blood-pressure decreased to about 120 mmHg. During this time pulmonary capillary wedge pressure (PCWP) was measured at ca. 1-min intervals. All measurements were performed prior to the beginning of aortocoronary bypass.

The course of systolic arterial pressure (SAP), mean arterial pressure (MAP), and heart rate (HR) is demonstrated in Fig. 1. Enflurane reduced systolic arterial pressure from 172 (±11) to 115 (±9) mmHg ($p < 0.005$). Mean arterial pressure was diminished by 25 mmHg to a final value of 87 (±5) mmHg ($p < 0.05$). Heart rate was decreased from 108 (±12) to 92 (±7) beats/min.

Cardiac index (CI) remained almost unchanged under enflurane (2.7 ± 0.3 to 2.8 ± 0.3 l/min · m^2; Fig. 2). As expected, systemic vascular resistance (SVR) decreased under enflurane. This decrease amounted to 21% ($p < 0.05$); PCWP fell slightly from 15 (±3) to 13 (±3) mmHg. There were no signs of impaired global myocardial function under enflurane administration and stroke volume had even increased.

Right heart function and pulmonary circulation were only very slightly affected by enflurane administration. The changes are presented in Fig. 3. Right atrial pressure (RAP) remained completely unchanged (9 ± 2 to 8.5 ± 2 mmHg). Mean pulmonary arterial pressure (PAP) fell from 24 ± 4 to 22 ± 3 mmHg. The fall in pulmonary resistance (PVR) was correspondingly slight (170 ± 30 to 160 ± 21 dyn × sec × cm^{-5}).

Under enflurane the arteriovenous O_2 difference ($CaO_2 - CvO_2$) was unchanged (Fig. 4). In five patients coronary sinus blood was withdrawn and the oxygen content was determined. A fall in arterio-coronary sinus O_2 difference ($CaO_2 - Cv \sin O_2$) of about 1 vol.% was observed in each individual patient.

The calculated and measured determinants of myocardial oxygen consumption in terms of percentage of control are presented in Fig. 5. Left ventricular work, calculated indirectly

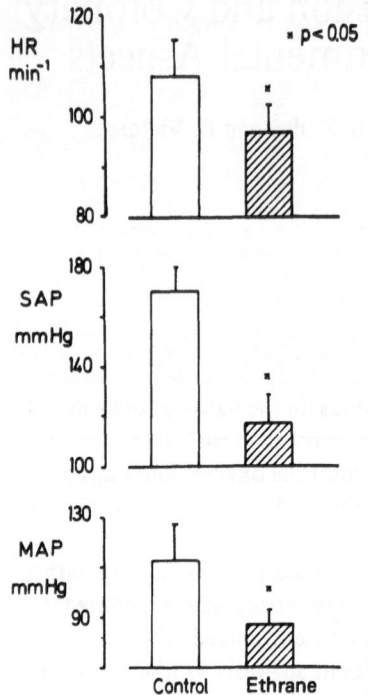

Fig. 1. Mean values of heart rate (*HR*), systolic arterial pressure (*SAP*), and mean arterial pressure (*MAP*) before (*Control*) and after enflurane (*Ethrane*) administration

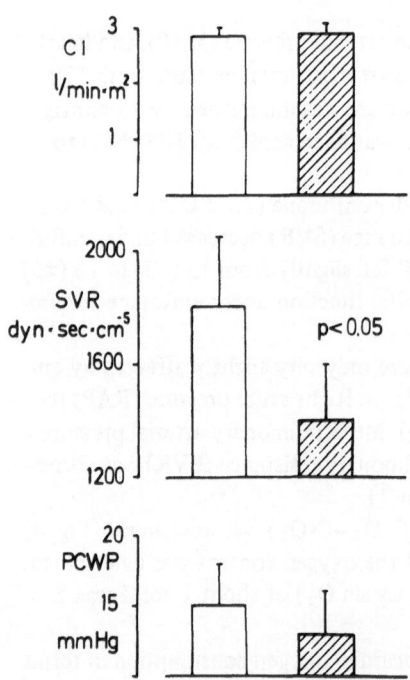

Fig. 2. Changes of cardiac index (*CI*), systemic vascular resistance (*SVR*), and pulmonary capillary wedge pressure (*PCWP*) after enflurane

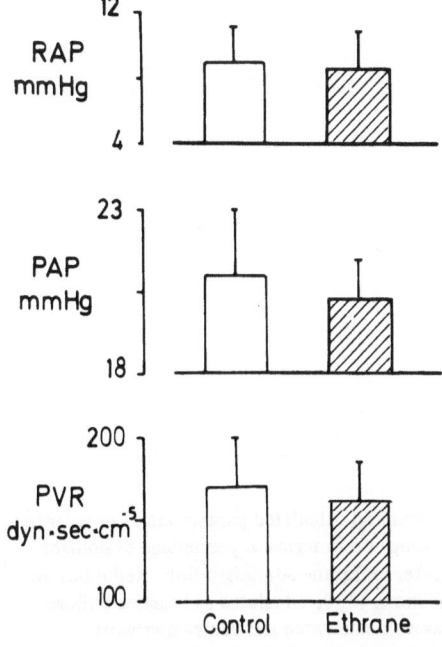

Fig. 3. Effects of enflurane on right atrial pressure (*RAP*), mean pulmonary pressure (*PAP*), and pulmonary vascular resistance (*PVR*)

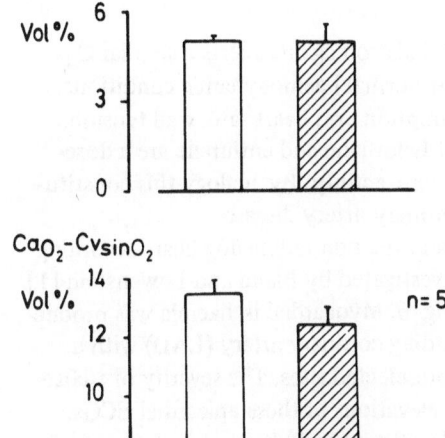

Fig. 4. Arteriovenous oxygen difference ($Ca_{O_2} - Cv_{O_2}$) in 12 patients and arteriocoronary sinus oxygen difference ($Ca_{O_2} - C_{vsinO_2}$) in five patients during hypertension (*Control*) and after reduction of blood-pressure produced by enflurane (*Ethrane*)

by multiplying cardiac output by systolic pressure, fell by 25% ($p < 0.05$). As already shown, heart rate was reduced by 16.5%. The decline in work and heart rate clearly indicated that myocardial oxygen consumption was reduced. This reduction was also verified by the fall in the heart rate pressure product, which was reduced by 41% ($p < 0.005$). The results of this study showed that hypertensive reactions could be successfully treated using enflurane. Enflurane-induced reduction of elevated blood-pressure and heart rate caused a decrease in myocardial oxygen demand without jeopardizing left ventricular function.

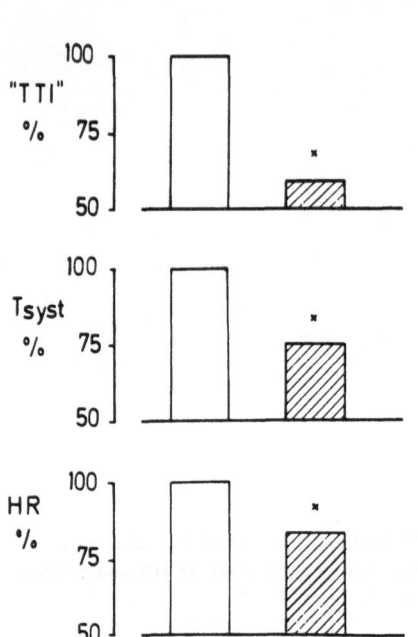

* p < 0.05

Fig. 5. Measured and calculated parameters of myocardial oxygen consumption in terms of percentage of control before and after enflurane administration: Reduction of tension-time index (*TTI*, calculated as heart rate times systolic pressure), calculated left ventricular work (*T syst.*, calculated indirectly by multiplying cardiac output by systolic pressure), and heart rate (*HR*)

The question is now whether administration of inhalation agents exerts a similiar O_2-saving effect on the ischaemic myocardium also under normal haemodynamic conditions. The major determinants of myocardial oxygen consumption are: heart rate, wall tension, and contractility. The main haemodynamic effects of halothane and enflurane are a dose-dependent reduction of heart rate, wall tension, and contractility. By analogy this constitutes the clinical concept of beta-blocker therapy in coronary artery disease.

The effect of halothane on myocardial ischaemia in the non-failing dog heart according to the method developed by Maroko et al. [3] was investigated by Bland and Lowenstein [1]. The method used is schematically demonstrated in Fig. 6. Myocardial ischaemia was produced in dogs by occlusion of a branch of the left descending coronary artery (LAD) with a tourniquet. Epicardial ECGs were determined at 15 preselected sites. The severity of ischaemia was considered to be the sum of the ST segment elevations of these epicardial ECGs.

Figure 7 demonstrates the sum of ST segment elevations (ΣST) before, during, and after 0.75% halothane administration in six dogs. Myocardial ischaemia produced by occlusion of the identical branch of the left anterior descending artery appeared to be significantly less severe during halothane anaesthesia.

A further study [8] elicited similar results with enflurane using the same animal model. Administration of 1 MAC enflurane, which is 2.2 vol% in dogs, produced a significant reduction of the sum of ST segment elevation in the ischaemic area (Fig. 8). In addition to Bland and Lowenstein's parameters [1], cardiac output and dp/dt_{max} were measured in this experiment. Enflurane administration resulted in a significant reduction of mean arterial pressure ($p < 0.005$) and systemic vascular resistance ($p < 0.005$; Fig. 9). Cardiac output remained almost unchanged. Heart rate was only slightly affected. Left atrial pressure (LAP)

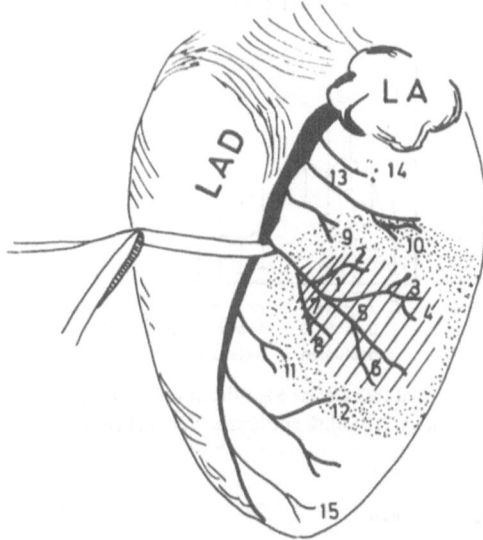

Fig. 6. Schematic graph of the experimental model. Regional myocardial ischaemia was produced by a temporary occlusion of a branch of the left descending coronary artery (*LAD*) with a tourniquet. Epicardial ECGs were recorded at 15 preselected sites: eight directly in the area supplied by the occluded branch (*1–8, hatched zone*), four in the adjacent area (*9–12, dotted zone*), and three in the non-affected area (13–15). The sum of the ST segment elevations was calculated from individual values determined at each site

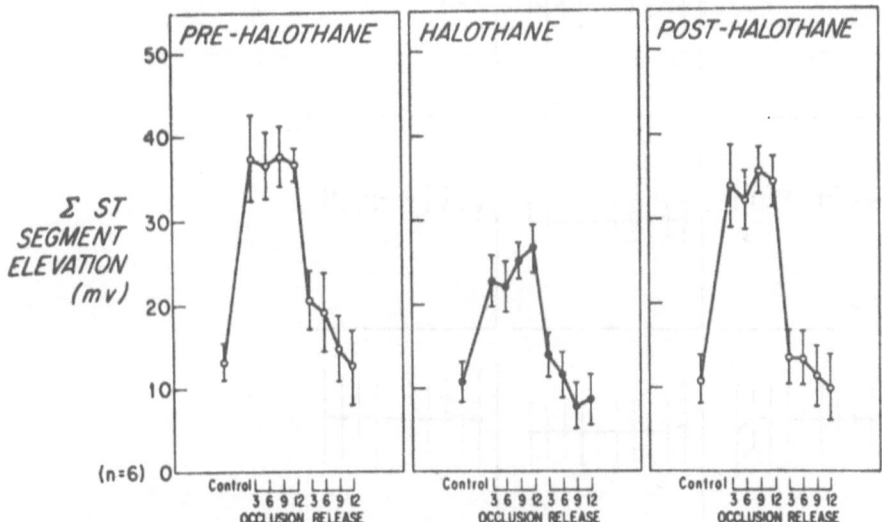

Fig. 7. Sum of ST segment elevations (Σ*ST*) before, during, and after 0.75 vol.% halothane in six dogs (Bland and Lowenstein [1]). The severity of regional ischaemia produced by occlusion of the identical branch of the LAD was significantly less during halothane administration

was unchanged, while left ventricular pressure (LVP) and dp/dt_{max} were decreased ($p <$ 0.05 and $p < 0.005$, respectively; Fig. 10). Left ventricular stroke work index (LVSW) was not significantly affected.

The decline in blood-pressure and dp/dt_{max} resulted in a decreased myocardial oxygen consumption, estimated by the heart rate pressure product ($p < 0.005$; Fig. 11) and in a reduced regional myocardial ischaemia. Although there are some disagreements on the value

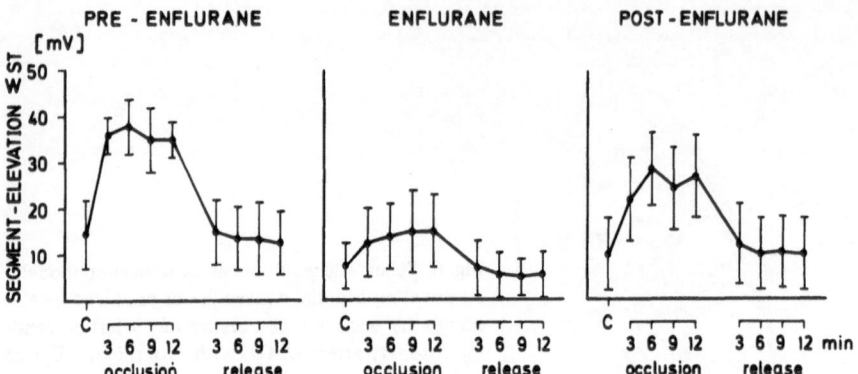

Fig. 8. Effects of enflurane administration on regional myocardial ischaemia: Significant reduction of the sum of ST segment elevations (ΣST) before, during, and after 2.2 vol.% enflurane. Van Ackern et al. [8]

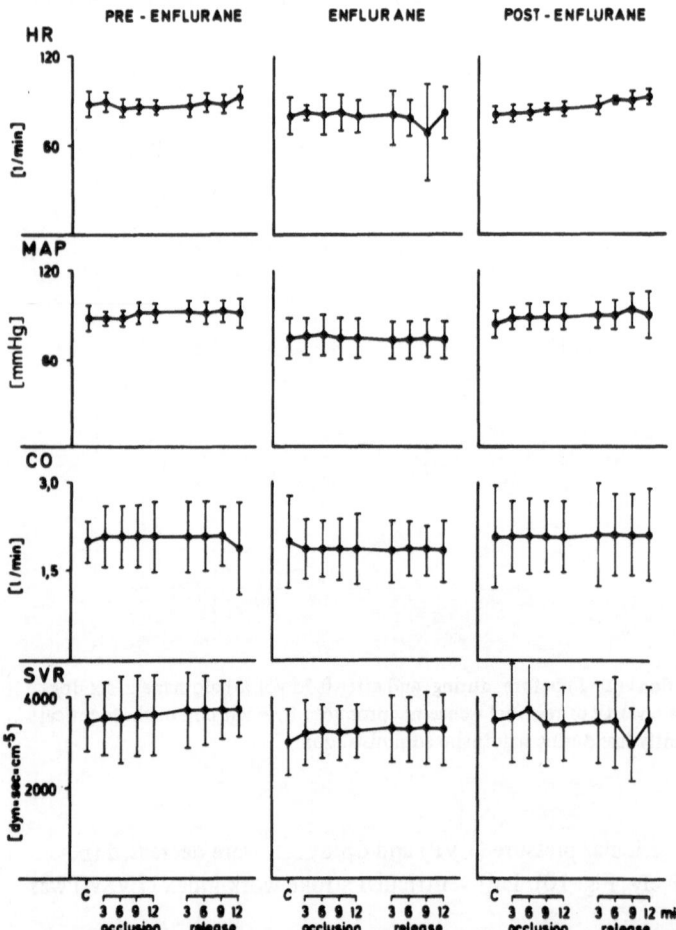

Fig. 9. Mean values of heart rate (*HR*), mean aterial pressure (*MAP*), cardiac output (*CO*), and systemic vascular resistance (*SVR*) before, during, and after 2.2 vol.% enflurane administration. Enflurane produced a significant reduction of MAP and SVR

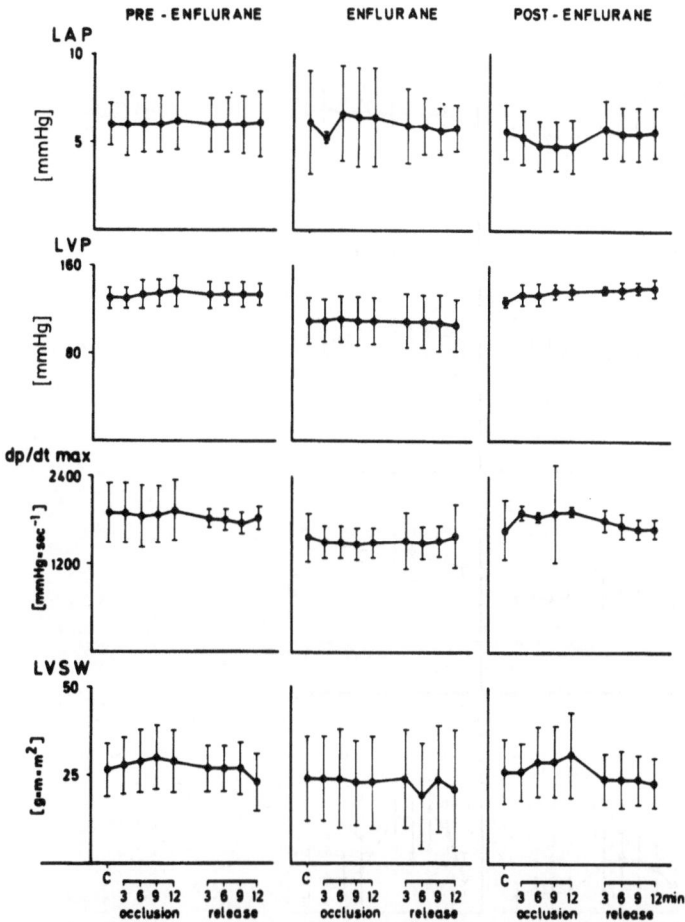

Fig. 10. Changes of left atrial pressure (*LAP*), left ventricular pressure (*LVP*), dp/dt$_{max}$, and left ventricular stroke work index (*LVSW*) before, during, and after enflurane. LVP and dp/dt$_{max}$ were significantly reduced

of this electrocardiographic indicator of myocardial injury [5], these results appear to indicate that myocardial oxygen balance of an ischaemic area in the non-failing heart can be improved by administration of halothane and enflurane.

In order to evaluate the influence of enflurane on regional myocardial function and oxygen uptake in myocardial ischaemia, the following experiments in dogs were performed by our group. Figure 12 demonstrates schematically the method used. The left anterior descending artery was carefully isolated near its origin. An electromagnetic flow probe and a micrometer constrictor were attached to the LAD. Myocardial ischaemia was produced by constriction of the LAD to a flow of 20% of control using the micrometer constrictor. Two opposing ultrasonic crystals were placed in the endocardium of the flow-constricted area for measuring regional wall motion.

An ECG electrode was inserted on the surface of the ischaemic area for measurement of ST segment elevations. A small catheter was introduced through the coronary sinus into the vena cordis magna for withdrawing blood mainly from the ischaemic area. A tip mano-

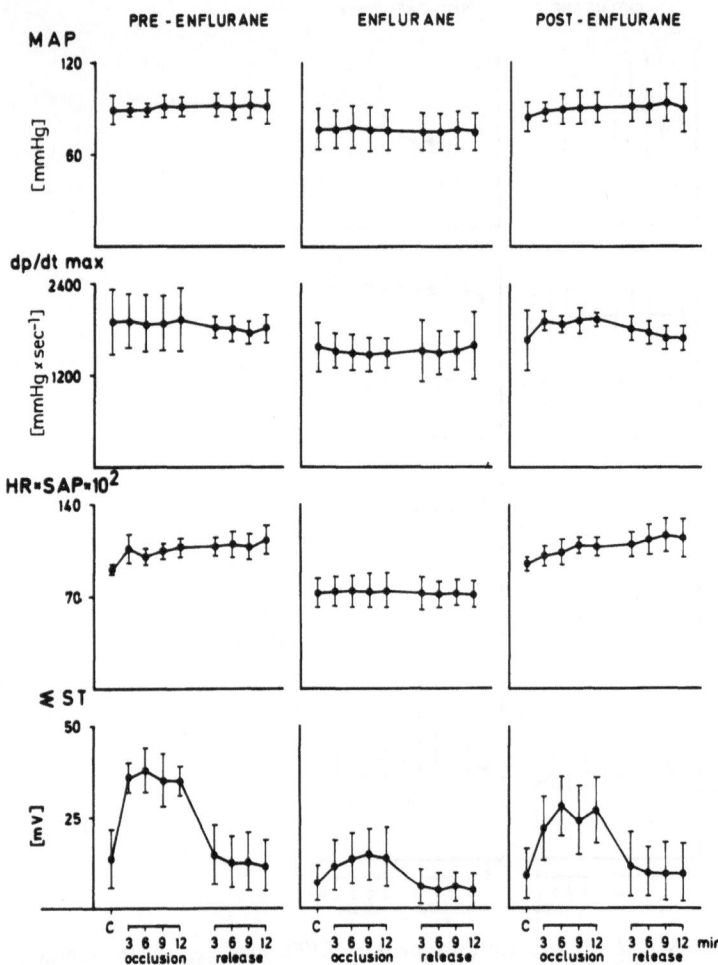

Fig. 11. Summary of MAP, dp/dt$_{max}$, HR, SAP, and ΣST before, during, and after enflurane administration. The decline in blood-pressure and dp/dt$_{max}$ resulted in a decreased myocardial oxygen consumption, calculated indirectly by the heart rate-systolic pressure product and in a reduced regional myocardial ischaemia

meter was inserted in the left ventricle for measuring left ventricular pressure and its derived parameters. Radioactive microspheres were injected via a small catheter into the left atrium. In Fig. 13 the course of mean arterial pressure, cardiac output, total systemic resistance and heart rate are demonstrated. On the abscissa the interventions are seen: After a control period of 10 min, reduction of LAD flow to 20% of control was performed for 60 min. After 20 min LAD constriction, 1 MAC enflurane was added to the inspired gas for 20 min. After 20 min enflurane was withdrawn and after further 20 min occlusion of LAD was released. The mean arterial pressure was not affected by LAD-constriction. Cardiac output, however, was reduced. Total systemic resistance ($p < 0.05$) and also heart rate ($p < 0.05$) were significantly increased. Administration of enflurane produced the well-known changes described in the literature [4]: Reduction in mean arterial pressure, cardiac index, total systemic resistance, and heart rate. In some experiments enflurane blood concentrations were measured.

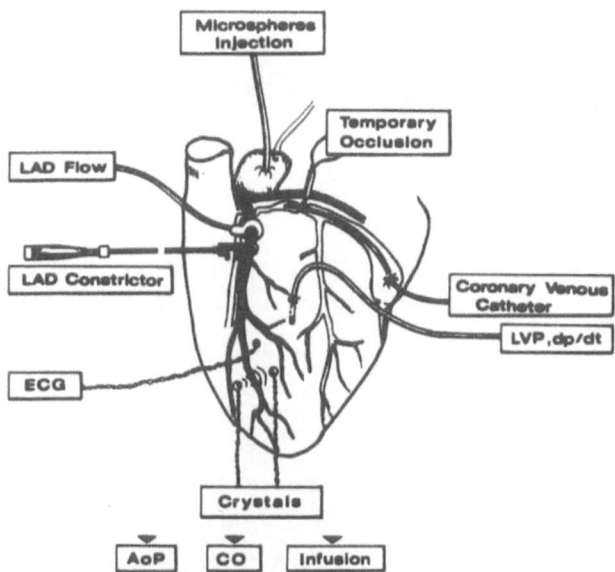

Fig. 12. Schematic diagram of the experimental model and the proceedings. An electromagnetic flow probe and a micrometer constrictor were placed on the left ascending coronary artery (LAD) near its origin. Regional myocardial ischaemia was produced by constriction of the LAD to a flow of 20% of control. Two opposing ultrasonic crystals were inserted into the endocardium for measuring wall motion. An ECG electrode was placed in the surface of the ischaemic area. A small catheter was introduced through the coronary sinus into the vena cordis magna for withdrawing blood mainly from the ischaemic area. A tip manometer was inserted in the left ventricle for measuring left ventricular pressure and its derived parameters dp/dt_{max} and V_{PM}

Blood concentrations 10 min after withdrawal of enflurane was still elevated. They were in a range similar to that measured after enflurane administration. Enddiastolic pressure (EDP) was unchanged; dp/dt_{max} and V_{PM} decreased after constriction and during enflurane administration, as demonstrated in Fig. 14.

In Fig. 15 the end-diastolic muscle length (EDL) and the regional contraction (Δl) measured by the ultrasonic crystals are shown. Acute reduction of LAD flow to 20% of control resulted in a decrease of regional myocardial contraction at increased fibre length. Additional administration of enflurane produced a further slight diminution of regional contraction at a reduced diastolic fibre length. After-load reduction and the negative inotropic effect of enflurane may be involved in this response. These effects of enflurane were reversible.

The electromagnetically measured flow in the LAD (CF_{LAD}) and the subendocardial flow (MBF_{ENDO}) in the ischaemic area measured with radioactive microspheres are demonstrated in Fig. 16. Enflurane reduced subendocardial flow in the non-affected part of the ventricle, which is not demonstrated in the figure. However, flow in the ischaemic area was apparently not altered by enflurane.

Acute LAD constriction resulted in an increase of the oxygen difference between arterial blood and blood from the ischaemic myocardium ($AVDO_2$), and in a marked elevation of the ST segment (Fig. 17). Additional enflurane administration reduced the ST segment elevation significantly, and the $AVDO_2$ showed a tendency to decrease. These effects were reversed on withdrawal of enflurane.

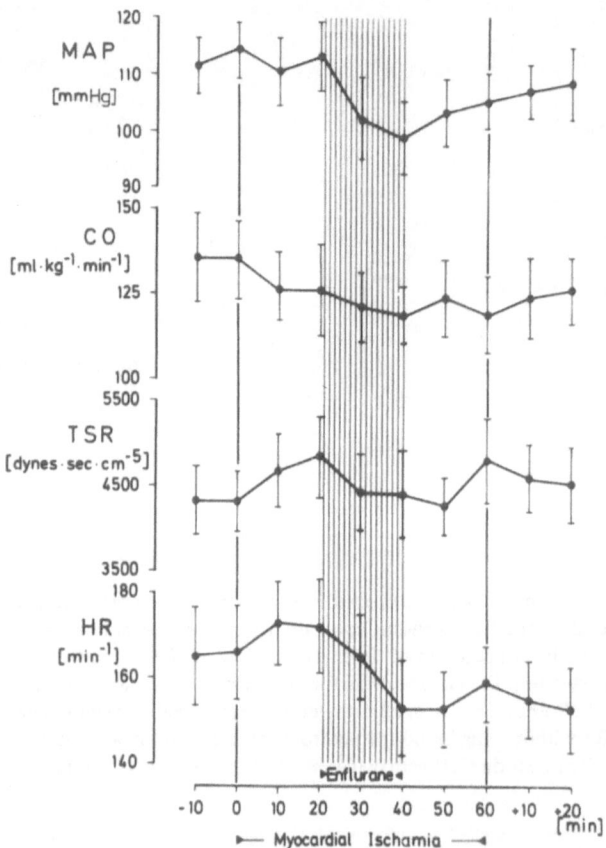

Fig. 13. The experimental protocol is demonstrated here and in the following figures on the abscissa. After a control period of 10 min (−10−0 min), reduction of left descending coronary artery (LAD) flow to 20% of control for 60 min (0−60 min). After 20 min of LAD constriction (0−20 min), administration of 1 MAC enflurane for 20 min (20−40 min, hatched area), withdrawal of enflurane and observation for 20 min (40−60 min); release of constriction and observation for 20 min (+10−+20 min). The course of mean arterial pressure (MAP), cardiac output (CO), total systemic resistance (TSR), and heart rate (HR) before, during and after constriction of the LAD and the effects of enflurane administration during regional myocardial ischaemia. Effects of enflurane were here and in the following parameters reversible after withdrawal of enflurane

The effects of enflurane under the condition of coronary artery constriction are demonstrated in summary in Fig. 18. There was no additional reduction in regional subendocardial flow. The increased end-diastolic fibre length in the ischaemic area was reduced under enflurane. The ST segment elevation was improved. The O_2 difference between arterial blood and blood from the ischaemic myocardium showed a tendency to decrease. Lactate extraction determined from arterial blood and blood mainly from the regional ischaemic myocardium was decreased after constriction of the LAD. After enflurane this reduced lactate extraction also showed a tendency to improve. Total left ventricular O_2 uptake estimated by the formula of Strauer et al. [6] was reduced under enflurane.

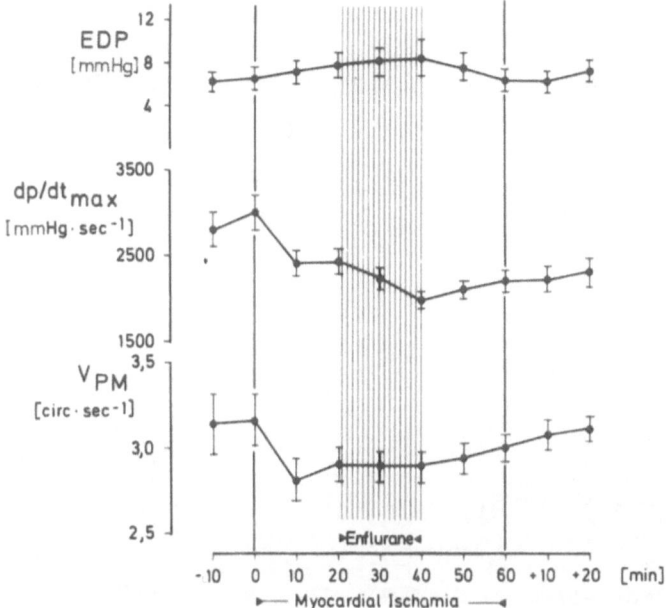

Fig. 14. Changes of end-diastolic pressure (*EDP*), dp/dt$_{max}$, and V$_{PM}$ of the left ventricle

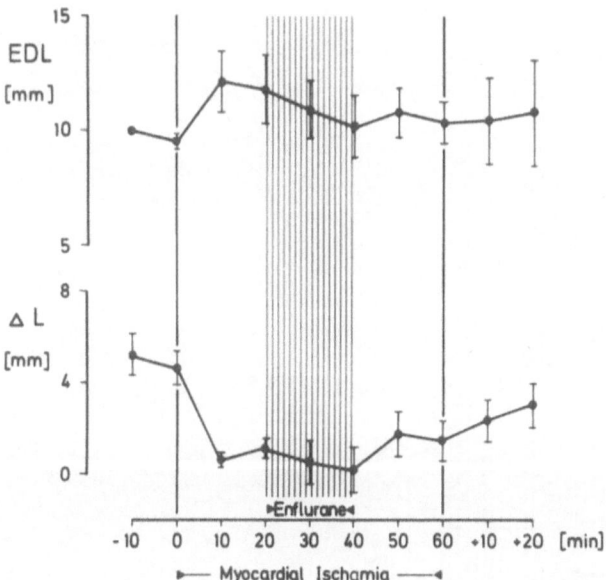

Fig. 15. Course of end-diastolic muscle fibre length (*EDL*) and regional myocardial contraction (*Σl*) measured by two ultrasonic crystals in the ischaemic area of the myocardium

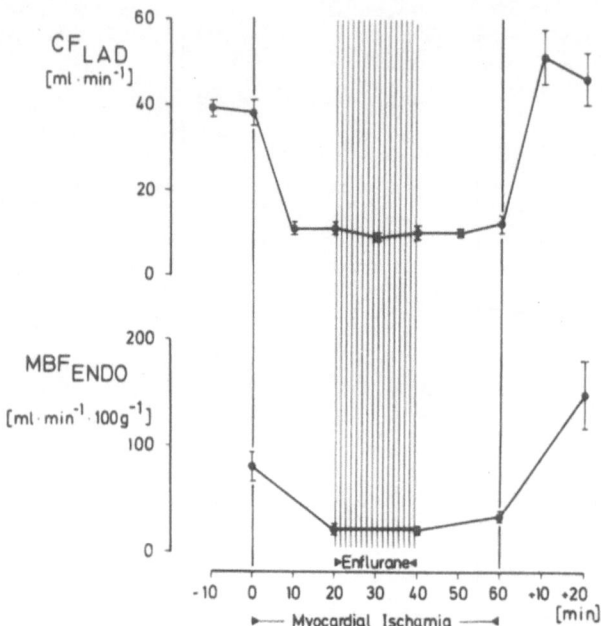

Fig. 16. Mean values of the electromagnetic measured flow in the left descending coronary artery (CF_{LAD}) and of the subendocardial flow in the ischaemic area measured with radioactive microspheres (MBF_{ENDO})

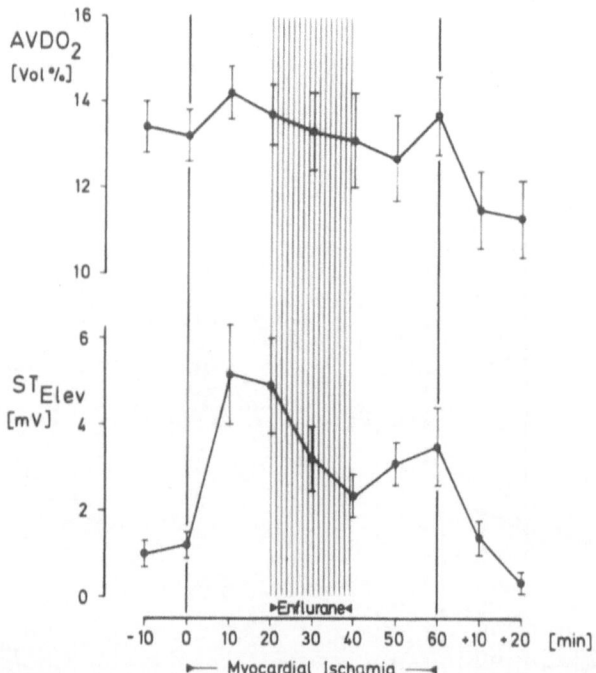

Fig. 17. The oxygen difference between arterial blood and blood mainly withdrawn from the constricted area ($AVDO_2$), and ST segment elevation in this zone (ST_{ELEV})

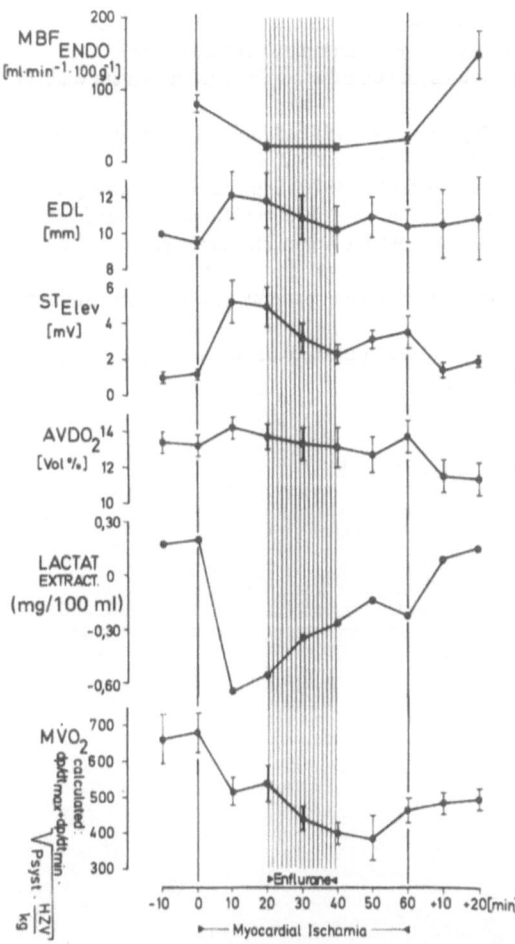

Fig. 18. Summary of some of the main changes after reduction of left descending coronary artery (LAD) flow to 20% of control and after enflurane administration: subendocardial flow (MBF$_{ENDO}$), end-diastolic muscle length (EDL), ST segment elevation (ST$_{ELEV}$), oxygen difference between arterial blood and blood from the ischaemic myocardium (AVDO$_2$), lactate extraction in the ischaemic area and calculated myocardial oxygen consumption (MVO$_2$)

In summary, our results suggest that besides unloading of the left ventricle, enflurane anaesthesia appears to have a beneficial O$_2$-saving influence on the ischaemic myocardium. The effects described may not be myocardial specific for the anaesthetic agent used, but rather they are likely to be caused by a myocardial and peripheral vascular action of enflurane.

References

1. Bland JHL, Lowenstein E (1976) Decrease in experimental myocardial ischemia by halothane anesthesia in the non-failing dog heart. Anesthesiology 45:287
2. Estefanous FG, Tarazi RC, Viljoin JF, Eltawil MY (1973) Systemic hypertension following myocardial revascularisation. Am Heart J 85:732

3. Maroko PR, Kjekshus JE, Sobel BE, Watanabe T, Covell JW, Ross J, Braunwald E (1971) Factors influencing infarct size following experimental coronary artery occlusions. Circulation 43:67
4. Peter K, Van Ackern K, Altstaedt F (1973) Kreislaufanalyse von Ethrane-Untersuchungen am wachen Tier. Z Prakt Anaesth 8:227
5. Sniderman A, Mickleborough L, Huttner I, Poirier N, Symes J (1979) Fallibility of the epicardial electrocardiogram in quantitation of myocardial necrosis. Cardiovasc Res 5:274
6. Strauer BE, Tauchert BM, Cott L, Kochsiek K, Bretschneider HJ (1970) Simultane Bestimmung des Sauerstoffverbrauchs und der Coronardurchblutung des linken Ventrikels bei Mitral- und Aortenklappenfehler mit einem neuen haemodynamischen Parameter und der Argon Fremdgasmethode. Verh Dtsch Ges Inn Med 76:217
7. Van Ackern K, Franke N, Peter K, Schmucker P (1979) Enflurane in patients with coronary artery disease. Acta Anaesth Scand [Suppl] 71:71
8. Van Ackern K, Jesch F, Forst H, Kreuzer E, Reichart B (1980) Influence of enflurane on experimental myocardial ischemia in dogs. Excerpta Medica 533:152

Inhalation Anaesthetics as Hypotensive Agents: Controversial Aspects

O. Hilfiker, D. Kettler, R. Larsen, J. Teichmann and H. Sonntag

Introduction

Deliberate hypotension has been controversial ever since it was introduced in 1946 by Gardner [1]. That it actually decreases blood loss has been reported by several authors, including Thompson et al. [2] as recently as 1978. Improved understanding of the cardiovascular physiology and the development of monitoring devices for continuous invasive monitoring in the past 2 decades have contributed to a more critical and safer use of controlled hypotension.

Controlled hypotension may be regarded as a well-established procedure applied by the anaesthesiologists in the following fields (after Tinker):

1. Neurosurgery
2. Cancer resection
3. Coarctation of the aorta
4. Major maxillo-facial surgery
5. Orthopaedic surgery
6. Religious blood refusal

Documented or suspected compromised blood supply to any vital organ and impaired cardiovascular function are considered to be contra-indications for controlled hypotension. Indications for blood pressure reduction other than reducing blood loss or facilitating surgery, e.g. intra-operative after-load reduction to treat cardiac dysfunction, are not considered in this paper.

Hypotension may be achieved either by lowering peripheral vascular resistance by vasodilators or by decreasing cardiac output by the administration of increasing concentrations of a negative inotropic-acting inhalation anaesthetic such as halothane or enflurane.

Induction of Hypotension by Inhalation Anaesthetics

General Haemodynamics

In a recent study in man by Sonntag et al. [3], increasing halothane concentration from 0 to 0.9% and then to 1.8% led to an almost linear reduction of mean arterial pressure, cardiac index, and contractility as reflected by dp/dt_{max}, whereas left ventricular end-diastolic pressure increased. Heart rate showed a slight tendency to bradycardia. Peripheral vascular resistance remained unchanged.

In animals and in part also in man, we have studied the effects of inhalation anaesthetic and vasodilator hypotension at a mean arterial blood pressure of 50 mmHg on perfusion and oxygen uptake of the heart and the brain, which are the organs most vulnerable to a decreased oxygen supply. The results of these studies will be presented here and discussed in the light of the recent literature.

Figure 1 shows the results of halothane hypotension in dog experiments. Inspiratory halothane concentration of 2.5% resulted in a reduction of mean arterial pressure to about 50 mmHg. Hypotension was the result of a decreased cardiac output, whereas peripheral vascular resistance remained unchanged.

Figure 2 shows similar results with enflurane hypotension in dogs. Hypotension resulted from a decreased cardiac output and in part also from a reduced peripheral vascular resistance. There seems to be little difference between halothane and enflurane in their action on peripheral vascular resistance.

Myocardial Blood Flow (MBF) and Myocardial Oxygen Uptake (MV̇O₂)

Halothane (Fig. 3) and enflurane (Fig. 4) produced a marked reduction in myocardial blood flow (MBF) and myocardial oxygen uptake (MV̇O₂), mainly due to their negative inotropic effects on the heart. In a study of halothane hypotension we found in four patients at an

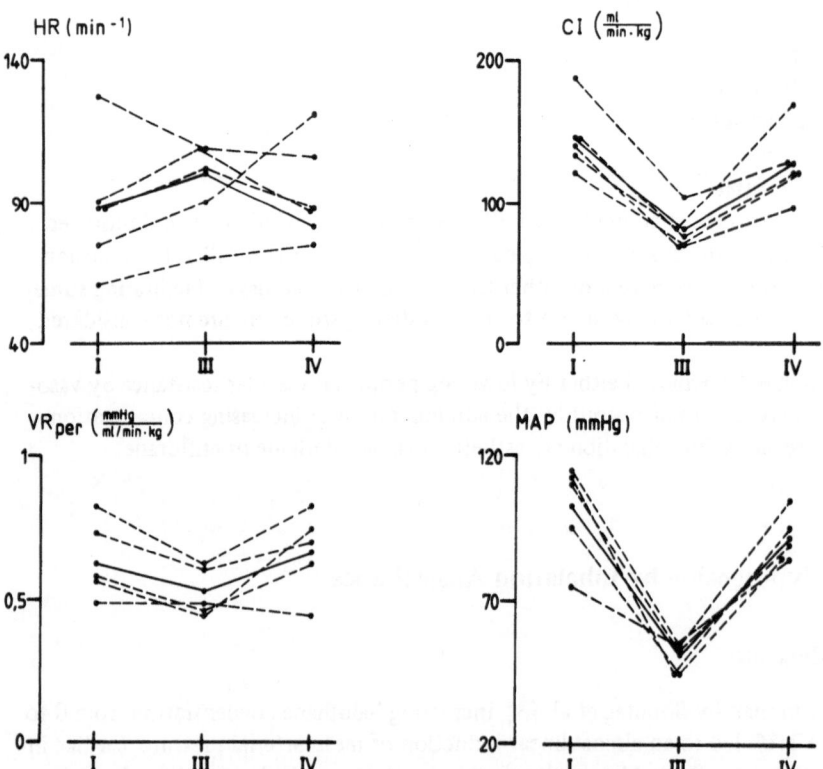

Fig. 1. Halothane hypotension in the dog (n = 5). Individual results in each animal before (*I*), during (*III*), and after (*IV*) halothane administration. *HR*, heart rate; *CI*, cardiac index; *VR_per*, peripheral vascular resistance; *MAP*, mean aortic pressure

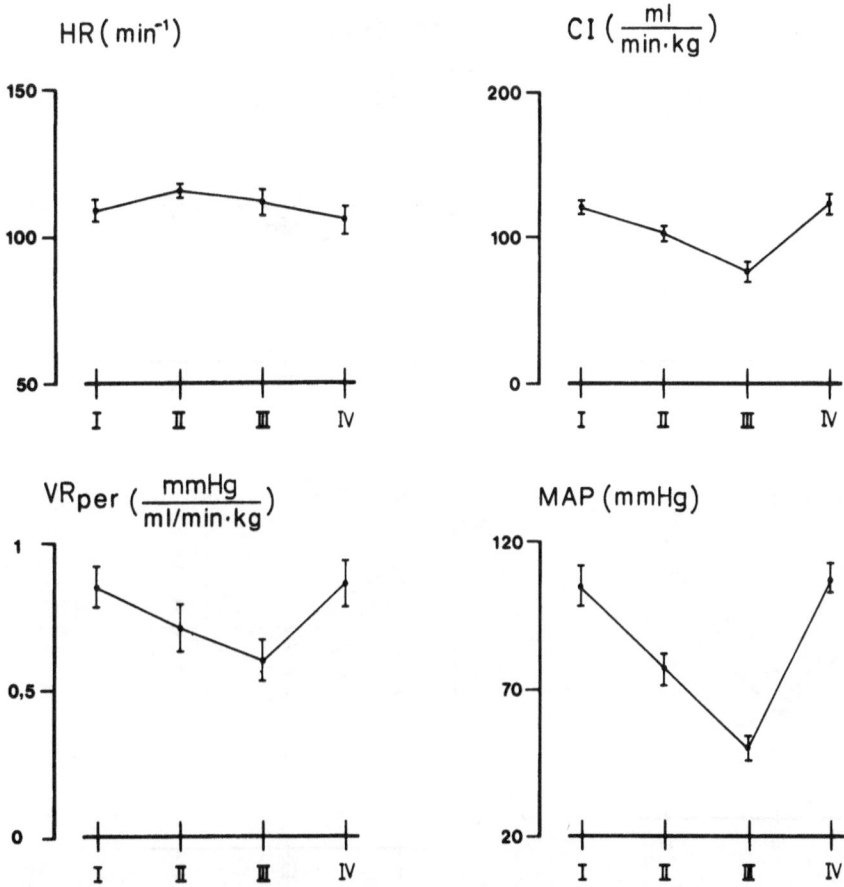

Fig. 2. Enflurane hypotension in the dog (n = 8). Mean values ± SEM. *I*, control, enflurane concentration 1.8% ± 0.3%; *II*, mean aortic pressure 25% of control, enflurane concentration 2.4% ± 0.3%; *III*, mean aortic pressure 50% of control, enflurane concentration 3.2% ± 0.1%; *IV*, control; *HR*, heart rate; *CI*, cardiac index; *VR*$_{per}$, peripheral vascular resistance; *MAP*, mean aortic pressure

average mean arterial pressure of 50 mmHg a reduction of $M\dot{V}O_2$ from 10 to 5.3 ml O_2/min/ 100 g heart wt. Myocardial blood flow fell from 87 to 56 ml/min/100 g (Fig. 5). Neither in the animal nor in the human study could lactate release from the myocardium be demonstrated.

Cerebral Blood Flow (CBF) and Cerebral Metabolic Rate for Oxygen ($CMRO_2$)

In the dog experiment halothane had little effect on CBF, but $CMRO_2$ decreased from 3.2 to 2.6 ml O_2/100 g brain wt. (Fig. 6). Cerebral vascular resistance and perfusion pressure dropped considerably. The decrease in the cerebral perfusion pressure was due to the reduced mean arterial pressure. Intracranial pressure as reflected by the epidural pressure remained essentially unchanged.

Enflurane effects differed from halothane insofar as $CMRO_2$ increased from 2.4 to 3.4 ml O_2/min/100 g with high inspiratory enflurane concentration (3.2 vol.%) (Fig. 7). The in-

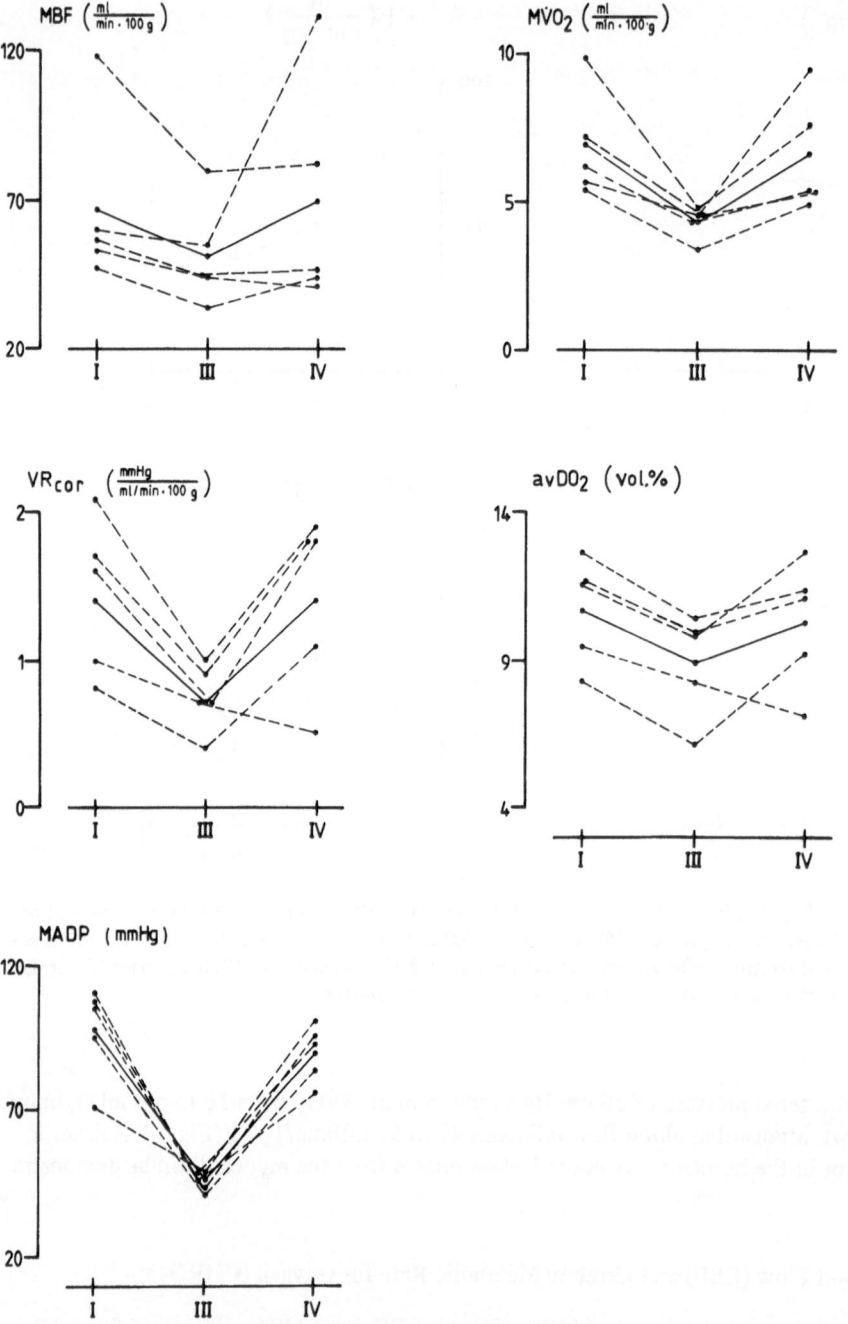

Fig. 3. Myocardial blood flow and myocardial oxygen uptake under halothane hypotension in the dog. Individual results for each animal: *I*, before; *III*, during; *VI*, after. *MBF*, myocardial blood flow; $M\dot{V}O_2$, myocardial oxygen uptake; VR_{cor}, coronary vascular resistance; $avDO_2$, arteriocoronary venous oxygen content difference; *MADP*, mean aortic diastolic pressure

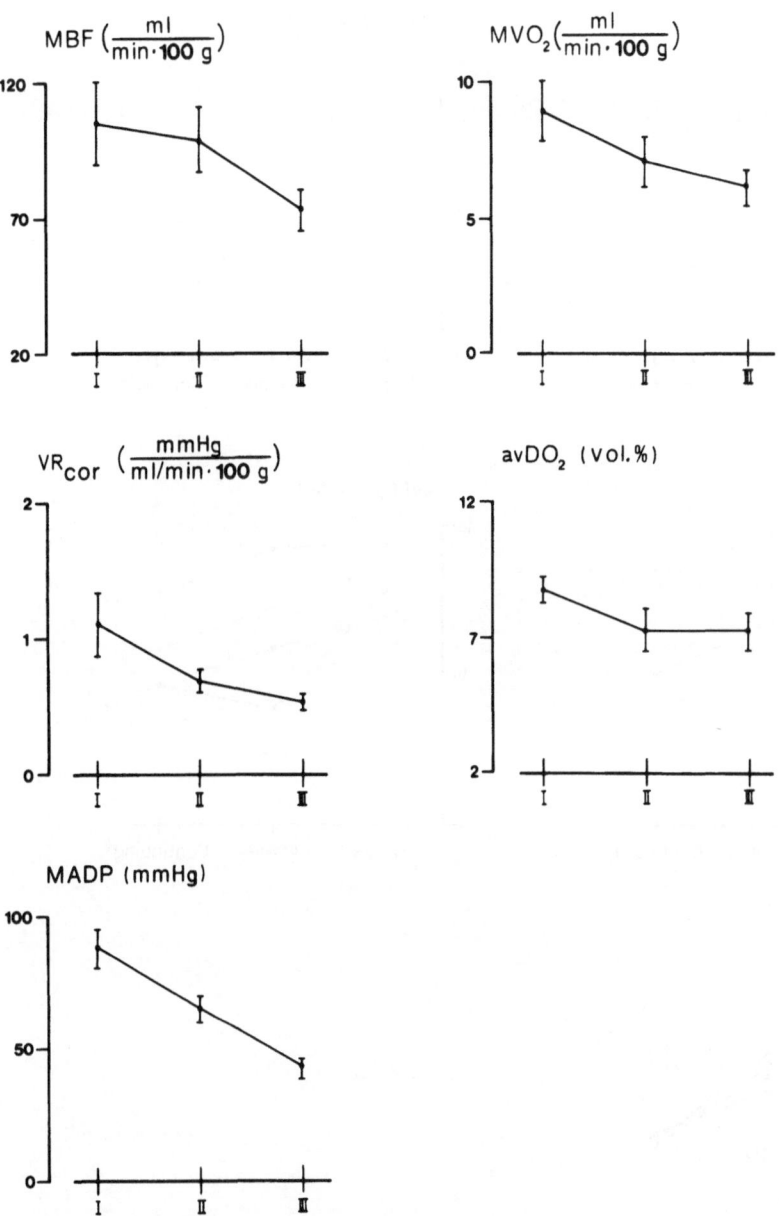

Fig. 4. Myocardial blood flow and myocardial oxygen uptake under enflurane hypotension in the dog. Mean values ± SEM; n = 7. *I*, control, enflurane concentration 1.8% ± 0.3%; *II*, mean aortic pressure 50% of control, enflurane concentration 3.2% ± 0.1%; *III*, control. *MBF*, myocardial blood flow; *MV̇O₂*, myocardial oxygen uptake; *VR꜀ₒᵣ*, coronary vascular resistance; *avDO₂*, arteriocoronary venous oxygen content difference; *MADP*, mean aortic diastolic pressure

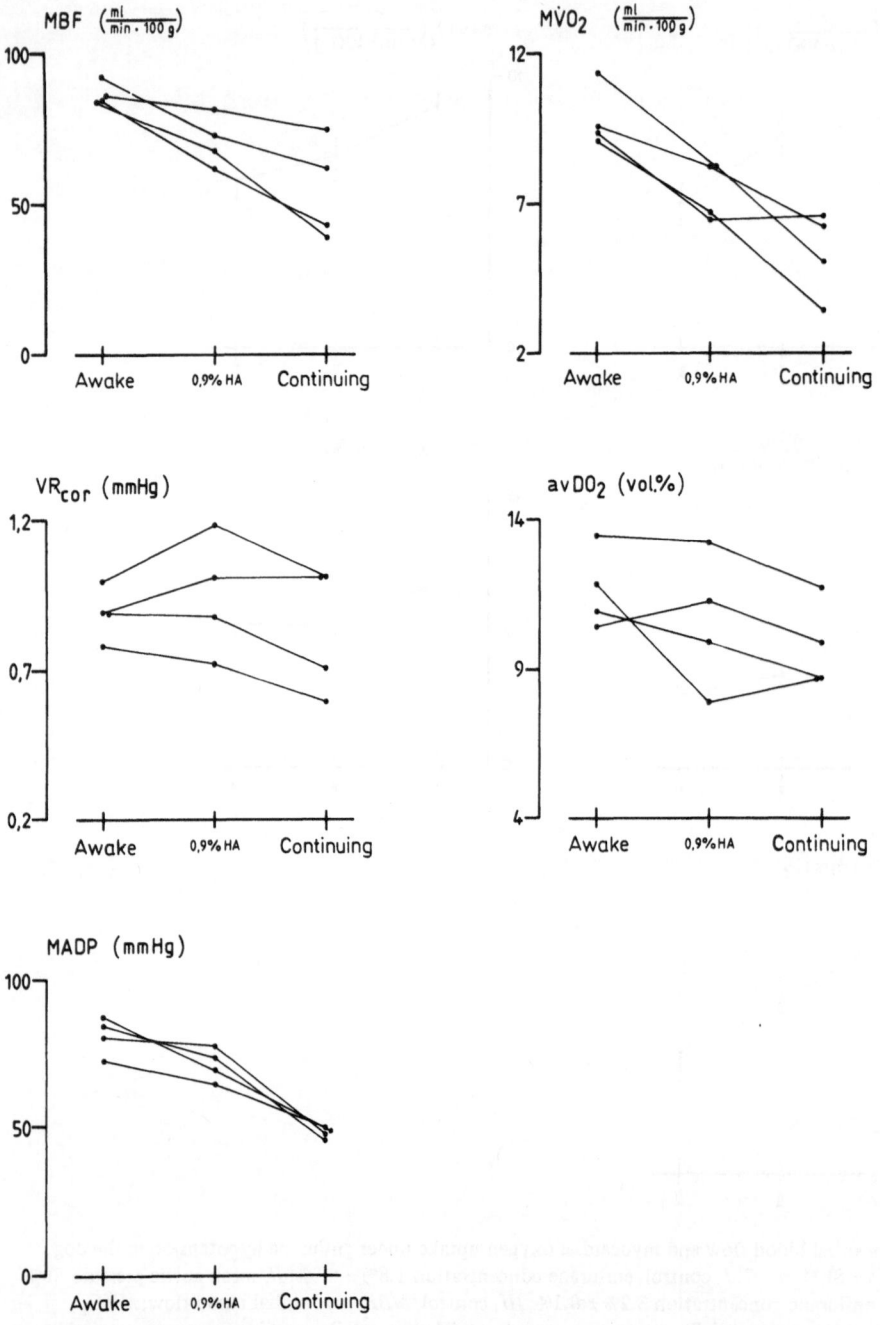

Fig. 5. Myocardial blood flow in man, awake and during halothane hypotension (0.9% and 1.8%). Individual results in four patients. *MBF*, myocardial blood flow; *MVO₂*, myocardial oxygen uptake; *VR_cor*, coronary vascular resistance; *avDO₂*, arteriocoronary venous oxygen content difference; *MADP*, mean aortic diastolic pressure

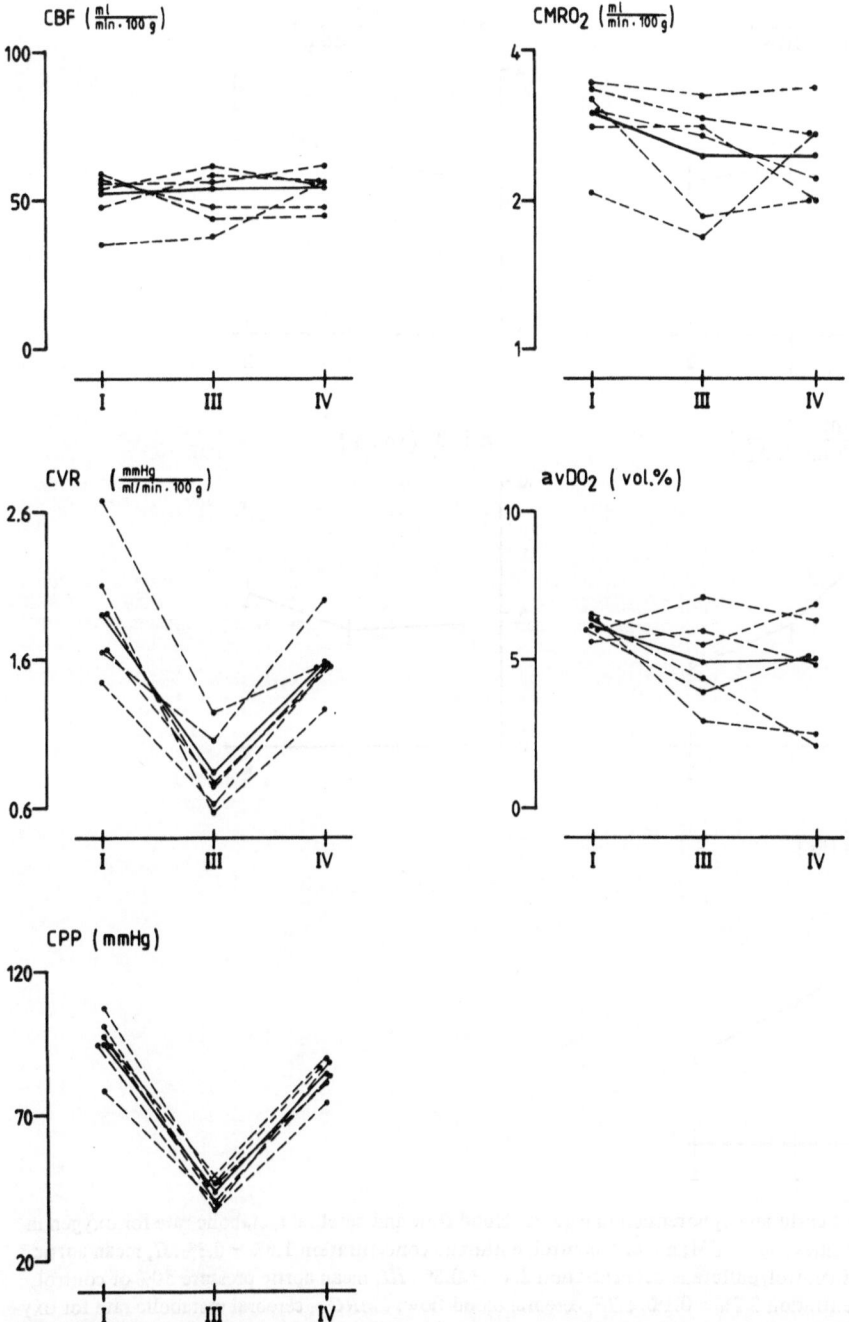

Fig. 6. Effects of halothane hypotension on cerebral blood flow and cerebral metabolic rate for oxygen. Individual results in six dogs before (*I*), during (*III*), and after (*IV*) halothane administration. *CBF*, cerebral blood flow; *CMRO₂*, cerebral metabolic rate for oxygen; *CVR*, cerebral vascular resistance; *avDO₂*, arteriovenous oxygen content difference; *CPP*, cerebral perfusion pressure

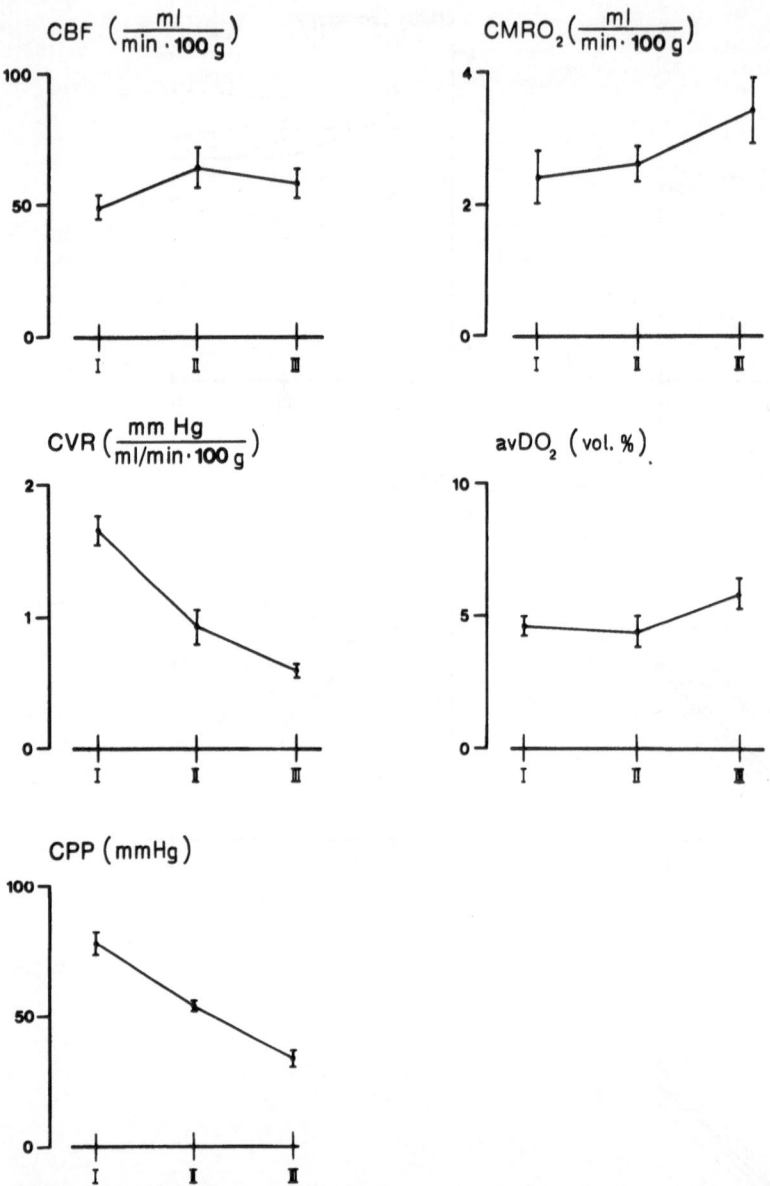

Fig. 7. Effects of enflurane hypotension in cerebral blood flow and cerebral metabolic rate for oxygen in the dog. Mean values and ± SEM; n = 6. *I*, control, enflurane concentration 1.8% ± 0.3%; *II*, mean aortic pressure 25% of control, enflurane concentration 2.4% ± 0.3%; *III*, mean aortic pressure 50% of control, enflurane concentration 3.2% ± 0.1%; *CBF*, cerebral blood flow; *CMRO₂*, cerebral metabolic rate for oxygen; *CVR*, cerebral vascular resistance; *avDO₂*, arteriovenous oxygen content difference; *CPP*, cerebral perfusion pressure

crease in $CMRO_2$ was accompanied by a sharp fall in relative brain oxygen tension from 100 to 52 mmHg measured with a pO_2 tissue microelectrode [4]. Although we did no electroencephalographic studies, seizure activity was likely to occur in some dogs at high inspiratory enflurane concentration.

Vasodilator Hypotension

The effects of sodium nitroprusside (SNP) were investigated by our group in animals and compared with the effects of the inhalation anaesthetics. A similar study in man is continuing.

General Haemodynamics

As one would expect, hypotension was caused by a decrease in peripheral vascular resistance (Fig. 8). Cardiac output rose slightly. There was a considerable increase in heart rate (up to 172 beats/min). Contractility as represented by dp/dt_{max} was unaffected by the counteracting effect of tachycardia to pre-load and after-load reduction.

MBF and $M\dot{V}O_2$ Under SNP Hypotension

Myocardial oxygen uptake remained constant, reflecting two opposing effects: after-load reduction and heart rate increase (Fig. 9). The pattern of O_2 supply changed considerably under SNP. Myocardial blood flow increased from 70 to 160 ml/min/100 g, and arteriocoronary venous O_2 difference decreased from 11 to 6.2 vol.%, pointing to a direct coronary vasodilation.

CBF and $CMRO_2$ Under SNP Hypotension

In the dog we found, despite a drop in perfusion pressure, an increase in CBF from 57 to 75 ml/min/100 g accompanied by a reduction of approximately 50% in the arteriovenous O_2 content difference (Fig. 10). The $CMRO_2$ fell from 3.6 to 2.6 ml O_2/min. The augmentation of CBF was still present when, 30 min after cessation of SNP infusion, arterial pressure was restored to normal values. It appears that SNP directly dilates the cerebral vessels and abolishes cerebral autoregulation. Propranolol administration before SNP hypotension modified this behaviour only in part.

Discussion

In summary, we can state the following when comparing the effects of (a) hypotension induced by inhalation anaesthesia and (b) SNP-induced hypotension: Hypotension by inhalation anaesthetics is achieved by reduction of cardiac output as a result of their negative inotropic action and venous pooling. Despite the fact that a reduction in cardiac output occurs during a short period of hypotension in otherwise healthy patients, oxygen supply to the vital organs, the heart and the brain, is not compromised. These findings are in agreement with the recent report by Thompson et al. [2]. Enflurane in high concentrations may have a sti-

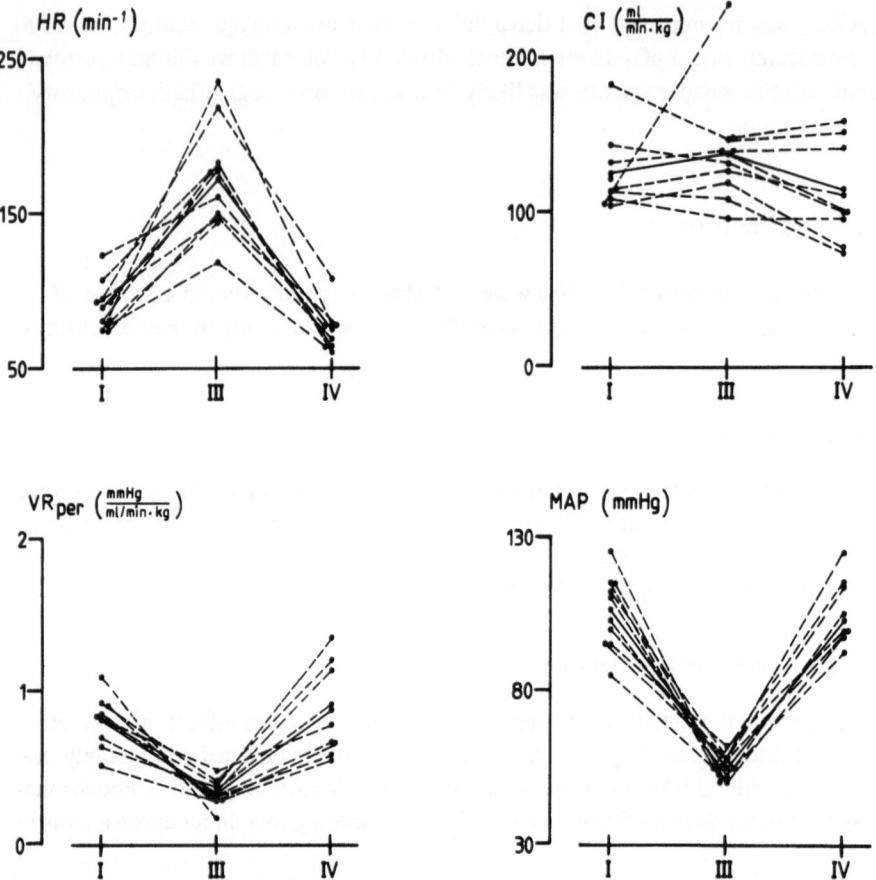

Fig. 8. General haemodynamics and SNP hypotension in the dog (n = 10). Individual results from each animal. (*I*) before, (*III*) during, and (*IV*) after SNP administration. *HR*, heart rate; *CI*, cardiac index; *VR*$_{per}$, peripheral vascular resistance; *MAP*, mean aortic pressure

mulating effect on brain metabolism, probably by inducing seizure activity or leading to inhomogeneous perfusion of the brain with malperfused areas [4].

In contrast, SNP hypotension is created by reduction of peripheral vascular resistance, leaving contractility and cardiac output almost unaffected. Tachycardia is frequently observed and does not allow pressure-dependent diminution of $M\dot{V}O_2$. Despite the fall in perfusion pressure, MBF and CBF increase to values well above the demand perfusion given by $M\dot{V}O_2$ and $CMRO_2$.

The data presented are derived mainly from animal experiments. The validity of the haemodynamic effects of halothane and enflurane reported in animal experiments has been confirmed in man by Sonntag and others [3, 5, 6]. The effects of the inhalation anaesthetics halothane and enflurane on CBF and $CMRO_2$ in our experiments are similar to those reported by other authors in man and animal [7]. High enflurane concentrations (more than 3 vol.%) are also reported to facilitate seizure activity in man [7]. The effects of SNP on vital organ perfusion and oxygen uptake have also been reported by Fan et al. [8] in the dog. These results are practically identical with our findings. Griffiths and co-workers reported no change

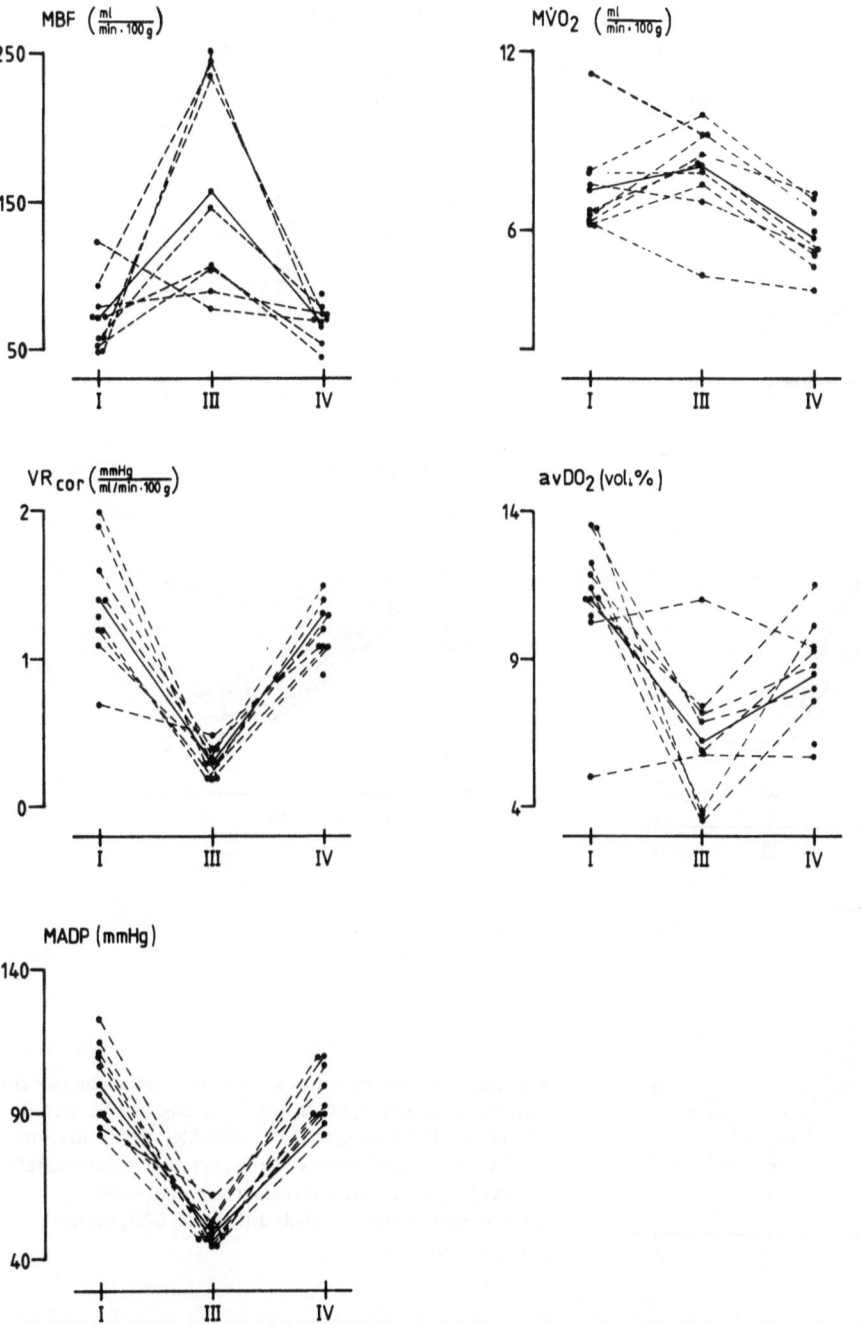

Fig. 9. Myocardial blood flow and myocardial oxygen uptake under SNP hypotension in the dog (n = 10). Individual results from each animal (*I*) before, (*III*) during, and (*IV*) after SNP administration. *MBF*, myocardial blood flow; $M\dot{V}O_2$, myocardial oxygen uptake; VR_{cor}, coronary vascular resistance; $avDO_2$, arteriocoronary venous oxygen content difference; *MADP*, mean aortic diastolic pressure

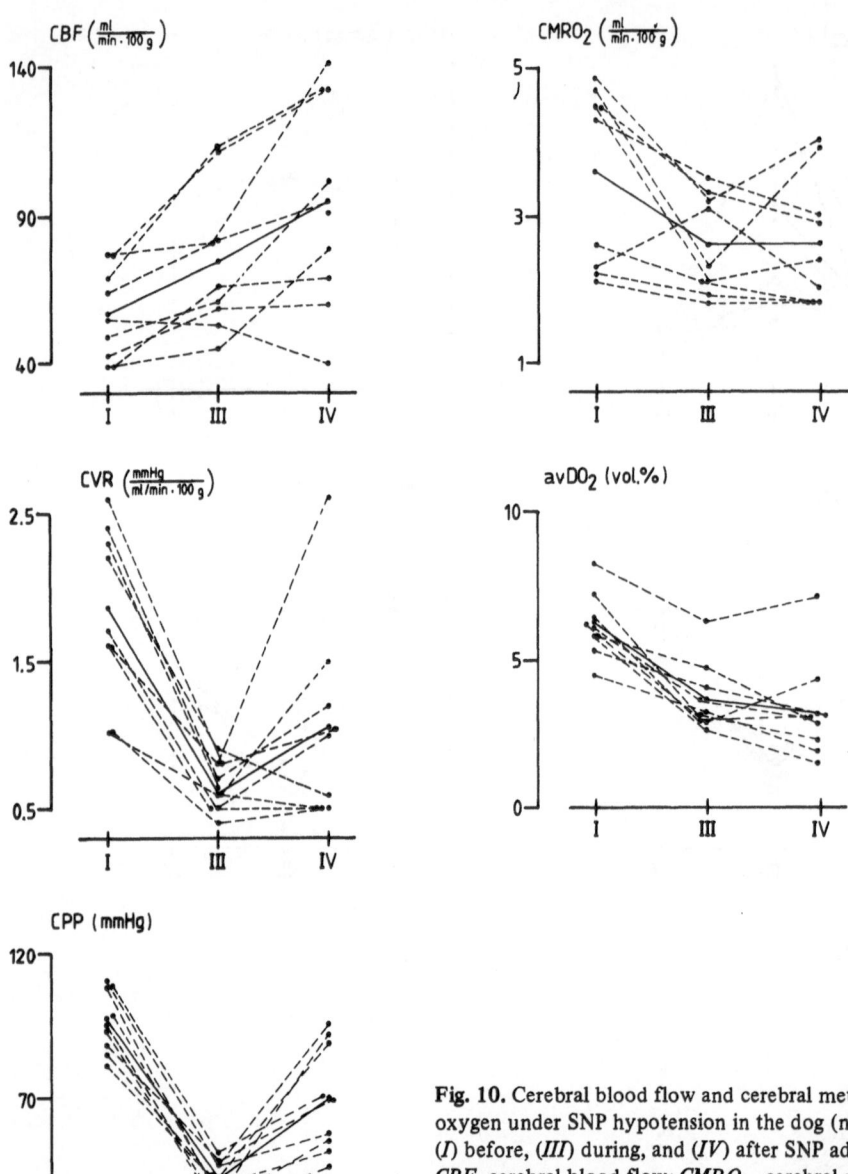

Fig. 10. Cerebral blood flow and cerebral metabolic rate for oxygen under SNP hypotension in the dog (n = 9). Results (*I*) before, (*III*) during, and (*IV*) after SNP administration. *CBF*, cerebral blood flow; $CMRO_2$, cerebral metabolic rate for oxygen; *CVR*, cerebral vascular resistance; $avDO_2$, arteriovenous oxygen content difference; *CPP*, cerebral perfusion pressure

in CBF and $CMRO_2$ under SNP hypotension in man [9]. In our patients (unpublished data) we found great variations in the responses of CBF and $CMRO_2$, depending on the SNP dose requirement. With small doses of SNP we found no changes in CBF and $CMRO_2$, whereas high doses of SNP may lead to an increase of CBF and $CMRO_2$. Reflex tachycardia and the need for high doses of SNP can also be a problem in the patient [10, 11]. Some authors advocate the use of beta-blocking agents [11]; others recommend their combination with inhalation anaesthetics to reduce the SNP dose requirement [10, 11]. Administration of SNP without the smoothing effect of inhalation anaesthesia on blood pressure can produce rebound hypertension on discontinuation of SNP [13]. In the light of our findings and the work of others [2, 10, 12], and despite the rapid development of new and old hypotensive drugs, we think the favourable properties of inhalation anaesthetics should not be forgotten when short and moderate hypotension is desired.

Conclusions

Inhalation anaesthesia can be safely used to induce short periods of moderate hypotension in patients without compromising blood supply to the vital organs. High inspiratory concentrations of enflurane should be avoided. Vasodilators should be added if the desired level of hypotension cannot be reached with inhalation anaesthesia. The addition of beta-blocking agents can limit both the reflex tachycardia and the vasodilator dose. For neurosurgery, in which any increase in brain volume must be avoided, other types of anaesthesia (e.g. barbiturates) may be preferable.

References

1. Gardner WJ (1946) The control of bleeding during operation by induced hypotension. JAMA 132: 572–574
2. Thompson GE, Miller RD, Stevens WC et al. (1978) Hypotensive anaesthesia for total hip arthroplasty: a study of blood loss and organ function (brain, heart, liver, and kidney). Anesthesiology 48:91–96
3. Sonntag H, Donath U, Hillebrand W et al. (1978) Left ventricular function in conscious man and during halothane anesthesia. Anesthesiology 48:320–324
4. Longnecker DE, Radke J, Schenk H-D et al. (1980) Cerebral oxygenation during deliberate hypotension (Abstr). Anesthesiology 53:3S–S91
5. Sonntag H, Merin RG, Donath U et al. (1979) Myocardial metabolism and oxygenation in man awake and during halothane anesthesia. Anesthesiology 51:204–210
6. Calverley RK, Smith NT, Prys-Roberts C et al. (1978) Cardiovascular effects of enflurane anesthesia during controlled ventilation in man. Anaesth Analg (Cleve) 57:619
7. Steen PA, Michenfelder JD (1979) Neurotoxicity of anesthetics. Anesthesiology 50:437–453
8. Fan FG, Kim S, Sunchon S et al. (1980) Effects of sodium nitroprusside on systemic and regional hemodynamics and oxygen utilisation in dog. Anesthesiology 53:113–120
9. Griffiths DPG, Cummins BH, Greenbaum R et al. (1974) Cerebral blood flow and metabolism during hypotension induced with sodium nitroprusside. Br J Anaesth 46:671–679
10. Csondgrady A, Mayr E, Kamp HD et al. (1979) Dosisprobleme mit Natriumnitroprussid bei kontrollierter Hypotension in der Hals-Nasen-Ohrenchirurgie. Anaesthesist 28:564–571
11. Lüben V, Patschke G, Hempelmann G (1978) Hämodynamische Untersuchung der kontrollierten Hypotension mit Natriumnitroprussid unter Betareceptorenblockade (Abstr). Zentral-Europäischer Anaesthesie-Kongreß Innsbruck K79
12. Bedford RF (1978) Increasing halothane concentration reduces nitroprusside dose requirement. Anesth Analg (Cleve) 57:457–462
13. Khambatta HJ, Stone JG, Khan E (1979) Hypertension during anesthesia on discontinuation of sodium nitroprusside induced hypotension. Anesthesiology 51:127–130

Inhalation Anaesthesia in Paediatrics

J.C. Rouge and G. Gemperle

Introduction

Anaesthesia with potent inhalation agents is often accepted as a first choice in paediatric surgery. Since methoxyflurane has disappeared from practice in our clinic, and isoflurane is not commercially available, it seems reasonable to review the effects and some clinical applications of halothane and enflurane in paediatrics. Before discussing the merits and the relative indications and contra-indications of these agents, it is essential to remember that children, and particularly infants, differ sharply from adults. Although the most apparent difference is the size, one should be fully aware that infants, children, and adults also differ in their response to anaesthesia and to drugs.

The uptake of volatile agents is much faster in infants and children than in adults. This difference is apparent with nitrous oxide, halothane, and enflurane. It is believed to be related to differences in the composition of body mass, and in respiratory and circulatory functions [12]. Children have a larger ventilatory volume, a higher cardiac output, and a proportionally larger percentage of highly perfused tissues in relation to their body weight than adults. An increased ventilation will hasten equilibration of the inhaled anaesthetic, and the greater cardiac output will increase total body uptake. As the well-perfused tissues receive a large portion of the cardiac output, anaesthetic equilibration of the inhaled anaesthetic, and the greater cardiac output will increase total body uptake. As the well-perfused tissues receive a large portion of the cardiac output, anaesthetic equilibration occurs sooner in children than in adults. This perfectly explains the clinical impression that induction of and recovery from inhalation anaesthesia are faster in children than in adults. It also explains how the fluctuation of anaesthetic level can be very rapid with both agents. Infants and children require a higher drug concentration to achieve a surgical plane of anaesthesia. The minimal alveolar concentration (MAC) for inhalation agents is highest in infants and declines throughout life [3, 5]. As blood and tissues become saturated more rapidly and as higher concentration of anaesthetic agents are needed to obtain surgical planes of anaesthesia, toxic concentrations of drugs can be reached rapidly, thus narrowing the margin of safety between the stage of surgical anaesthesia and that which may precipitate respiratory arrest or severe hypotension. If one changes rapidly from spontaneous to controlled ventilation without reducing the inhaled concentration, many more molecules of the anaesthetic gas are pushed into the lungs and the circulation. Under these circumstances, cardiovascular collapse can develop within a few minutes. Early recognition of such changes can easily be detected with the use of a precordial stethoscope and by measurement of arterial blood-pressure.

Under clinical use, myocardial depression appears to be less with enflurane than that caused by halothane, but during controlled studies performed under steady state, this is not true. Both halothane and enflurane depress cardiovascular activity, the mean blood-pressure falling in proportion to the depth of anaesthesia. The dynamic response to rapid changes in inspired concentration of these two drugs is, however, considerably different. Smith and co-workers have studied this response in dogs [13]; they demonstrated that a bolus of enflurane depresses arterial pressure twice as much as a bolus of halothane, but much of the difference is probably due to the more rapid action of enflurane, which in turn is due to its lower blood/gas partition coefficient. Using a non-invasive echocardiographic technique to evaluate cardiac function in children, Barrash et al. [1, 2] demonstrated that both halothane and enflurane significantly depress ventricular performance in a dose-related fashion. At equipotent concentration, no significant difference was noted between these two anaesthetics. They emphasize the importance of using atropine when giving these drugs in order to prevent vagal activity. Acute augmentation of heart rate by intravenous atropine results in a significant improvement of cardiac index.

Cardiac arrhythmias are frequently observed during halothane anaesthesia, particularly during operation on the face. The use of epinephrine may not be entirely contra-indicated, but should be limited. In comparison, the incidence of cardiac arrhythmias is significantly less when enflurane is used, with and without exogenous epinephrine [6].

Both enflurane and halothane depress ventilation. With increasing depth of anaesthesia, they decrease tidal volume and increase arterial carbon dioxide tension; there is a direct relation between the MAC multiples and the arterial carbon dioxide tension. There is also a linear inverse relationship between the MAC concentration and the reduction of slope of the ventilatory response to carbon dioxide. With both agents, anaesthesia should be assisted or controlled, particularly in paediatrics.

Muscular tonic-clonic twitching of the face and of the limbs has been observed during deep levels of enflurane anaesthesia and could be induced by hyperventilation [10]. Spike and dome complexes with burst suppression can be terminated readily by lightening the level of anaesthesia and reducing the minute ventilation. These signs were clearly observed during induction and attempt at endotracheal intubation without the use of muscle relaxants. We agree with Rosen and Soderberg that only concentrations of enflurane greater that 3% cause signs of central nervous system excitation in children [11]. Hyperventilation, which is easily caused in children with very compliant chest and lungs, should then be avoided when using enflurane.

Anaesthesia in the Neonate

The newborns who require immediate operation have usually made little or no recovery from birth. Many of these have one or more congenital defects in addition to their presenting illness. Potent inhalation anaesthetics are not without risk in this situation. Studies in premature infants and in newborn animals [7, 8, 9] have demonstrated severe cardiac and circulatory depression when using enflurane or halothane at 1 MAC. In clinical practice, these two agents may be used, but with great caution.

Awake intubation is often performed as a first step. Inspred concentration of the anaesthetic should be increased very progressively, with particular attention paid to heart rate and blood-pressure. Clinical signs of anaesthesia are difficult to assess in neonates, and a systolic blood-pressure lower than 60 mmHg is a strong indication to reduce the inspired concentration. We often prefer the use of a low inspired concentration of enflurane, and to add muscular relaxant and/or analgesic drugs to avoid high anaesthetic concentration, which may interfere with cardiac function. Halothane and enflurane also interfere with the maintenance of normal body temperature. Normothermia is, however, easily achieved by maintaining the temperature of the operating-room as high as the operating team will tolerate, by placing the child on a circulating water mattress, and by heating the inspired gas.

Anaesthesia in Infants and Children

Choice of an anaesthetic technique in infants and children will depend on several factors, such as the age of the patient, his physical and emotional status, the type of surgery to be performed, and the special need of the surgeon. Induction of anaesthesia is a crucial event in both physical and emotional development of the child. Induction should be handled very carefully with much consideration. Psychologically, this should not be traumatic. Inhalation induction is actually very popular, since venipuncture is often difficult in infants, and children fear needles. Some children are easily talked to sleep, with the involvement of some degree of hypnosis. Some require a premedication and rectal methohexital is currently used. Some are very happy with an intravenous injection, providing a vein can be found! If this is not the case, on no account should any child be submitted to numerous venipunctures prior to losing consciousness, and an inhalation induction should then be preferred.

Using a high concentration of nitrous oxide and relatively early introduction of a more potent drug, induction is rapidly performed. Halothane or enflurane is gradually increased every 2–3 breaths. Both agents are usually well accepted by the child. Irritability, as manifested by breath-holding or coughing on induction, is somewhat greater with enflurane than with halothane. To avoid this complication, an airtight mask fit should be maintained, as well as a moderate positive pressure during the entire respiratory cycle. This technique hastens induction and prevents airway obstruction.

Endotracheal intubation can be carried out under general anaesthesia alone, but adequate plane of anaesthesia is sometimes difficult to achieve. Yakaitis et al. have shown that the end-tidal concentration for endotracheal intubation in children is 30% greater than MAC for both halothane and enflurane [14, 15]. With both agents, a too-early attempt may induce severe anoxic obstruction with laryngospasm. A too-late attempt may result in complications: with halothane, one comes close to overdosage, with bradycardia and hypotension; with enflurane, bradycardia is not observed, but one comes close to a level known to produce signs of central nervous system excitation. With both agents, endotracheal intubation should be performed with the aid of a muscular relaxant.

Minor surgical precedures are performed in about 50% of all children. Most of these could be done on an outpatient basis. At the Geneva Children's Hospital, this practice represents 25%–30% of our everyday work. This attitude has several advantages for the child, but should not increase the risk of the procedure. When performed under general anaesthesia, this type of surgery should have a predictable post-operative course and the inhalation technique has increasing popularity. Simple anaesthetic techniques are preferred and inhalation agents are more commonly used. With enflurane, it is sometimes difficult to prevent reflex movements in response to surgery. Supplementation with a short-acting analgesic such as fentanyl, given either intramuscularly during induction or intravenously, will avoid this type of reaction.

For more extensive surgical procedures our actual trend is to use several drugs instead of one to achieve anaesthesia. Midazolam, a new water-soluble benzodiazepine, is actually under clinical investigation in our service. This drug appears to potentiate the effects of inhalation agents and of analgesic drugs. As shown by Melvin et al., Midazolam slightly decreases MAC for halothane in a dose-related fashion [4]. Used in paediatrics, Midazolam associated with an analgesic drug decreases the need for high concentrations of enflurane. Such a technique is used for surgical procedures of 1—3 h duration. When this technique is used for plastic surgery on the face, particularly for cleft lip and cleft palate repair, recovery begins usually 15 min after stopping the administration of enflurane. Awakening is quiet, with minimal respiratory depression and no airway obstruction. For procedures of longer duration, flunitrazepam is used in place of midazolam and appears to have the same properties on the MAC of inhalation agents.

Children undergoing neurosurgical procedure are often under 1 year of age. Some of them have elevated intracranial pressure pre-operatively. Extensive studies of neurophysiology and neuropharmacology in animals and in adults have established rules that may be applied to children. In patients with pre-operatively normal intracranial pressure, the use of an inhalation anaesthetic is permissible. In infants, in whom veins are difficult to find, induction with nitrous oxide and inhalation agents is acceptable. Patients with no elevation of intracranial pressure prior to induction need special consideration, since any straining is to be avoided. The use of thiopental or of methohexital by rectum is particularly advantageous; induction is subsequently continued with nitrous oxide, halothane, or enflurane by mask. Hyperventilation prior to the introduction of inhalation agents has been shown to improve intracranial compliance and attenuate the increase of intracranial pressure produced by halothane and enflurane. In children, hyperventilation prior to the use of these agents is, however, extremely difficult to manage correctly. In the presence of significant elevation of intracranial pressure, we then prefer the use of a nitrous oxide relaxant technique with analgesic drugs.

Choice of anaesthetic agents for paediatric cardiac surgery is mostly influenced by the pathophysiology of the cardiac defect. In patients with left-to-right shunt, anaesthesia is induced with inhalation techniques or intravenously. In patients with right-to-left shunt, however, inhalation agents lead to a slow induction; minor periods of excitement can trigger anoxic spells. Any reduction of left ventricular function or decrease in peripheral resistance will cause the right-to-left shunt to increase, thus worsening the hypoxaemia. Inhalation induction should then be avoided.

Anaesthesia is maintained using nitrous oxide, oxygen, and enflurane in low concentrations. At least 50% of nitrous oxide is required to provide analgesia, and there is a relative contra-indication to its use in patients with hypoxaemia. For extracardiac palliative operations in cyanotic patients, we frequently use oxygen and low concentrations of enflurane to achieve anaesthesia. This technique is supplemented with fentanyl and pancuronium. Prompt awakening is expected, and extubation usually performed in the operating-room.

For infants in whom profound hypothermia with circulatory arrest is intended, the pre-bypass period includes surface cooling to 30 °C. The use of enflurane during cooling has considerably shortened the time required to reach the desired temperature, without producing marked depression of cardiac function. We never observed cardiac arrhythmias, even in strongly digitalized infants.

Conclusion

Today anaesthesia with inhalation agents is still the technique of choice for minor surgical precedures in infants and children. This technique will probably remain the same tomorrow. For major surgical procedures, however, our actual trend is to use several drugs instead of one. Short- and long-acting benzodiazepines supplemented with nitrous oxide and short-acting analgesics are used today, sometimes with inhalation agents. It may be that such a technique could replace inhalation agents tomorrow.

References

1. Barash PG, Glanz S, Katz JE et al. (1978) Ventricular function in children during halothane anesthesia; an echocardiographic evaluation. Anesthesiology 49:79
2. Barash PG, Katz JD, Firestone S et al. (1979) Cardiovascular performance in children during induction: an echocardiographic comparison of enflurane and halothane (Abstr). Anesthesiology 51:315
3. Gregory GA, Eger EI, Munson ES (1969) The relationship between age and halothane requirement in man. Anesthesiology 30:348
4. Melvin MA, Johnson BH, Quashe AL, Eger EI (1980) Induction of anesthesia with Midazolam decreases halothane MAC in man (Abstr). Anesthesiology 53:10
5. Nicodemus HF, Nassiri-Rahimi C, Bachman L, Smith TC (1969) Median effective doses (ED$_{50}$) of halothane in adults and children. Anesthesiology 31:344
6. Reisner LS, Lippman M (1975) Ventricular arrhythmias after epinephrine injection in enflurane and in halothane anesthesia. Curr Res Anesth Analg 54:468
7. Robinson S, Gregory GA (1980) Circulatory effects of anesthesia in the developing sheep. I halothane (Abstr). Anesthesiology 53:330
8. Robinson S, Gregory GA (1980) Circulatory effects of anesthesia in the developing sheep. II enflurane (Abstr). Anesthesiology 53:331
9. Robinson S, Gregory GA (1980) Fentanyl-air oxygen anesthesia for patient ductus arteriosus ligation in infants less than 1500 gr. Curr Res Anesth Analg 59:557
10. Rouge JC, Hemmer M, Gemperle G (1974) Enflurane (Ethrane) in pediatric anesthesia. Acta Anaesthesiol Belg 25:223
11. Rosen I, Soderber M (1975) Electroencephalographic activity in children under enflurane anesthesia. Acta Anaesth Scand 19:361
12. Salanitre E, Rackow H (1969) The pulmonary exchange of nitrous oxide and halothane in infants and children. Anesthesiology 30:388
13. Smith NT, Rampil IJ, Sasse FJ et al. (1980) The dynamic pressure response to enflurane and halothane (Abstr). Anesthesiology 53:37
14. Yakaitis RW, Blitt CD, Angiulo JP (1977) End tidal halothane concentration for endotracheal intubation. Anesthesiology 47:386
15. Yakaitis RW, Blitt CD, Angiulo JP (1979) End tidal enflurane concentration for endotracheal intubation. Anesthesiology 50:59

Inhalation Anaesthesia in Geriatric Patients

G. Haldemann

Introduction

It is a world-wide phenomenon that the proportion of young people is progressively decreasing, and the intermediate age group of working people remains virtually unchanged, while the number of persons over 65 years of age continues to increase. According to the Federal Bureau of Social Insurance, it may be expected that by the year 2000 there will be more than one million persons over the age of 65 in Switzerland, in a total population of somewhat over 5 million.

In 1980, of a total of 11 000 anaesthetics at the Cantonal Hospital, Aarau, 30% of the patients were assigned to risk categories III–V. Of these patients 70% were over 65 years of age. The anaesthetic risk was determined with the aid of the checklist of Lutz et al. [13], which permits a more precise evaluation than the ASA method because of a point system allowing for factors such as pre-operative preparation, operative time, and type of procedure, as well as the patient's physical status.

Intra-operatively, anaesthetic risk in the elderly is determined by the cardiovascular reserve. Post-operatively, on the other hand, morbidity and mortality are influenced primarily by pulmonary and thrombo-embolic complications. It follows that during anaesthesia the best feasible monitoring of the heart and circulation should be sought, though this should be as non-invasive as possible, in the interests of broad applicability. The question may be raised to what extent monitoring the systolic time interval (STI) complies with these prerequisites. Furthermore, it should be determined what general measures are possible in order to achieve pre-anaesthetic improvement of cardiovascular performance in these elderly patients. The importance of guaranteed normovolaemia has been pointed out on many occasions, since elderly persons show significant immobilizational hypovolaemia even after short periods of confinement to bed, and this leads to extreme sensitivity to anaesthetic agents.

Methods

The effects of halothane, enflurane, and neurolept anaesthesia on STI were measured using the Myocard Check 970 of List [11]. Various newer induction agents were tested using the same method. The measurements were performed on patients between 65 and 95 years of age who required anaesthesia and intubation for lesser surgical procedures. Patients with manifest cardiac failure, coronary sclerosis, hypertension and renal insufficiency, anaemia, and electrolyte disturbances were excluded from the study. In order to determine the STI, it was necessary to monitor the electrocardiogram (ECG), the phonocardiogram, and the carotid pulse wave. The Q wave on the ECG represents the beginning of electromechanical systole, the second heart tone the closure of the aortic valve and hence the end of this phase (Q–S_2).

The left ventricular ejection time (LVET) is the interval from the beginning of the steep rise to the dicrotic notch in the carotid pulse curve. The pre-ejection period (PEP) is obtained when the ejection time is subtracted from the total electromechanical systole: PEP = ($Q - S_2$) – LVET (Fig. 1). In the computer employed (Fig. 2), a microprocessor selects the impulses; arrhythmias and beats which deviate greatly from the mean are discarded. The average STIs are the means of ten artefact-free signals after the two extremes of 12 accumulated cardiac cycles have been discarded [14]. From (Q–S_2) and LVET, the computer calculates PEP and $1/(PEP)^2$ or the pulse wave velocity, the electromechanical diastole (S_2–Q), and the Weissler coefficient Q [20]. The latter is probably the most suitable single parameter for the bloodless determination of myocardial function. It is independent of sex and is applicable to a range of rates from 40 to 120 per min. Good correlations have been found for the various

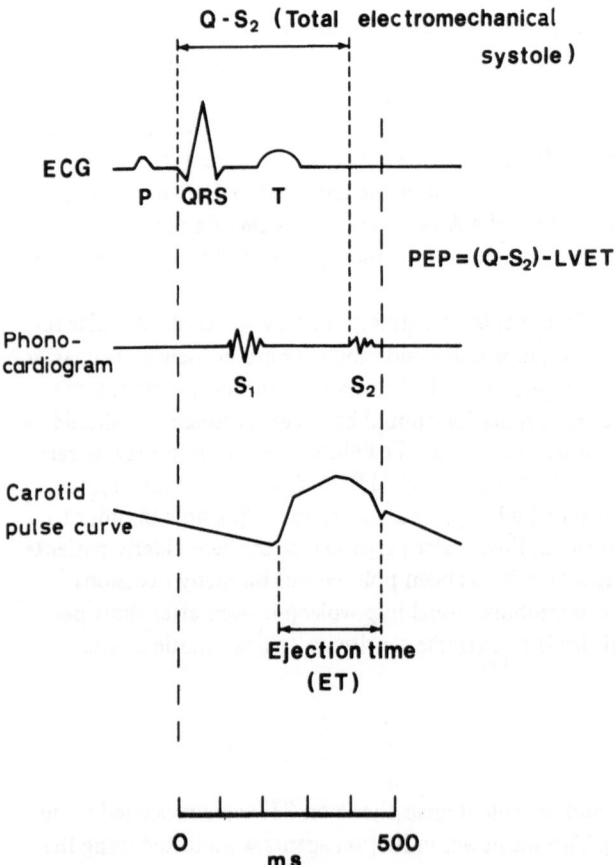

Fig. 1. Measurement of the systolic time interval using electrocardiogram (*ECG*), phonocardiogram, and carotid pulse curve. *Q–S₂*, total electromechanical systole; *LVET* (left ventricular ejection time), from the beginning of the steep rise to the notch in the carotid pulse curve; *PEP* (pre-ejection period), (Q–S₂) – LVET

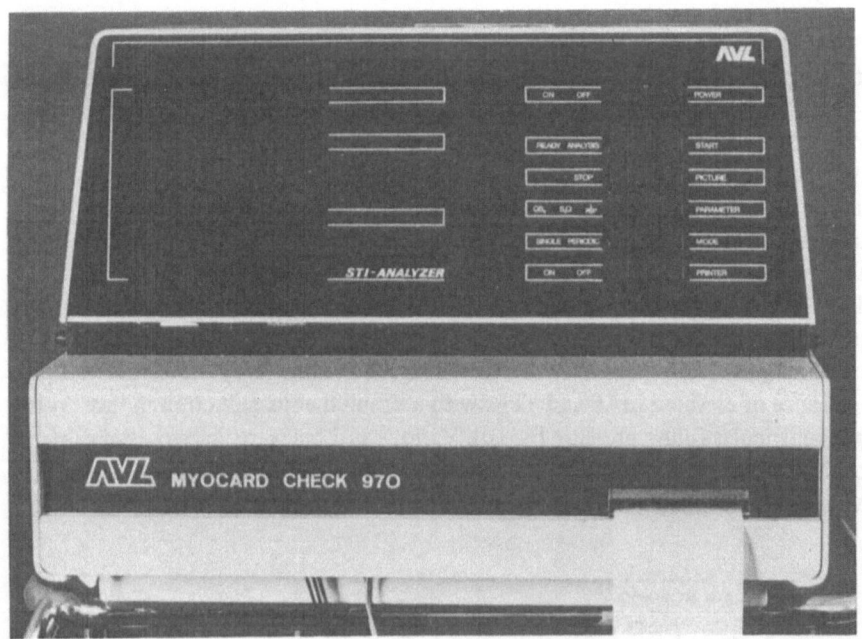

Fig. 2. Myocard Check 970 of List [11]. Analytical computer for systolic time intervals from the AVL Co., Schaffhausen, Switzerland

non-invasively measured parameters of STI, particularly the Q, and the myocardial function values measured by intravascular methods [1, 7, 15, 20].

The effects of 3% dextran/Ringer lactate and 6% HES on blood volume (BV) and plasma volume (PV) were determined in the same patient population by the Volemetron technique (Ames Corp., Elkhardt. USA) [18] using radioiodine human serum albumin (RISHA). Ready-to-use 2-ml injections each containing 10 mg human serum albumin with a specific activity of 0.5 μCi/mg albumin were used. Regular checks with test sets and in vitro dilutional studies were carried out to ensure correct functioning of the Volemetron.

Serum protein levels were determined by means of the biuret reaction, as modified by Appel et al. [2] to prevent dextran-induced turbidity. The protein fractions were identified by cellulose acetate electrophoresis. The total circulating albumin (TPA) is the product of PV and albumin concentration. The serum dextran and HES concentrations were determined using the anthron method of Roe [17]. The haematocrit (Hct) was measured in both pre-mix and post-mix samples from the central venous catheter. Colloid osmotic pressure (COP) was measured using the Weil et al. oncometer [19].

The mean ($\bar{x}$), the standard error of the mean (SEM), and the variance (V) were determined for all measured and calculated values. In addition, the Z test [16] was used to detect significant differences from the control values and among the means of the various groups.

Results

The relevant changes in STI during halothane, enflurane, and neurolept anaesthesia pre-operatively, 15–30 min after intubation, and intra-operatively (at the earliest 10 min after incision) in normoventilated patients on 1:1 N_2O/O_2 are shown in Fig. 3. Q-prolongation, at
+17.9% ± 2.9% for halothane, 22.1% ± 3.0% for NLA, and 23.8% ± 2.7% for enflurane, lay
within the same order of magnitude for all three techniques pre-operatively. The reduction
in myocardial function remained essentially the same intra-operatively. After the incision, on
the other hand, an increase in total peripheral resistance (TPR) caused the mean arterial
pressures (MAP) to increase to their initial values. Thus, no differences in effect on the STI
could be found among the three techniques.

A typical finding in elderly patients is decreased stroke volume (SV) and cardiac output
(CO) in the presence of elevated MAP and TPR, with a simultaneous reduction in heart rate
(HR) and right ventricular filling pressure [8, 10]. Various authors were able to diminish
markedly the circulatory depression from the inhalation anaesthetics by adequate direct pre-
anaesthetic volume replacement. Thus, using enflurane in geriatric patients, we could not de-

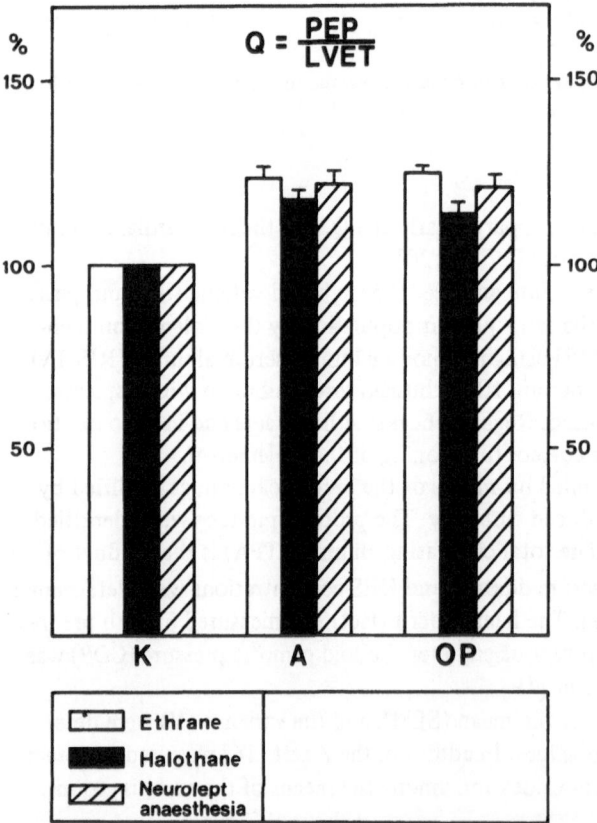

Fig. 3. Relative changes in pre-ejection period/left ventricular ejection time (PEP/LVET) quotient in geriatric patients. *K*, control value in conscious patient; *A*, anaesthesia prior to surgery; *OP*, anaesthesia during
surgery. Mean ± SEM; n = 8 in each group

tect any significant reduction in CO and SV after the administration of 15 ml/kg body wt. 1.8% dextran-70 solution in Ringer lactate. When no fluid load was administered, the CO decreased by 37% ± 5% and the SV by 35% ± 7% [9]. The rapid administration of this volume led to increases in MAP of 5.6% ± 2.1%, in CO of 10% ± 3.6%, and in SV of 14.8% ± 4.9%, and decreases in HR of 5% ± 3.6%, TPR 12% ± 4.6%, and Hct 5.2% ± 1.3% with a rise of 6.5 ± 1.4 cmH$_2$O in right ventricular filling pressure (CVP). Helms et al. [10] found an average increase in pulmonary capillary pressure (PCP) of 10 mmHg, to 15.5 ± 3 mmHg, after a similar dextran load and infusion rate in the same type of patients. We have recently begun using a 3% dextran/Ringer lactate solution for the pre-anaesthetic volume load, or 6% HES solution if the effect of dextran on coagulation is not desired. As seen in Fig. 4, the volume effect 10

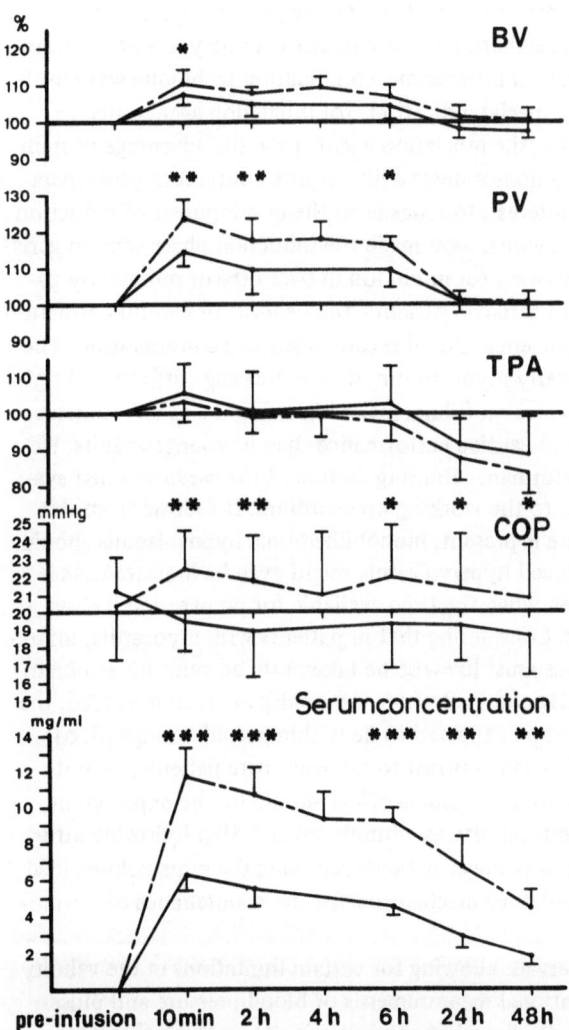

Fig. 4. Effects of 800 ml 3% dextran-70/Ringer lactate (– – –) and 800 ml 6% HES (–·–) on blood volume (*BV*), plasma volume (*PV*), total plasma albumin (*TPA*), colloid osmotic pressure (*COP*), and serum concentration in elderly patients. Serum concentration and COP are indicated in mmHg or mg/ml. Mean ± SD; n = 8 in each group. * p < 0.05; ** p < 0.01; *** p < 0.001

min after infusion of 15 ml/kg of HES, with a 123.5% ± 5.2% increase over the initial values, was significantly greater than that of 3% dextran (+ 114.8% ± 3.9%), particularly for the PV. The BV and PV remained significantly above the control values for up to 6 h after the plasma substitutes were infused. The COP increased slightly after HES, but fell continuously after dextran. Although the Hct decreased from an average of 43% to 37% after the infusions, the values never fell below the critical limit for adequate oxygen transport advocated by Lundsgaard-Hansen [12]. The TPA lay significantly below the initial values 24 h, and even more 48 h, after the administration of both plasma expanders.

Discussions

Inhalation anaesthetics cannot be considered unimportant for the geriatric age-group. In 1980, for example, 70% of all general anaesthetics in our patients over 65 years of age were performed using halothane and enflurane; an intravenous combination technique was employed in only 25% of cases. Aside from special indications for inhalation agents such as out-patient surgery, short procedures, etc., the inhalation agents have the advantage of minimal respiratory after-effects, so that they do not necessarily require continuous post-operative supervision in a recovery-room. Of interest, too, has been the development of induction agents with negligible circulatory effects, which have made the induction phase safer in geriatric risk patients. In 1980, etomidate was used for induction in over 60% of our elderly patients. When inhalation agents are used in geriatric patients, the benefits of careful correction of the common immobilizational hypovolaemia should receive adequate consideration. The pathological-anatomic changes in the elderly myocardium, with increasing stiffness and rigidity and with the stroke volume dependence on filling, make higher right and left ventricular filling pressures necessary for increased cardiac performance than in younger adults. We agree with Helms et al. [10] that the performance-limiting factors of the cardiovascular system in elderly persons are often external to the working myocardium. It follows from this that when no indication of cardiac failure is present, immobilizational hypovolaemia should at the least be corrected; short-term induced hypervolaemia might even be indicated. As is apparent from Fig. 4, this is possible even when the time available for preparation is short, thanks to the modern plasma expanders. Considering that in patients with myocardial infarctions whose increased ventricular stiffness must likewise be taken into account for circulatory stabilization, CVP values of 6—8 mmHg and PCP of 16—18 mmHg are recommended, the optimal values for geriatric patients might be expected to lie within a similar range [3, 6]. Since the majority of these elderly patients, in contrast to intensive care patients, do not have diminished protein reserves, an insufficient volume effect should not be expected in this patient population [4, 5]. The fall in total plasma albumin 24 and 48 h following infusion is on the same general order as that in younger patients receiving the same volume load, and should be regarded as one of the regulatory mechanisms for the maintenance of normovolaemia.

The monitoring of systolic time intervals, allowing for certain limitations in the validity of the method, complements the conventional measurements of blood-pressure and pulse-rate in patients at risk. The problem for its clinical applicability is not so much the data processing, which is made rapid and reliable by the computer, but rather the registering of the impulses, particularly adequate recording of the carotid pulse curve. Progress has been made in a practical sense by amplification of the pulse curve, which simplifies localization of the ideal cut-off point, adjustment of the input voltage, with the possibility of using intra-arterial pressure instead of the pulse curve, and devising a test program which facilitates the rapid identification of causes of artefacts.

The haemodynamic effects of both enflurane and halothane in geriatric patients differ only slightly from those in younger patients when the decreased anaesthetic requirement is allowed for and normovolaemia is ensured. As in the other age-groups, the advantages of enflurane are its low rate of biotransformation and excellent regulability.

The expired wastes of volatile anaesthetics do, indeed, represent a problem for chronically exposed operating-room personnel. That we are not powerless to prevent the contamination of our working areas was demonstrated in a study performed by the Department of Industrial Medicine of the Federal Bureau of Industry, Business and Labor at our hospital in 1978. The anaesthetic concentrations in the operating-rooms of the old buildings differed substantially from those in the newly constructed operating suite with 4- to 6-fold air exchange and efficient extraction of the anaesthetic gases. The average levels of N_2O were 142–239 ppm as compared with 2–8 ppm and for halothane 12–22 ppm versus 1–3 ppm. This shows that it is technically possible to continue offering patients the advantages of inhalation anaesthetics without having to accept excessive contamination of the working area.

Summary

The effects of halothane, enflurane, and neurolept anaesthesia on the quotient pre-ejection period/ejection time = Q in geriatric patients were studied for the purpose of evaluating the systolic time interval as a supplement to conventional methods of haemodynamic monitoring. Halothane exerted the smallest influence on this non-invasive parameter of myocardial function, but the difference was not significant in comparison with the other techniques.

In geriatric patients, the negative effects of anaesthetic agents may be substantially diminished by correction of the immobilizational hypovolaemia which is frequently present, and by adjusting the right and left ventricular filling pressures to conform with the altered dynamics of the aging myocardium. Colloidal plasma expanders such as dilute dextran and HES solutions are suitable for this purpose.

It may be assumed that inhalation anaesthetics will continue to hold their own thanks to their particular advantages: controllability, minimal post-operative respiratory effects, etc. When the pathophysiological organ changes associated with aging are allowed for, the negative cardiovascular effects can be kept within limits. In addition, the development of haemodynamically indifferent induction agents has made the induction phase safer in patients at risk.

References

1. Ahmed SS, Levinson GE, Schwartz CJ, Ettinger PO (1972) Systolic time intervals as measures of the contractile state of the left ventricular myocardium in man. Circulation 46:559
2. Appel W, Wirmer V, Ebenezer S (1968) Beeinflussung klinisch-chemischer Untersuchungen durch Dextran. Anaesthesist 17:95
3. Crexells C, Chatterjee K, Forrester JS, Dikshit K, Swan HJC (1971) Optimal level of filling pressure in the left side of the heart in acute myocardial infarction. N Engl J Med 285:190

4. Draxler V, Wagner H, Zekert F, Sporn P, Watzek C, Steinbereithner K (1975) Studies on a modified dextran-Ringer's-lactate mixture in intensive care patients. Eur J Intens Care Med 1:43
5. Draxler V, Sporn P, Steinbereithner K, Wagner M, Walzer R (1979) Einfluss einer 3,6%igen Dextran-Ringer-Azetatlösung auf mässig hypovolämische Intensivpatienten. Infusionstherapie 6:162
6. Forrester JS, Diamond G, McHugh TJ, Swan HJC (1971) Filling pressures in the right and left sides of the heart in acute myocardial infarction. N Engl J Med 285:190
7. Garrard CL, Weissler AM, Dodge HT (1970) The relationship of alterations in systolic time intervals to ejection fraction in patients with cardiac disease. Circulation 42:455
8. Granath A, Jonsson B, Strandell T (1961) Studies on the central circulation at rest and during exercise in the supine and sitting body position in old men. Acta Med Scand 169:125
9. Haldemann G, Wüst HP, Hossli G, Schaer H (1976) Die Auswirkungen einer Volumenrestitution mit Dextran-Ringerlaktat auf den kreislaufdepressorischen Effekt von Ethrane bei geriatrischen Patienten. Anaesthesist 25:522
10. Helms U, Weihrauch H, Jacobitz K (1978) Auswirkungen der raschen Volumensubstitution auf hämodynamische Parameter bei geriatrischen Patienten. Anaesthesist 27:298
11. List WF (1978) Monitoring of myocardial function with systolic time intervals. Acta Anaesthesiol Belg 29:271
12. Lundsgaard-Hansen P (1979) Component therapy of surgical haemorrhage: red cell concentrates, colloids and crystalloids. Symposium über Chirurgische Haemotherapie, Bern, 28.–30. Aug 1979
13. Lutz H, Klose R, Peter K (1976) Die Problematik der praeoperativen Risikoeinstufung. Anaesth Info 7:342
14. Marsoner HJ, Savora G, Moser W, List WF (1980) An instrument for the on-line determination of systolic time intervals. In: List WF, Gravenstein JS, Spodick DH (eds) Systolic time intervals. Vol 110. Springer, Berlin Heidelberg New York, pp
15. Reitan JA, Smith NT, Kadis LB (1969) The correlations between cardiac pre-ejection period and ascending blood flow acceleration (Abstr) ASA meeting, San Francisco, 1969, Abstract No. 13
16. Riedwyl H (1978) Angewandte mathematische Statistik in Wissenschaft, Administration und Technik. Haupt, Bern Stuttgart
17. Roe JH (1954) The determination of dextran in blood and urine with anthrone reagent. J Biol Chem 208:889
18. Siewert R (1968) Messmethoden und klinische Bedeutung des Blutvolumens. Méd Lab (Stuttg) 21:1
19. Weil MH, Henning RJ, Morisette M, Michaelis S (1978) Relationship between colloid osmotic pressure and pulmonary artery wedge pressure in patients with acute cardiorespiratory failure. Am J Med 64:643
20. Weissler AM, Harris WS, Schoenfeld CD (1969) Bedside technics for the evaluation of ventricular function in man. Am J Cardiol 23:577

Balanced Anaesthesia as an Alternative Concept

O. Norlander

Introduction

While most anaesthetic procedures today involve some kind of "balance" between several agents, in this paper I have aimed to present some personal opinious about current methods of anaesthesia involving such combinations as intravenous anaesthetics plus nitrous oxide and conduction blocks plus inhalational anaesthesia.

The intriguing aspect of the discussion of the advantages and disadvantages of different anaesthetic methods is that we do not really know very much about the possible harm caused by, for example, changes in endocrine metabolic response or certain changes in sympathetic stimulation. It is logical to assume that abnormal changes evoked by anaesthesia and surgery are potentially hazardous, but positive proof is lacking in most cases. What is the importance of anaesthesia in relation to surgery? There are certain risk patients in whom we may anticipate rather dangerous side-effects, e.g. sympathetic stimulation during anaesthesia and surgery, as well as the stress responses.

Definitions

The concept of balanced anaesthesia was introduced by Lundy in 1926 [8]. Balanced anaesthesia was a method of providing pain relief and establishing conditions suitable for surgery adequate. It involved combining premedication and local anaesthesia, conduction block and agents to provide attional analgesia and sedation, and differed from other methods in which only one anaesthetic agent, e.g. ether or chloroform, was used. The aim of the method, shown to have been achieved by later experience, was to create greater safety for the patient, both during the procedure and post-operatively. Although Lundy popularized this technique, making it well known to many anaesthesiologists, it had already been advocated by the famous surgeon George Crile (1900–1911). Crile's [1] defined anaesthesia as "anoci-association" on the basis of a series of clinical observations in patients who had not received wht he called toxic concentrations of the most common inhalational agents, ether or chloroform. Crile observed that unpleasant auditory, olfactory, and visual sensations could be abolished with low-dose concentrations of inhalation anaesthetics, but that this was not the case with surgically evoked pain. For this he used local anaesthesia and blocks. Crile therefore recommended the use of combinations of drugs to achieve what he reported as *anoci-association, and to prevent all efferent reflexes to the brain.* The techniques and methods of Crile and Lundy were later generally accepted, and with newer, more effective anaesthetic agents and other drugs, e.g. cyclopropane and thipentone, the method could be further developed. The term "combined" anaesthesia is now generally used in preference to "balanced" anaesthesia [7]; it is basically the same method as that advocated by Crile and Lundy, but with more modern agents, and especially muscle relaxants.

Neurolept Analgesia and Neurolept Anaesthesia

Neurolept analgesia and neurolept anaesthesia were launched as new concepts and techniques by de Castro and Mundeler in 1959 [2]. The original method of neurolept analgesia has been replaced by the technique of neurolept anaesthesia, which is an integration of hypnotics, analgesics, and relaxants supplemented by nitrous oxide. The neurolept technique is often talked about as a "new" method, but is in fact a further development of the techniques of Laborit and Huguenard from 1954 [6]. The neurolept effect is achieved by a number of potent drugs of which droperidol is the best known, and is supposed to relax and calm the patient. It also has certain alpha-receptor-blocking properties and is a powerful anti-emetic drug. However, quite a few patients experience various degrees of anxiety, fright, and unpleasant sensations in spite of what seems to be calm behaviour to the observing physician. The drug is therefore not as harmless as is generally stated. In clinical practice there are many variations of neurolept anaesthesia and it is not always quite clear what precisely the terms neurolept anaesthesia and analgesia mean. One problem with the method is the rather large variation in the dose-response to the most commonly used analgesic, fentanyl, and the neurolept component. This has resulted in techniques involving repeated dosage of fentanyl during the operation without exact knowledge about the threshold of pain, or, in certain situations, awareness, due to insufficient neurolept and hypnotic effects during the intervention. It has also been observed in several investigations that sympathetic stimulation is usually persistent during neurolept anaesthesia even when dosage of fentanyl is sufficient to abolish pain as such. In the light of new information we know that very high dosage of fentanyl is necessary in order to avoid vegetative reactions. Stress-free response during fentanyl anaesthesia necessitates high dosages — 50 μg/kg body wt. has recently been reported [4]. Stanley [11] found in coronary patients that unresponsiveness was achieved at 25 μg/kg body wt. and at 13 μg/kg body wt. in patients with septic shock [12]. Such doses are higher than those used in general anaesthesia and usually require either prolonged post-operative ventilation, or the use of naloxone with its own risk of sympathetic stimulation involving increase of metabolism and secondary effects on the circulation.

It is obvious that our methods for providing safe anaesthesia still have to be improved and that neurolept anaesthesia is no general solution to an anaesthetic problem. This has led us to re-examine the current widespread use of neurolept techniques, and we are reverting increasingly to the old balanced anaesthesia techniques according to Crile and Lundy. This means that we are trying to combine the advantages of the strong narcotic type drugs such as fentanyl, supplementing them with low fractions of inhalation anaesthesia using nitrous oxide/oxygen. In suitable patients we use complementary conduction blocks, especially epidural, to relatively high levels.

Rationale Behind Combining Narcotic-Type Drugs with Inhalation Anaesthesia

The advantages of intravenous drugs include rapid action and ease of administration, which make them extremely useful for induction. Combination of an intravenous barbiturate with a reasonable loading dose of a narcotic such as fentanyl, oral spraying of the cords, and, if necessary, low-dose enfluran in oxygen makes intubation a non-stimulatory procedure in most patients, without extreme side-effects due to sympathetic stimulation (tachycardia, increased blood pressure). The anaesthesia is then continued with efrane and nitrous oxide in MAC concentrations and supplemented with muscle relaxants if necessary. In this way the depth of anaesthesia is controlled by the inhalational agent in low fractions (3/4−1 MAC).

Serious side-effects are seldom seen and no analgesic antidotes are necessary for stimulation of respiration after the end of the procedure. Furthermore, this technique is independent of the length of surgery, as delivery of the inhalational agent can be stopped at any time. We have found that this technique is particularly suitable in high-risk patients in whom a possible small decrease in myocardial contractility caused by enflurane is not critical. In patients with hypertension and/or ischaemic heart disease, we believe this method to be superior to the high-dose narcotic methods. The absence of sympathetic stimulation improves the ratio between oxygen demand and supply to the myocardium. Recent studies by Järnberg (1981, personal communication) from our department have clearly demonstrated that the amounts of plasma adrenaline and noradrenaline are significantly lower in enflurane-nitrous oxide anaesthesia than in the classic neurolept technique.

Epidural Block in Combination with General Anaesthesia

Although inhalational anaesthesia with enflurane or halothane is associated with less sympathetic reaction than neurolept analgesia, a stress-free response is not completely achieved [13]. For this it is necessary to use an epidural block extending from T_4 to S_5 [3]. The lower block from T_6 to S_5 will partially inhibit the stress response. This has recently been confirmed by Reiz (1980, personal communication) in patients undergoing cholecystectomy. High epidural block in dogs has demonstrated an improved distribution of coronary blood flow to the endocardium when coronary flow was decreased and after infarction [5, 9]. This effect is probably due not to systemic effects of the epidural block but to changes in sympathetic tone of the coronary vessels [10]. Thus the classic good results with high epidural block and general anaesthesia in patients with major vascular surgery can partially be explained by a direct myocardial effect as well as the general haemodynamic effect due to a reduction of after-load, reduced oxygen demand, and the decrease in wall tension, all factors leading to a better balance between oxygen demand and supply to the myocardium. The decrease in mean arterial (and diastolic) pressure and the resulting effect on coronary blood flow are well compensated for by a better diastolic coronary blood flow and less susceptibility to subendocardial ischaemia due to a left ward shift in the coronary prefusion flow curve with a concomitant higher coronary reserve [14]. The epidural technique allows for the post-operative use of morphine − epidural pain control − an important aspect in the care of the patient.

In summary, it is time to re-examine our widespread standard methods with analgesics and neurolept drugs in the light of new information on stress and metabolism related to anaesthetic techniques. Furthermore, the newer concepts of the regulation of coronary blod flow in ischaemic heart disease during anaesthesia make it logical to convert to combinations with inhalational agents and even high epidural blocks.

References

1. Crile GW, Lower WE (1921) Surgical shock and the shockless operation through anoci-association. Saunders, Philadelphia
2. De Castro J, Mundeleer P (1959) Anaesthesia sans sommeil, 'La neuroleptanalgesia'. Acta Chir Belg 58:69
3. Engqvist A, Brand MR, Fernandez A, Kehlet H (1977) The blocking effects of epidural analgesia on the adrenocortical and hyperglycæmic responses to surgery. Acta Anaesth Scand 21:330
4. Kehlet H, Brand MR, Prauge-Hansen A, Alberti K (1979) Effect of epidural analgesia in metabolic profiles during surgery. Br J Surg 66:543
5. Klassen GA, Braunwell RS, Bromage P, Zborowska-Shnis DT (1980) Effects of acute sympathectomy by epidural anaesthesia in the canine coronary circulation. Anaesthesiology 52:8
6. Laborit H, Huguenard P (1954) Pratique de l'hibernotherapie en chirurgie et en medecine. Paris Masson
7. Little DM, Stephen CR (1954) Modern balanced anaesthesia. A concept. Anaesthesiology 15:246
8. Lundy JS (1942) Clinical anaesthesia. Saunders, Philadelphia
9. Ottesen S, Renck H, Jynge P (1979) Cardiovascular effects of epidural analgesia. Acta Anaesth Scand 23: [Suppl] 69
10. Reiz S (1980) Haemodynamic and cardiometabolic effects of thoracic epidural block. Anaesthesia and betablockade. Lindgren & Söner, Gothenburg
11. Stanley T, Berman L, Green O, Robertson D, Roizen M (1979) Fentanyloxygen anaesthesia for coronary artery surgery: Plasma catecholamine and cortisol responses. Anaesthesiology 5:139
12. Stanley T, Reddy E (1979) Fentanyl-oxygen anesthesia in septic shock. Anesthesiology 51:100
13. Traynor C, Hall GM (1981) Endocrine and metabolic changes during surgery: anaesthetic implications. Br J Anaesth 53:153
14. Verrier ED, Edelist G, Consigny PM, Robinson S, Hoffman JIE (1980) Greater coronary vascular reserve in dog anaesthetized with halothane. Anaesthesiology 53:445

Subject Index

Anaesthesiologie und Intensivmedizin

Anaesthesiology and Intensive Care Medicine

vormals „Anaesthesiologie und Wiederbelebung"
begründet von R. Frey, F. Kern und O. Mayrhofer

Herausgeber: H. Bergmann (Schriftleiter),
J. B. Brückner, M. Gemperle, W. F. Henschel,
O. Mayrhofer, K. Peter

Band 141
Experimentelle Anaesthesie – Monitoring – Immunologie
Band 3
ZAK Innsbruck 1979: Freie Themen: Experimentelle und klinisch-experimentelle Anaesthesie, Technik und Monitoring, Anaesthesie und EEG. Panel I: Immunologische Aspekte.
Freie Themen: Immunologie
Herausgeber: B. Haid, G. Mitterschiffthaler
1981. 183 Abbildungen, 32 Tabellen.
XIII, 252 Seiten (7 Seiten in Englisch).
DM 98,-. ISBN 3-540-10944-7

Band 142
Herz Kreislauf Atmung
Band 4
ZAK Innsbruck 1979: Freie Themen: Kontrollierte Blutdrucksenkung, Anaesthesie bei Cardiochirurgie, Haemodynamik, Atmung
Herausgeber: B. Haid, G. Mitterschiffthaler
1981. 263 Abbildungen, 51 Tabellen. XIV, 335 Seiten. DM 128,-. ISBN 3-540-10945-5

Band 143
Intensivmedizin – Notfallmedizin
Band 5
ZAK Innsbruck 1979: Hauptthema II: Anaesthesie und Notfallmedizin. Hauptthema III: Grenzen der Intensivmedizin. Freie Themen: Intensivmedizin, Parenterale Ernährung und Volumenersatz, Säure-Basen-Haushalt
Herausgeber: B. Haid, G. Mitterschiffthaler
1981. 269 Abbildungen, 95 Tabellen. XV, 373 Seiten (13 Seiten in Englisch). DM 148,-.
ISBN 3-540-10946-3

Band 144
Spinal Opiate Analgesia
Experimental and Clinical Studies
Editors: T. L. Yaksh, H. Müller
1982. 55 figures, 54 tables.
ISBN 3-540-11036-4

Band 145
J. D. Beyer, K. Messmer
Organdurchblutung und Sauerstoffversorgung bei PEEP
Tierexperimentelle Untersuchungen zur regionalen Organdurchblutung und lokalen Sauerstoffversorgung bei Beatmung mit positiv-endexspiratorischem Druck
1982. 17 Abbildungen, 18 Tabellen. X, 84 Seiten. DM 54,-. ISBN 3-540-11220-0

Band 146
H. Harke
Massivtransfusionen
Hämostase und Schocklunge
1982. 78 Abbildungen, 50 Tabellen.
XIV, 196 Seiten. DM 65,-. ISBN 3-540-11467-X

Band 148
Regionalanaesthesie
Zentraleuropäischer Anaesthesiekongreß 1981
Berlin „ZAK 81"
Herausgeber: J. B. Brückner
1982. Etwa 123 Abbildungen, etwa 45 Tabellen.
Etwa 390 Seiten. DM 83,-. ISBN 3-540-11744-X

In Vorbereitung
Band 147
L. Tonczar
Kardiopulmonale Wiederbelebung
1982. ISBN 3-540-11760-1

Band 149
K. Peter, F. Jesch
Inhalations-Anaesthesie
1982. ISBN 3-540-11756-3

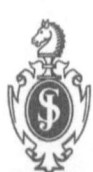

Springer-Verlag Berlin Heidelberg New York

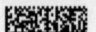